ROCKVILLE CA

AIDS

PROFILE OF AN EPIDEMIC

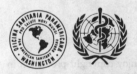

Scientific Publication No. 514

PAN AMERICAN HEALTH ORGANIZATION
Pan American Sanitary Bureau, Regional Office of the
WORLD HEALTH ORGANIZATION
525 Twenty-third Street, N.W.
Washington, D.C. 20037, USA

1989

AAV7240

Published also in Spanish (1989) with the title:
SIDA: perfil de una epidemia
ISBN 92 75 31514 0

ISBN 92 75 11514 1

©Pan American Health Organization, 1989

CONTRIBUTORS

A. Adrien
Infection Control Service, Department of Community Health,
Montreal General Hospital, Montreal, Canada

Laura Astarloa
Department of Microbiology, Faculty of Medicine, University of
Buenos Aires, Buenos Aires, Argentina

C. Bartholomew
Department of Medicine, University of the West Indies, General
Hospital, Port of Spain, Trinidad and Tobago

David C. Bassett
Caribbean Epidemiology Center, Port of Spain, Trinidad and Tobago

Nicolás E. Bianco
National Reference Center on Clinical Immunology (WHO
Collaborating Center for Clinical Immunology), Caracas, Venezuela

Isaac Blanca
National Reference Center on Clinical Immunology (WHO
Collaborating Center for Clinical Immunology), Caracas, Venezuela

Lydia S. Bond
Education, Information, and Counseling, PAHO/WHO Global
Program on AIDS in the Americas, Pan American Health
Organization, Washington, D.C., United States of America

Jorge Boshell S.
Virology Group, National Institute of Health, Bogotá, Colombia

Martha Boxaca
Department of Microbiology, Faculty of Medicine, University of Buenos Aires, Buenos Aires, Argentina

Rosalba de Cabas
National Blood Bank, Colombian Red Cross, Bogotá, Colombia

Miguel Angel Calello
Department of Microbiology, Faculty of Medicine, University of Buenos Aires, Buenos Aires, Argentina

Pedro Chequer
Epidemiology Service, National Division for the Control of Sexually Transmitted Diseases and AIDS, Ministry of Health, Brasília, Brazil

James Chin
Surveillance, Forecasting, and Impact Assessment Unit, Global Program on AIDS, World Health Organization, Geneva, Switzerland

A. J. Clayton
Federal Center for AIDS, National Health and Welfare, Ottawa, Ontario, Canada

F. Cleghorn
Caribbean Epidemiology Center, Port of Spain, Trinidad and Tobago

Susan Scholle Connor
Office of Legal Affairs, and PAHO/WHO Global Program on AIDS in the Americas, Pan American Health Organization, Washington, D.C., United States of America

Leopoldo Deibis
National Reference Center on Clinical Immunology (WHO Collaborating Center for Clinical Immunology), Caracas, Venezuela

Marcelo Díaz Lestrem
Francisco J. Muñiz Hospital, Buenos Aires, Argentina

José Luis Domínguez Tórix
National Blood Transfusion Center, Mexico City, Mexico

Gloria Echeverría de Pérez
National Reference Center on Clinical Immunology (WHO Collaborating Center on Clinical Immunology), Caracas, Venezuela

Hugo Fainboim
Francisco J. Muñiz Hospital, Buenos Aires, Argentina

María Mercedes Fergusson
Virology Group, National Institute of Health, Bogotá, Colombia

Jair Ferreira
Sanitary Dermatology, Secretariat of Health and Environment, State of Rio Grande do Sul, Brazil

J. Peter Figueroa
Epidemiology Section, Ministry of Health, Jamaica

Manuel G. Gacharná
Epidemiology Section, Ministry of Health, Bogotá, Colombia

Enrique Galbán García
Ministry of Public Health, Havana, Cuba

Bernardo Galvão-Castro
Department of Immunology (WHO Collaborating Center on AIDS), Fundação Oswaldo Cruz, Rio de Janeiro, Brazil

Carmen Silvia García
National Reference Center on Clinical Immunology (WHO Collaborating Center for Clinical Immunology), Caracas, Venezuela

Marcela García
National Blood Bank, Colombian Red Cross, Bogotá, Colombia

María de Lourdes García García
General Directorate of Epidemiology, Secretariat of Health, Mexico City, Mexico

A. J. Garrett
National Institute for Biological Standards and Control (WHO Collaborating Center on AIDS), South Mimms, Potters Bar, Hertsfordshire, England

Stella González
Meta Department of Laboratory Health Services, Villavicencio,
Colombia

K. O. Habermehl
Institute for Clinical and Experimental Virology (WHO Collaborating
Center on AIDS), Free University of Berlin, Berlin (West)

H. Hampl
Institute for Clinical and Experimental Virology (WHO Collaborating
Center on AIDS), Free University of Berlin, Berlin (West)

C. Hankins
Montreal Regional Sexually Transmitted Disease Control Program,
Montreal, Canada

C. J. Hospedales
Caribbean Epidemiology Center, Port of Spain, Trinidad and Tobago

B. Hull
Caribbean Epidemiology Center, Port of Spain, Trinidad and Tobago

Jairo Ivo-dos-Santos
Department of Immunology (WHO Collaborating Center on AIDS),
Fundação Oswaldo Cruz, Rio de Janeiro, Brazil

José Antonio Izazola L.
General Directorate of Epidemiology, Secretariat of Health, Mexico
City, Mexico

Luz Socorro Jaramillo
Virology Group, National Institute of Health, Bogotá, Colombia

Warren Johnson, Jr.
Division of International Medicine, Cornell University Medical
College, New York, New York, United States of America

Osvaldo Libonatti
Department of Microbiology, Faculty of Medicine, University of
Buenos Aires, Buenos Aires, Argentina

S. Mahabir
Caribbean Epidemiology Center, Port of Spain, Trinidad and Tobago

Gladys Márquez
Virology Group, National Institute of Health, Bogotá, Colombia

Merly Márquez
National Reference Center on Clinical Immunology (WHO Collaborating Center for Clinical Immunology), Caracas, Venezuela

A. S. Meltzer
Bureau of External Cooperation, Federal Center for AIDS, National Health and Welfare, Ottawa, Ontario, Canada

Nora Méndez
Francisco J. Muñiz Hospital, Buenos Aires, Argentina

Jai P. Narain
Caribbean Epidemiology Center, Port of Spain, Trinidad and Tobago

Tania Olaria
National Reference Center on Clinical Immunology (WHO Collaborating Center for Clinical Immunology), Caracas, Venezuela

Jean W. Pape
Division of International Medicine, Cornell University Medical College, New York, New York, United States of America

Elsa Y. Prada
Social Security Institute, Meta Department, Villavicencio, Colombia

Thomas C. Quinn
Laboratory of Immunoregulation, National Institute of Allergy and Infectious Diseases, Bethesda, Maryland, and Johns Hopkins University School of Medicine and School of Public Health and Hygiene, Baltimore, Maryland, United States of America

Rosana de Rangel
Bogotá Department of Health Services, Bogotá, Colombia

R. Remis
Montreal Regional Infectious Disease Control Office, Montreal, Canada

Blanca Rico G.
National Committee for AIDS Prevention, Mexico City, Mexico

Lair Guerra de Macedo Rodrigues
National Division for the Control of Sexually Transmitted Diseases
and AIDS, Brasília, Brazil

Rodolfo Rodríguez Cruz
Ministry of Public Health, Havana, Cuba

G. C. Schild
National Institute for Biological Standards and Control (WHO
Collaborating Center on AIDS), South Mimms, Potters Bar,
Hertsfordshire, England

V. Seagroatt
National Institute for Biological Standards and Control (WHO
Collaborating Center on AIDS), South Mimms, Potters Bar,
Hertsfordshire, England

Jaime Sepúlveda Amor
General Directorate of Epidemiology, Secretariat of Health, Mexico
City, Mexico

E. M. Supran
Division of Microbiological Reagents and Quality Control, Central
Public Health Service Laboratory (WHO Collaborating Center on
AIDS), Colindale, London, England

Daniel Tarantola
Global Program on AIDS, World Health Organization, Geneva,
Switzerland

Hector Terry Molinert
Ministry of Public Health, Havana, Cuba

José Luis Valdespino Gómez
General Directorate of Epidemiology, Secretariat of Health, Mexico
City, Mexico

Mercedes Weissenbacher
Department of Microbiology, Faculty of Medicine, University of
Buenos Aires, Buenos Aires, Argentina

Fernando Zacarías
PAHO/WHO Global Program on AIDS in the Americas, Pan
American Health Organization, Washington, D.C., United
States of America

CONTENTS

PHOTOGRAPHS

All photographs were taken by Carlos Gaggero, Pan American
Health Organization. The patients depicted are AIDS victims from
Brazil, Haiti, and the United States.

PREFACE

Faced with the growing threat of acquired immunodeficiency syndrome (AIDS), communities and institutions throughout the world are responding gradually, but firmly and concertedly. In just seven years, gains in scientific research have surpassed every expectation, with the exploration of new frontiers in knowledge of the structure and pathologic mechanisms of the human immunodeficiency virus (HIV), the infectious agent of the disease. These gains, in turn, have made it possible to develop new, reliable diagnostic tests and to entertain the first hopes of finding an effective treatment for HIV infection. Like science, society is working to meet the challenge posed by the alarming vulnerability of some of its members to this disease: daily there emerge new community organizations—governmental and nongovernmental, public and private—that offer support, comfort, advice, and information to people afflicted with HIV infection or AIDS, to those who are at risk of suffering them, and to the general population.

Given the serious situation stemming from this epidemic, the Pan American Health Organization has joined forces with those of the WHO Global Program on AIDS and is collaborating with all the governments of the Americas in planning and carrying out national and regional prevention and control activities. Notwithstanding, there continues to be a need for urgent action: the 85,000 cases of AIDS reported in the Americas by 1 October 1988 represent only a fraction of the actual number; moreover, they are the result of infections transmitted five to ten years ago and do not reflect the current spread of the virus. Consequently, as health workers and as members of society, our responsibility is enormous. It is time for us to act decisively, vigorously, and with commitment, and we should spare neither effort nor resources. Clearly, whatever we do—or fail to do—will inevitably affect the magnitude of the AIDS epidemic and its grave economic and social consequences in the approaching millenium.

Carlyle Guerra de Macedo, *Director*
Pan American Health Organization

INTRODUCTION

This publication reflects the interest and concern of the community of workers and scientists in the health field in the face of the problem caused by acquired immunodeficiency syndrome (AIDS) in the Region of the Americas. It constitutes what could be considered an epidemiologic mosaic of the similarities and differences of AIDS and human immunodeficiency virus (HIV) infection in various countries and subregions of the Hemisphere. The North American experience, in which transmission among homosexuals and by contaminated needles and syringes predominates, contrasts with the rapid changes observed in the distribution of cases in the English-speaking Caribbean and Haiti, where an increasing number of women are affected by AIDS, and with the persistence of blood transmission in countries of Latin America.

The first part of this publication provides a descriptive and analytic sample of the epidemiology of AIDS that—ranging from the northern to the southern end of the Hemisphere—comprises Canada, the United States of America, Mexico, Colombia, and Brazil, as well as Cuba and the English-speaking Caribbean. Interestingly, some of the articles not only document what has happened with the disease, but venture projections, derived from various premises and forecasting techniques, about the future of the epidemic. Withal, the consensus is that the problem will get considerably worse in the near future.

The changing nature of the epidemiology of HIV infection and the importance of factors associated with these changes are pointed out by Narain et al. in their article on the situation in the Caribbean and by Díaz Lestrem et al. in theirs about the growing risk of the disease among intravenous drug users in Argentina. The latter article demonstrates how the modes and mechanisms of transmission of the hepatitis and AIDS viruses point up a common social problem. The article by Bartholomew and Cleghorn serves as a reminder that we are barely beginning to understand and deal with the spread of HIV and other human retroviruses. The importance of defining the clinical and immunologic parameters of the infection is signaled in the article by Echeverría de Pérez et al., and the urgent need to develop sensitive and appropriate technologies for HIV testing is the underlying message of the article by Ivo-dos-Santos and Galvão-Castro. Pape and Johnson, who explain perinatal transmission of HIV, provide a glimpse of the threat posed to newborns and infants if action is not taken to contain sexual transmission among adults. Analyzing the experience gained in four countries of the Americas, Bond shows that public education about AIDS has not been sufficient, despite the fact that it represents an essential first step in preventing the disease. AIDS transcends the field of biomedicine and poses thorny ethical and legal dilemmas that society must face, as Scholle Connor points out in her essay. Sepúlveda Amor et al. present an account of the efforts undertaken in Mexico to detect and attack the specific problem of HIV in blood banks. In the last article in this section, Clayton and Meltzer delineate the structure of the scientific-technical center on AIDS created by the Government of Canada to support health services in the provinces—an example of what can and should be done in other countries.

In the second part, the ideas expressed by the eminent dean of epidemiology, Alexander Langmuir, serve as a basis for the round table in which the future of the AIDS epidemic is debated from various national and international perspectives. While at present, when we are scarcely beginning to understand the natural history of retroviral infection, it is obviously impossible to make reliable projections about the consequences that AIDS will have for individuals, groups, and large populations, it is also obvious that we need to reflect, discuss, and prepare ourselves to deal with any foreseeable possibility.

The third part of this publication consists of reports and abstracts from numerous sources that complement the information provided in the articles and that deal with various aspects, positions, and activities in the fight against AIDS. Included among the subjects are the regional and global responses to the problem; the results of the First Pan American Teleconference on AIDS, which provided up-to-date scientific information and afforded an opportunity for more than 45,000 health workers in the Americas to participate; guidelines and aspects to be considered in prevention activities; reports of research underway; and, finally, evidence that it is necessary and possible to bring together worldwide political will to combat the epidemic, as has been seen in the success of the World Summit of Ministers of Health, held in London in January 1988, which strengthened the foundation from which countries can progress from concept to action and from promise to reality.

Among the articles some discrepancies and duplication may be apparent. These are due, in part, to the promptness with which the authors responded to our urgent appeal to provide information on the AIDS situation in the countries of the Americas. To a greater degree, they may reflect the difficulty of assimilating immediately and efficiently the vertiginous explosion of new knowledge; the history of AIDS is being written as the epidemic evolves. Similarly, and for the same reasons, the contents do not represent a perfect balance of subjects nor an exactly proportional representation of countries and subregions. There is not, for example, any article dedicated exclusively to an analysis of the economic impact of AIDS on communities and health services (which is currently being carried out in Brazil) nor a description of the changing epidemiology of the infection in the Central American isthmus. Nor are there included examples of the important clinical and virologic studies underway in the Southern Cone, nor of the community-based prevention approaches aimed at individuals with high-risk behavior in the Spanish- and French-speaking Caribbean. The time limits inherent to publishing dictate that these and other studies yet to be described and written will have to await dissemination.

Notwithstanding, this publication serves as a dual testimony: on the one hand, it shows the readiness of our colleagues throughout the Region—from Ottawa and Baltimore to Buenos Aires, Rio de Janeiro, and Havana—to make known their national experiences; on the other, it is a document which, covering subjects as diverse as molecular biology and the ethical and legal aspects of AIDS, clearly reflects both the multidisciplinary importance of the subject and the coalescing role of epidemiology and public health.

Finally, this volume, which seemed to materialize in no time, would not have been possible without the expert involvement of the excellent groups of editors that work in the Pan American Health Organization: thanks to them, what had been merely an idea became, in six months, a tangible and important publication.

Fernando R. K. Zacarías, *Regional Adviser*
PAHO/WHO Global Program on AIDS in the Americas

Errata

<u>AIDS: PROFILE OF AN EPIDEMIC</u>

The indicated passages should be corrected to read
as follows:

Page 147, last paragraph

. . .The degree of test sensitivity—100% sensitivity means that
all true positives are identified—is over 99%; but if a large
population is tested, even one false negative result in every
hundred tests can add up to a substantial number.

Page 148, first paragraph

By the same token, the degree of test specificity—100%
specificity means that all true negatives are identified—while
approaching 99%, will still lead to a number of false positive
results. . .

Part I

ARTICLES

CANADIAN EXPERIENCES WITH AIDS AND HIV INFECTION

A. ADRIEN, C. HANKINS, & R. REMIS

The human immunodeficiency virus (HIV) epidemic began in Canada in the late 1970s. As a result, Canadians are now experiencing the consequences—an increasing number of acquired immunodeficiency syndrome (AIDS) cases with their concomitant political and social repercussions.

As the extent of this epidemic becomes more evident throughout the world, we all benefit from learning about the initiatives of individual countries and by comparing cultural differences in the control of HIV transmission. The article presented here describes Canadian experiences with AIDS and HIV infection.

Epidemiology of HIV Infection in Canada

AIDS Cases

The first patient with AIDS in Canada was diagnosed in 1978, and in 1982 the Laboratory Center for Disease Control established a reporting system to monitor the emerging Canadian AIDS epidemic. AIDS is now a notifiable disease in all of Canada's 10 provinces and two territories.

As of September 1988, 2,003 cases of AIDS had been reported in Canada with 90% of these occurring in the provinces of Ontario,

Table 1. Reported cases of AIDS in Canada, by province and risk category, up to 19 September 1988.

| | Province or area | | | | | | | | |
| | Ontario | | Quebec | | British Columbia | | Other | | Total | |
Category	No.	(%)	No.	(%)	No.	(%)	No.	(%)	No.	(%)
Adult cases in:										
Homosexual and bisexual men	696	(89.9)	396	(66.9)	391	(94.0)	184	(83.3)	1,667	(83.2)
I.V. drug abusers	8	(1.0)	4	(0.7)	1	(0.2)	1	(0.5)	14	(0.7)
Recipients of clotting factors	11	(1.4)	16	(2.7)	2	(0.5)	10	(4.5)	39	(1.9)
Heterosexual immigrants from endemic regions	5	(0.6)	89	(15.0)	0	(0.0)	1	(0.5)	95	(4.7)
Others with heterosexual contact	10	(1.3)	28	(4.7)	7	(1.7)	4	(1.8)	49	(2.4)
Transfusion recipients	22	(2.8)	11	(1.9)	8	(1.9)	10	(4.5)	51	(2.5)
Persons with no identified risk	20	(2.6)	19	(3.2)	6	(1.4)	6	(2.7)	51	(2.5)
Pediatric cases	2	(0.3)	29	(4.9)	1	(0.2)	5	(2.3)	37	(1.8)
Total cases	774	(100)	592	(100)	416	(100)	221	(100)	2,003	(100)

Quebec, and British Columbia. Specifically, Ontario had reported 774 cases (for a cumulative incidence of 83 per million inhabitants), Quebec had reported 592 (89 per million inhabitants), and British Columbia had reported 416 (142 per million inhabitants). As would be expected, most of the Canadian cases reported were found among residents of the major urban centers—with Toronto, Montreal, and Vancouver alone accounting for about two-thirds of the cases.

The rate of occurrence of new AIDS cases has changed over the course of the Canadian epidemic. In the initial period, from 1982 to 1986, the epidemic curve was exponential with a doubling time of under one year. Since 1986, however, the rate of increase has diminished, and the epidemic curve is now approximated by use of a polynomial equation. This change is normal in the course of a new epidemic and does not indicate that the epidemic is peaking at this time.

Adults between the ages of 20 and 49 years account for 88% of the cases. Among all of the 1,966 adult cases, 1,863 (95%) have occurred among males, yielding a male:female ratio of 18 to 1. Also, 1,667 (83%) of the cases have occurred among homosexual and bisexual men, 95 (4.7%) among immigrants from endemic regions, and 90 (4.5%) among recipients of blood and blood products. This latter group includes those presumably infected via blood transfusions and those who received contaminated clotting factors (Table 1).

However, the distribution by risk factor varies from province to province. In particular, the distribution among risk categories in the province of Quebec is different from distributions in other provinces. As of 19 September 1988, Quebec men admitting to homosexual or bisexual contact accounted for 67% of the cases, immigrants from endemic regions 15%, others with heterosexual contact 4.7%, and pediatric cases 4.9%. In contrast, the proportions in these risk categories in the rest of Canada were as follows: men with homosexual or bisexual contact 90%, immigrants from endemic regions 0.4%, others with heterosexual contact 1.5%, and pediatric cases 0.6%. However, the number of cases among immigrants from endemic regions in Quebec has remained relatively stable since mid-1984, and hence they account for a declining share of overall AIDS cases, a share currently representing about 10% of the new cases in Quebec.

HIV Infection

Knowledge of the epidemiology of HIV infection in Canada is inadequate. Only limited seroprevalence studies among homosexual men have been carried out to date. Nevertheless, on the basis of several independent epidemiologic and mathematical approaches, we estimate that approximately 30,000 Canadians were infected with HIV as of early 1988. This estimate is necessarily crude, and the true number could be as low as 10,000 or as high as 50,000 individuals.

Trends

Empirical models have provided a basis for tentatively projecting the future of the Canadian AIDS epidemic. As mentioned above, a polynomial model currently provides the best empirical fit for the epidemic curve. On the basis of this model, the Department of National

Health and Welfare's Federal Center for AIDS has estimated that
something like the following numbers of new cases will emerge in the
next five years: 1988, 1,061; 1989, 1,407; 1990, 1,805; 1991, 2,252; and
1992, 2,748. The cumulative total reached by the end of 1992 would be
approximately 11,000 cases.

Costs

A recent study by the Royal Society of Canada reported its findings in
April 1988. According to this study (1), the personal direct cost associated with a case of AIDS in Canada is about Can$82,500 per year. The
cumulative indirect costs of mortality range from Can$300,000 to
Can$1,000,000 for a person 20 to 39 years old.

On this basis, the investigators estimated that the hospital costs for
AIDS cases diagnosed from 1979 to November 1987 were approximately Can$76 million, and that the personal direct costs would total
nearly Can$165 million by 1992. The indirect costs are probably much
higher but are difficult to estimate. It was the conclusion of the study
that the cost of caring for AIDS patients is considerable and will
represent a substantial and growing proportion of health care
expenditures in the future.

Canadian Responses

Surveillance

Surveillance of AIDS and HIV infection is critical to successful public
health efforts designed to prevent transmission and care for those
infected. As with other communicable diseases, effective surveillance
permits evaluation of the nature and scope of the infection, facilitates
rational planning of health services, and provides grounds for the
appraisal and appropriate modification of preventive programs.

Monitoring the occurrence of AIDS provides a highly specific surveillance tool, but one limited by the infection's long incubation
period. Thus, the current AIDS incidence reflects transmission patterns of five to seven and more years ago. The other main limitation
of AIDS surveillance is its inability to assess the full spectrum of
morbidity and even mortality associated with HIV infection. Thus,

although AIDS surveillance must be continued and strengthened, it alone cannot completely answer all our questions.

Other approaches to surveillance of HIV infection include monitoring sexually transmitted diseases with short incubation periods (e.g., gonorrhea and syphilis), studying high-risk sexual behaviors in our population, and conducting large-scale seroprevalence studies. Regarding the latter, anonymous unlinked studies of population-based serum samples provide the most unbiased estimates of underlying seropositivity and have the additional advantage of being rapid and affordable. These surveys are currently being planned for different regions of Canada. Although usually initiated as research studies, they can easily be modified for ongoing use as a surveillance system monitoring the spread of HIV infection.

HIV Testing

HIV antibody tests are available free of charge to any Canadian who requests the test. Whether a test is clinically indicated or patient-initiated, all three prerequisites advocated by the World Health Organization for the testing of individuals must be fulfilled. These conditions are informed consent, adequate pre-test counseling combined with appropriate post-test counseling, and confidentiality.

HIV testing facilities were created in each province in 1985 to provide an alternative to the Red Cross Blood Transfusion Service Testing Program for determining infection status. This step was taken in order to discourage use of the Red Cross program by individuals at high risk, who might test negative during the period shortly after exposure to HIV, thereby potentially exposing patients transfused with their blood to the virus. The initial test is an enzyme-linked immunosorbent assay (ELISA) test that is both sensitive and simple. Positive specimens are subsequently checked using a confirmatory test such as the immunofluorescent assay (IFA). Specimens that are equivocal or indeterminant on IFA testing undergo Western blot testing or the radioimmunoprecipitation assay (RIPA). In general, the confirmatory tests are more specific than ELISA, but they are also complex and require expert interpretation. In Canada, seropositive results are not released to the physician without having been confirmed, a process that causes some delay.

In seven of Canada's 10 provinces, HIV seropositivity is reportable to public health authorities. One of these provinces conducts a contact tracing program based on traditional sexually transmitted disease control principles. The other six provinces use some form of passive system that places prime responsibility on the patient for notifying his or her partners, with support from the public health service.

Since 1985, seropositivity rates among the individuals tested in all risk categories have fallen as the demand for testing has increased. Since the people coming in are self-selected, it is not possible to draw conclusions about the overall infection rate in Canada from testing service data.

No mandatory testing of anyone has been approved. Both the National Advisory Committee on AIDS (2) and the Royal Society of Canada (1) have recommended against screening immigrants, prisoners, and surgical patients, among others. The only people who are systematically screened are donors of blood, sperm, tissues, and organs. Hence, at present a system of voluntary testing of individuals for personal or clinical reasons, combined with anonymous screening of populations for epidemiologic purposes, comprises the HIV testing program in Canada.

Proposals have recently been developed for anonymous seroprevalence surveys (especially of women of childbearing age) in order to obtain an epidemiologic picture of HIV's penetration among the general population. In 1987 the National Advisory Committee on AIDS approved the following conditions for conducting these surveys: (1) Ethically justified studies should only be conducted in a blinded, anonymous fashion. (2) In general, ethically justified studies should only be done on specimens that have been obtained for other routine tests. (3) Only demographic information that is routinely attached to specimens should be collected. (4) Voluntary HIV antibody testing under conditions of informed consent, pre-test and post-test counseling, and confidentiality must be accessible to people who are being seen in the proposed study setting. (5) Finally, all cell sizes used for purposes of analysis must be large enough to preclude any possible intentional or inadvertent linkage to any individual by deduction.

Education

AIDS is a behavioral disease, and the main risk behaviors are well-documented: unprotected sexual intercourse with an infected individual and sharing contaminated needles and syringes with an infected person. Although it is too early to fully evaluate the impact of AIDS education efforts, those that have been successful are those that have been carefully targeted, using specific messages and appropriate language. These initiatives have also gone beyond simple transfer of knowledge to provide motivation and emphasize the need to change attitudes and beliefs.

In Canada, where Can$48 million will be spent on educating the public over the next five years, the first initiatives in AIDS education were taken by volunteer groups. They started community-based activities and health-promoting education programs in the early 1980s. Most major Canadian cities now have volunteer AIDS support committees conducting education, advocacy, and support activities. The education programs of these groups usually include information and "safer sex" campaigns, news releases, documentation centers, information kiosks, speaker's bureaus, and telephone services providing information on AIDS. Thirty community-based volunteer organizations are now active members of the Canadian AIDS Society, working together nationally for the prevention of HIV infections.

Municipal and provincial efforts vary in their intensity and funding commitments. The provinces with the highest AIDS incidence have not always been the most aggressive in their education strategies; and the Federal Government has been innovative in giving part of the mandate for improving Canadian AIDS education and awareness to a nongovernmental organization, the Canadian Public Health Association.

This organization's AIDS program has a clearinghouse function, in that it provides a resource center and publishes a bimonthly newsletter, *The New Facts of Life*. Consultation, coordination, and research activities constitute a large part of the program. Seminars and conferences have been organized for professionals, workers, students, and the general public; and educational projects (such as production of a video and workbook on AIDS risk reduction in collaboration with the Canadian Labor Congress) have been set up. The program has been most visible in the media and advertising field, where it has launched a national public service campaign that has included development of four television and radio service announcements.

Although formal evaluation of most of these interventions is still pending, and although many other factors are involved, there is now some evidence of behavior changes in the gay population. For instance, among a cohort of 600 homosexual men followed at an average interval of 19.4 months between March 1984 and September 1986, the average annual number of sex partners declined from 7.7 to 6.4 (3). The seroconversion rates in this same cohort during five successive nine-month periods from November 1982 to July 1986 were 4.4%, 9.1%, 5.2%, 4.3%, and 1.7% (4). The observed decline in the infection rate has continued since then, the 1987 rate being estimated at 0.9% (5). Recent documentation of reduced rectal gonorrhea rates in Quebec beginning in 1986 (data from Regional Infectious Diseases Office, Montreal) and in Alberta (6) also provide evidence of sexual behavior changes in the gay community. In addition, overall reductions in the incidence of sexually transmitted disease in Canada in 1986 could also point to rising public awareness of the danger and of the safer sex practices that tend to prevent infection (7).

Research

Over the past five years, research on AIDS-HIV infection in Canada has occurred primarily in the three major urban centers with the highest AIDS incidence: Toronto, Montreal, and Vancouver. Research teams are now forming in other centers as the epidemic progresses.

AIDS research has placed new demands on institutional ethics review committees for critical scrutiny—not only of confidentiality provisions but also of methodologic issues. Also, perhaps more than any other disease in recent history, AIDS has stimulated the development of teams providing multidisciplinary care.

Canadian scientists have made important contributions in the AIDS field. Among other things, they obtained the first confirmatory evidence of antepartum vertical transmission (8), provided a risk analysis demonstrating that oral sex is low-risk (4), and performed animal model testing of a promising envelope glycoprotein 160 vaccine (9).

Canadian research is funded by various entities including the Federal Government, provincial governments, and private organizations. Federal research support is administered mainly by the National Health Research Development Program (NHRDP), to which Can$35 million has been allocated for AIDS-related projects over the five-year period 1988–1992. This sum reflects a significant increase in the Federal Government's annual level of spending on AIDS research, which previously stood at approximately Can$3.52 million. Other federal agencies funding Canadian researchers include the Medical Research Council (MRC), the International Development Research Center (IDRC), and the Social Sciences and Humanities Research Council (SSHRC).

Combining federal funding with that of provincial and nonprofit private agencies, the total funding provided in fiscal year 1987–1988 was Can$4.26 million. Analysis of the allocation of funds from all these sources by area of research during the two-year period 1986–1988 shows that 37% of these funds were spent on epidemiologic studies; 30% went for virology studies (most of this being spent to establish or improve laboratory facilities); and the remainder was distributed between immunologic (13%) and clinical (14%) investigations, with only 5% of the total going to research in economics and the other social sciences (10).

Current priorities of the major federal agency funding research (NHRDP) include encouragement of joint agency funding—such as NHRDP-IDRC funding of cooperative research initiatives in the developing world and NHRDP-SSHRC funding of social sciences research. Also, researchers who are new to AIDS are being encouraged to join established AIDS researchers in collaborative projects.

In general, Canadian researchers are looking forward to the opportunity for receiving their colleagues from around the world that will be offered by the Fifth International Conference on AIDS, which is to be held during June 1989 in Montreal.

International Cooperation

Canada has important contributions to make in the international effort to prevent HIV infection. It possesses a long tradition of overseas commitments, and its bilingual heritage is an important asset.

However, AIDS has only recently come to receive priority among the overseas health commitments of Canadian institutions, and the funds involved are limited. For example, it is estimated that as of 1987 a total of Can$15 million had been used to support Canadian international initiatives compared to Can$2 billion spent on international AIDS research and training by the United States (R. Wilson, personal communication). However, in 1987 the Canadian International Development Agency (CIDA) contributed Can$5 million to WHO's Global Program on AIDS, a further Can$5 million was allocated for 1988, and an additional Can$6 million is to be spent over the next five years.

We have also noted increasing collaboration between the Federal Center for AIDS, the Canadian Public Health Association, and Canadian funding agencies—these latter including the International Development Research Center, the National Health Research and Development Program, and various Canadian nongovernmental organizations. This collaboration has allowed better coordination in conducting AIDS awareness programs overseas. A good example of easing collaboration is provided by a research project on chil- d HIV infection that is jointly funded by IDRC and NHRDP, having been developed by Spanish and Canadian scientists.

Regarding human resource development in developing countries, there is a priority need for AIDS-related training in a broad range of fields including epidemiology, nursing care, laboratory work, health education, communications, service management, and evaluation (11). At this point the best approach to the problem through international cooperation would appear to be an integrated one directed at training primary health care workers and emphasizing partnerships with developing countries.

Conclusions

Since there is still no treatment and no vaccine for AIDS, and since HIV is transmitted by human action, the principal way of preventing transmission and subsequent disease is through aggressive educational measures designed to change human behavior. In the past, public health interventions of this sort have proven effective in dealing with smoking, cardiovascular diseases, drug abuse, and other sexually transmitted diseases. There is some evidence that the HIV epidemic in Canada will not grow to be the same relative size as that found in the United States (1); but we can certainly learn from past experiences so as to improve our strategies for changing sexual behavior, thereby improving our chances for controlling the political and social consequences of this pandemic.

References

1. Royal Society of Canada. *AIDS: A Perspective for Canadians*. Ottawa, 1988.
2. Somerville, M. A., and N. Gilmore. Human Immunodeficiency Virus Antibody Testing in Canada. Federal Center for AIDS, Ottawa, January 6, 1988.
3. Willoughby, B., M. T. Schechter, W. J. Boyko, K. J. P. Craib, M. S. Weaver, B. Douglas, et al. Sexual Practices and Condom Use in a Cohort of Homosexual Men: Evidence of Differential Modification Between Seropositive and Seronegative Men. Paper presented at the III International Conference on AIDS held in Washington, D.C., 1–5 June 1987.

4. Schechter, M. T., W. J. Boyko, M. S. Weaver, et al. Progression to AIDS, Predictions of AIDS, and Seroconversion in a Cohort of Homosexual Men: Results of a Four-year Prospective Study. Paper presented at the III International Conference on AIDS held in Washington, D.C., 1–5 June 1987.

5. Willoughby, B., M. T. Schechter, B. Douglas, K. J. P. Craib, P. Constance, M. Maynard, et al. Risk Reduction and Seroconversion in a Cohort of Homosexual Men. Paper presented at the IV International Conference on AIDS held in Stockholm, 12–16 June 1988.

6. Romanowski, B., and J. Brown. AIDS and changing sexual behavior. *Can Med Assoc J* 134:872, 1986.

7. Todd, M. J., J. Doherty, A. G. Jessamine, and K. S. Hutchinson. Sexually transmitted disease in Canada, 1986. *Canada Diseases Weekly Report* 14:85–88, 1988.

8. Lapointe, N., J. Michaud, D. Peskovic, J. Chausseau, and J. M. Dupuy. Transplacental transmission of HTLV-III. *N Engl J Med* 312:1325–1326, 1985.

9. O'Shaughnessy, M. V., M. Cochran, and G. Smith. HIV Verification Testing: A Comparative Study of the Immunoreactivity of a Cloned Envelope Protein (gp160) and Commercially Available Viral Lysate. Paper presented at the III International Conference on AIDS held in Washington, D.C., 1–5 June 1987. Washington, D.C., 1987.

10. Heathcote, G. M. Research on AIDS and HIV in Canada: recent and current funding. In: Background Papers—*AIDS: A Perspective for Canadians*. Ottawa, 1988.

11. Canadian Society for Tropical Medicine and International Health. Canadian Human Resource Development Against AIDS in Developing Countries: Summary Report. Ottawa, February 1988.

PERSPECTIVES ON THE AIDS EPIDEMIC: THE EXPERIENCE WITHIN THE UNITED STATES

THOMAS C. QUINN

Shortly after initial recognition of the acquired immunodeficiency syndrome (AIDS) in the United States in 1981, additional cases were reported from Europe with similar clinical, immunologic, and epidemiologic features. By 1983–1984, it was apparent that AIDS was also present in some areas of Central Africa, the Caribbean, and South America (1, 2). Since then AIDS has become a global pandemic, with 96,433 cases of AIDS from 136 countries being reported officially to the World Health Organization as of June 1988 (Table 1).

Over 70,000 of these cases had been reported from 40 countries of the Americas, over 12,000 cases from 28 European countries, and over 11,500 from 43 African countries. The fact that slightly fewer than 900 cases had been reported from Oceania and only 254 cases had been reported from 21 Asian countries makes it appear possible that AIDS was introduced into these areas at a later time. In that case, given the right epidemiologic conditions, these areas could witness the same exponential increases in AIDS cases that other areas experienced during the first five years of this disease.

In some areas of the world, such as Africa, the official figures may be gross underestimates of the actual number of AIDS cases due to inaccurate reporting arising from secondary weaknesses in health infrastructure and from difficulties with the CDC/WHO case definition of AIDS (3) that typically requires sophisticated diagnostic equipment. However, using the limited serologic surveys and selected AIDS surveillance studies available, the World Health Organization estimated in 1988 that there had been over 150,000 cumulative cases of AIDS worldwide, approximately 500,000 cases of individuals with

Table 1. Numbers of countries reporting AIDS cases to the World Health Organization and the numbers of cases reported, by continent.[a]

Continent	No. of countries reporting one or more cases	No. of cases
Africa	43	11,530
The Americas	40	71,343
Asia	21	254
Europe	28	12,414
Oceania	4	892
Total	136	96,433

[a] As of June 1988 (World Health Organization, Global Program on AIDS). See updated case numbers (through 30 September 1988) on pp. 217–220.

AIDS-related conditions, and five to ten million people asymptomatically infected with the etiologic agent of AIDS, the human immunodeficiency virus (HIV) (2). It is from this latter pool of asymptomatically infected individuals that additional cases of AIDS will eventually develop, and from which thousands of additional individuals will be infected with HIV through sexual or parenteral exposure.

Unfortunately, it appears that the vast majority of infected individuals reside in developing countries, where the economic and social impact of this disease will be greatest. Furthermore, in the absence of any curative drug or effective vaccine, it is likely that the AIDS epidemic will continue to spread, killing 80% of the diagnosed AIDS patients within two years of diagnosis and exerting its effects on the people of all countries.

Many issues have been raised concerning the future of the AIDS epidemic. There are uncertainties about how many people within a given population are infected with HIV, how many will progress to symptomatic AIDS, whether drug intervention will delay AIDS fatalities, and whether educational efforts aimed at prevention and control of HIV infection will have a dramatic impact on slowing the spread of HIV and AIDS. There are also questions as to whether the epidemiologic features of HIV witnessed over the past several years will change, and what effect such changes might have on the overall distribution of AIDS cases.

For example, there is some evidence that the HIV epidemic has slowed among homosexual men—due either to saturation of the susceptible population or adherence to preventive measures such as "safe sex" recommendations. Similarly, there is some evidence that

HIV infection and AIDS have increased among intravenous drug abusers, raising yet another set of questions regarding heterosexual transmission of HIV to the sexual partners of these individuals; possible increases in the numbers of infected women spreading HIV infection to newborns via perinatal transmission; and eventual establishment of HIV infection as a sexually transmitted disease like syphilis, gonorrhea, or herpesvirus infection—thereby increasing the risk for promiscuous heterosexuals.

All of these issues have generated a great deal of debate and speculation that only time may be able to address. However, given nearly a decade of experience to date with this viral infection, it is possible to examine the available epidemiologic data from some countries with an eye to making some reasonably valid projections of epidemic trends over the next several years. These projections are needed to guide intensive educational and preventive control programs among selected high-risk populations, to plan financial assistance for medical research in some areas, and to conduct health planning designed to meet the AIDS-generated demand for medical care. Within that context, this article reviews the currently available data on HIV infection and AIDS in the United States, and presents some projections of the future of the AIDS epidemic there.

Epidemiologic Features of AIDS in the U.S.

As of 13 June 1988, a cumulative total of 64,896 AIDS cases had been reported to the U.S. Centers for Disease Control (CDC); of those afflicted, 36,480 (56%) had died. Also, 26,200 of these cases had been reported in the preceding 12 months, representing a 71% increase over the previous year. (AIDS ranked eighth among all diseases in 1986 with respect to years of potential life lost before age 65—4).

Most (63,880) of the 64,896 cases occurred among adults, 58,744 (92%) among men and 5,136 (8%) among women (Table 2). Homosexual and bisexual men accounted for 63% of these cases, intravenous drug users for 19%, and homosexual men who were also I.V. drug users for 7%. Three per cent of those afflicted had received blood transfusions contaminated with HIV, and 1% were hemophiliacs who had received infected factor 8 or factor 9 concentrates. Four per cent were heterosexuals who were either in sexual contact with people who had AIDS or were at risk for AIDS, or else were born in countries where heterosexual transmission of HIV is common. The remaining

Table 2. Cases of AIDS reported in the United States as of 13 June 1988, listed hierarchically.

Transmission categories	Males		Females		Total	
Adults:						
Homosexual and bisexual males	40,228	(68%)	0	(0%)	40,228	(63%)
I.V. drug users	9,343	(16%)	2,650	(52%)	11,993	(19%)
Homosexual males and I.V. drug users	4,740	(8%)	0	(0%)	4,740	(7%)
Hemophiliacs	602	(1%)	18	(0%)	620	(1%)
Heterosexuals[a]	1,163	(2%)	1,482	(29%)	2,645	(4%)
Blood transfusion recipients	1,034	(2%)	567	(11%)	1,601	(3%)
Undetermined[a]	1,634	(3%)	419	(8%)	2,053	(3%)
Subtotal	58,744	(100%)	5,136	(100%)	63,880	(100%)
Children:						
Hemophiliacs	55	(10%)	3	(1%)	58	(6%)
Parents with or at risk of AIDS	397	(71%)	385	(84%)	782	(77%)
Blood transfusion recipients	85	(15%)	52	(11%)	137	(13%)
Undetermined[a]	20	(4%)	19	(4%)	39	(4%)
Subtotal	557	(100%)	459	(100%)	1,016	(100%)
Total	59,301		5,595		64,896	

[a] See text for full description.

3% were patients for whom risk factor information was incomplete—because they had died, refused to be interviewed, were lost to follow-up, were still under investigation, were men reported to have had only heterosexual contact with a prostitute, or were interviewed patients for whom no specific risk was identified.

Of the 1,016 children with AIDS, 77% were born to a parent who had AIDS or who was at risk of AIDS; 13% had received infected blood transfusions; and 6% were hemophiliacs who had received infected factor 8 or factor 9 concentrates. The remaining 4% included patients for whom risk information was incomplete.

Sixty-two per cent of the reported adult AIDS cases and 23% of the pediatric cases occurred among whites. Blacks accounted for 25% of the adult cases and 56% of the pediatric cases, while Hispanics accounted for 13% of the adult cases and 20% of the pediatric cases. Since blacks and Hispanics, respectively, account for only 11.6% and 6.5% of the U.S. population, the percentages of AIDS cases among them are disproportionately high, particularly for black and Hispanic women and children with AIDS. Overall, the relative risk of AIDS for blacks and Hispanics is between two and ten times greater than for whites, suggesting that AIDS is becoming an increasing health

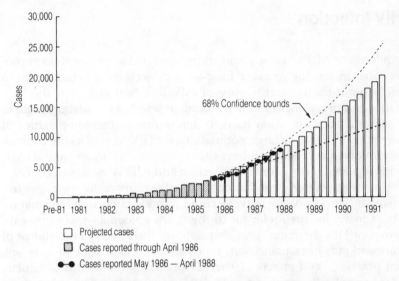

Figure 1. AIDS cases in the United States, showing projections through 1991 calculated from the known cases reported through April 1986 (adapted from ref. 6). Cases reported from May 1986 through April 1988 are shown for comparison.

problem for minorities—especially among inner-city populations where intravenous drug abuse is common.

In 1986 the U.S. Public Health Service made a tentative projection of the number of AIDS cases that might occur between 1986 and 1991, a projection based on statistical extrapolation of trends and cases reported to the CDC through April 1986 (5). Specifically, it was predicted that a cumulative total of about 270,000 AIDS cases would be diagnosed by the end of 1991 using current surveillance criteria, and that these would have caused approximately 180,000 deaths (Figure 1). The actual number of cases diagnosed using the foregoing criteria in 1986 and 1987 was 15,900 and 20,600, after adjusting for reporting delays. The total of these figures amounted to 94% of the 15,800 and 23,000 cases that were foreseen by the projection (6). Incomplete reporting, reporting delays, and recent changes in the AIDS case definition all affect the accuracy of these projections, but it is clear that the projections closely approximated the actual number of cases reported through 1987. (Obviously, reporting delays, as well as changes in diagnostic practices and therapeutic regimens, must be carefully evaluated in interpreting future trends of reported AIDS cases.)

HIV Infection

While these AIDS case extrapolations are reliable for short-term projections, in seeking to make long-term projections it is important to understand the natural history of HIV infection and both the incidence and prevalence of HIV infection in selected population groups. These statistics are often hard to derive due to the complexities of screening and testing large populations for HIV, as well as the difficulties involved in trying to follow these populations on an annual basis with repeated testing for HIV infection and AIDS case development.

However, properly conducted national seroprevalence surveys followed by seroincidence surveys could provide important information about many features relevant to the AIDS epidemic—including estimates of HIV infection rates and data on the relative importance of various kinds of transmission, types and frequencies of various sexual practices, and effects of various prevention and control efforts. More specifically focused serologic surveys could supplement these national surveys in order to more clearly define the natural history of HIV, the spread of HIV infection, and HIV risk factors in selected high-risk populations.

It is thought that retroviruses generally have long incubation periods between the time of infection and the development of symptoms. In the case of HIV, the mean incubation period following infection from a blood transfusion has been estimated at 8.23 years for adults and 1.97 years for children under five years old (7). Another study (6) has estimated the mean incubation period of AIDS in homosexual men to be 7.8 years.

Perhaps the best cohort study from which incubation times can be extrapolated is the San Francisco City Clinic Cohort Study. This investigation enrolled 6,700 homosexual and bisexual men in studies of hepatitis B virus infection between 1978 and 1980. Since 1983 these men have been followed for the development of AIDS, and sera collected from them as early as 1978 have been analyzed retrospectively for HIV infection (8). It was found that after 88 months of known HIV infection, 36% of the infected study subjects had developed AIDS and over 40% had other signs and symptoms of HIV infection; only 20% remained completely asymptomatic (Figure 2) (6).

It is clearly evident from this and other studies that the risk of disease progression increases with the duration of infection, and that a mean estimated incubation period of eight years is probably conservative, an estimate closer to 10 years being more realistic.

A large number of serologic surveys on selected populations have

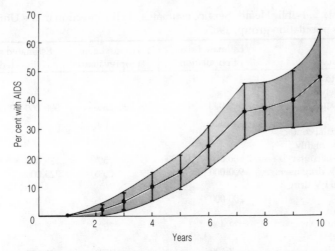

Figure 2. A Kaplan-Meier survival curve showing the proportions of homosexual men developing AIDS by estimated duration of HIV infection in the San Francisco City Cohort Study. The shaded area defines the 95% confidence interval (adapted from ref. 6).

provided important information about the extent of HIV infection in these high-risk groups, and the CDC has recently reviewed the extent of HIV infection in the U.S. in an effort to estimate the number of infected individuals within the country (9). Many of the studies included in this CDC review differ in their sampling methods, inclusion and exclusion criteria for study subjects, the rigor with which they ascertain risk information, and the resulting bias. Consequently, the results cannot always be validly compared, and significant gaps exist in the information. However, the review did manage to develop a description of the patterns and trends of HIV infection.

For homosexual men, over 50 surveys in 22 cities in 15 states found HIV antibody prevalences ranging from under 10% to 70%, with most prevalences being between 20% and 50% (Table 3) (9). The highest prevalences of HIV infection were found in cohorts of homosexual men in San Francisco; otherwise, the prevalences varied geographically, without major peaks in any one region.

The prevalence of HIV antibodies among I.V. drug users varied markedly by geographic region. Overall, 90 studies in 53 cities in 27 states and territories found rates ranging from 50–60% of I.V. drug users in New York City, New Jersey, and Puerto Rico to less than 5% in most areas of the country not on the East Coast. Most data were obtained from surveys at drug abuse treatment facilities that treat

Table 3. U.S. Public Health Service estimates of HIV infection in the United States by population group, 1987.

Population	Estimated size of population	Approximate seroprevalence	Estimated total infected
People who are exclusively homosexual	2,500,000	20–25%	500,000–625,000
Others with homosexual contact, including highly infrequent contact	2,500,000–7,500,000	5%	125,000–375,000
Regular I.V. drug users	900,000	25%	225,000
Occasional I.V. drug users	200,000	5%	10,000
People with hemophilia A	12,400	70%	8,700
People with hemophilia B	3,100	35%	1,100
Heterosexuals without specific identified risks	142,000,000	0.021%	30,000
Others (heterosexual partners of people at high risk, heterosexuals born in Haiti and Central Africa, transfusion recipients, etc.)			45,000–127,000[a]
Total			945,000–1,400,000

Source: Centers for Disease Control (9). See text for more details.
[a] Five to ten percent of the total number infected in other groups.

mainly heroin addicts. Patients undergoing drug treatment are believed to represent only about 50% of the estimated 1.1 million I.V. drug users in the United States. While some evidence suggests that many of those not in treatment are habitual users who may have an even higher risk of HIV infection, an estimated 200,000 intermittent users may have a lower prevalence of infection because of less frequent exposure to contaminated needles or equipment.

Regarding the estimated 15,500 persons with hemophilia, approximately 70% of the hemophilia A subjects tested and 35% of the hemophilia B subjects tested were seropositive.

Only a few studies have been performed that deal with people who are heterosexual partners of HIV-infected persons but who have no other identified risk factors for acquiring HIV infection. The prevalences of HIV infection observed among such groups range from under 10% to 60%. These wide ranges may reflect such things as different degrees of infectiousness of the index infected partner, differences in the frequency or type of sexual exposure, the duration of infection in the index partner, coexisting infections such as genital ulcers in one or both partners, or the clinical status of the index partner. Recent evidence suggests that infectiousness increases as the index partner's immune system deteriorates (10), and the relative efficiency of male-to-female versus female-to-male HIV transmission may also be an important factor in heterosexual infection. As yet there is insufficient information to definitively evaluate these differences (11).

Data from seroprevalence studies of the general U.S. population are even more limited, since these studies were only initiated in 1987. However, serologic screening of blood donors, civil applicants for military service, sexually transmitted disease (STD) clinic patients, newborn infants, women of reproductive age, and sentinel hospital patients has been under way for several years.

With respect to the highly selected population of blood donors, the prevalence of HIV infection was found to be 0.02% in 12.6 million American Red Cross blood donations made between April 1985 and May 1987 (9). (The overall level declined from 0.035% in mid-1985 to 0.012% in mid-1987, primarily as a result of eliminating previously identified seropositive people from the donor pool.) The overall prevalence among first-time donors in the period 1985–1987 was 0.043%.

Regarding military recruits, over 0.15% of 1,250,000 military applicants screened between October 1985 and September 1987 were HIV seropositive (12). As in other surveys, HIV seroprevalence varied considerably with the subjects' age, sex, race/ethnicity, and geographic area of residence.

Concerning patients attending STD clinics, review of 23 studies from 16 states indicated that 1,047 (4.6%) of 22,624 clinic attendees were HIV seropositive (9). In general, the seropositivity rate was higher among men (6.6%) than among women (1.6%). Seropositivity rates ranged from 0.5% to 15.2%, reflecting in part the proportion of attendees who were homosexual or bisexual, I.V. drug users, or heterosexual partners of bisexual men or I.V. drug users.

In these studies, nearly 90% of all HIV-seropositive persons belonged to recognized risk groups. Surveys conducted in six cities found the seroprevalence in heterosexual men and women without a history of I.V. drug abuse or known sexual contact with persons at risk to range from 0% to 2.6%, depending upon the population studied and the interview method used (6, 9, 13).

To sample a non-self-selected general population, the CDC developed a network of sentinel hospitals in collaboration with the participating institutions in September 1986. Based on the first 8,668 test results, the overall prevalence of infection was 0.32% (9). Higher rates were documented in selected areas such as Baltimore, Maryland, where over 5% of the emergency room patients studied were HIV-positive (14).

Another technique for determining levels of infection among sexually active women consists of filter-paper blood testing of newborns to measure maternal antibody passively transferred to the child. One study in Massachusetts found the weighted average prevalence of infection among 30,078 childbearing women to be 0.21% (9, 15), the prevalence varying from 0.09% for women delivering at suburban and rural hospitals to 0.80% for those delivering at inner-city hospitals. Additional information has been provided by 27 studies of women in female health and childbearing settings. Among other things these studies (conducted in 19 cities in 12 states and territories) documented infection in anywhere from 1% to 2.6% of study subjects in the New York City area and Puerto Rico.

Obviously, the epidemic of HIV infection and AIDS cases is a composite of many individual, overlapping, smaller epidemics, each of which has its own dynamics and time frame (6). Whereas the overall incidence of new infection as well as the incidence among certain subgroups such as homosexual men and Red Cross blood donors may have declined slightly, in the absence of specific information incidence rates cannot be assumed to have declined among all subgroups or in all geographic areas. In fact, HIV infection rates among I.V. drug users and heterosexually active people appear to be increasing in localized areas such as inner cities, especially on the East Coast. (Two studies among originally seronegative I.V. drug users in the New York City area showed seroconversion in 3% and 19%, respectively, between 1985 and 1986.)

On the basis of the available data presented in its review, the CDC estimated that the number of HIV-infected Americans ranged from 945,000 to 1,400,000 (Table 3) (6). The major factors limiting the precision of this estimate are the unknown size of the population of homosexual and bisexual men, the unknown distribution by frequency and type of various risk-related practices within this population, and the unknown overall seroprevalence rate among the general heterosexual population without any specific identified risk (a rate estimated at 0.021% based on the rate of infection in military applicants with no identifiable risk factors).

While there is no substitute for carefully obtained HIV antibody incidence and prevalence data, certain inferences can be derived from these past studies. First, it seems clear that HIV infection is widely prevalent among selected high-risk groups in our society, such as homosexual and bisexual men, intravenous drug abusers, hemophiliacs, and heterosexual partners of these at-risk individuals. Second, while the incidence of HIV infection may be slowing in homosexual men, it is continuing to increase in intravenous drug users and their heterosexual partners. Third, HIV infection rates appear to be increasing among minority populations, particularly in the inner cities along the Eastern Seaboard. Fourth, the natural history of HIV infection suggests that the mean incubation period from the time of infection to the time of developing AIDS is at least eight to ten years.

Together, these facts indicate that the AIDS epidemic has not yet peaked, and that the number of AIDS cases is not likely to decline within the next several years. Rather, it appears that the number of AIDS cases will continue to increase for at least five years and possibly longer. For even if we were 100% successful in preventing further transmission today, the number of AIDS cases would continue to rise on an annual basis because of the large number of people already infected with HIV.

AIDS Projections

At a recent meeting of the U.S. Public Health Service, the number of AIDS cases were projected by year for 1988–1992 using two methods. The first method, referred to as the extrapolation approach, statistically fit an empirical model to past trends and projected those trends into the future (5). This approach is reasonable because HIV's long and variable incubation time yields a distribution that will smooth trends and AIDS incidence even though the underlying trends in HIV infection may be changing. The total number of cumulative cases projected through 1992 using the extrapolation method was 365,000 (Table 4, Figure 3).

A second method, known as back-calculation, estimates future AIDS cases from the historical trends in HIV infection, AIDS incidence data, and knowledge of the incubation time distribution assuming that those infected continue to develop AIDS according to that distribution (16). Although the method as originally proposed does not account for new infections (such as those occurring within

Table 4. AIDS case projections by year, 1988–1992.[a]

| Years | Extrapolation method | | Back-calculation method |
	Estimated no. of cases	Interval (68% confidence)	
1981–1987	69,000		66,000
1988	39,000	32,000–41,000	41,000
1989	46,000	32,000–56,000	52,000
1990	60,000	28,000–73,000	63,000
1991	71,000	21,000–94,000	74,000
1992	80,000	13,000–111,900	84,000
Cumulative total	365,000	205,000–440,000	380,000

[a]Data provided by Mead Morgan, Ph.D., at the CDC (personal communication); and Ronald Brookmeyer, Ph.D., at Johns Hopkins University (personal communication).

two to three years), it gives reasonable near-term projections (two to three years) because of the long incubation time of HIV. (Additional adjustments can also be made to allow for new infections.) Utilizing the back-calculation method with the current estimate of infected people (Table 3), a cumulative total of 380,000 cases was estimated through 1992. It should be noted that the projected numbers of AIDS cases increased annually throughout the time period.

Each of these methods has certain limitations. The extrapolation model is purely empirical and assumes that diagnostic and reporting trends remain unchanged. The model does not depend upon or use quantitative data on the natural history of HIV infection. Despite these limitations, over the past three years the model has performed well in projecting relatively short-term AIDS trends (e.g., the number of future cases arising in two years—Figure 1, 6).

In contrast, the back-calculation method requires accurate information about HIV's incubation time distribution. Additional follow-up of selected cohorts is continually needed to more precisely estimate the shape of this distribution, and additional adjustments are required to account for new infections. While these matters have relatively little impact on short-term projections, they become increasingly important over time irrespective of the model used.

Conclusions

HIV infection and AIDS have become a major cause of morbidity and mortality in the United States. Since over a million U.S. residents are thought to be infected with HIV, morbidity and mortality can be

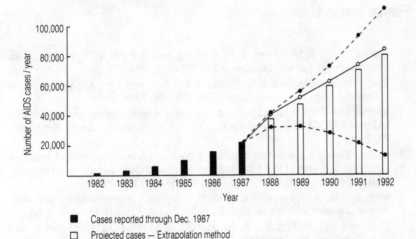

Figure 3. Revised projection of the number of AIDS cases anticipated in the United States through 1992, calculated from the known reported cases through 1987. The two projections shown were obtained using extrapolation and back-calculation (68% confidence limits for the projection based on extrapolation are also shown). The expected numbers of cases predicted by the two methods are remarkably similar.

expected to increase over the next few years, and the number of AIDS cases will continue to rise. While the social and medical impact of this disease will be profound, with medical care alone costing billions of dollars, the greatest tragedy will be the loss of thousands upon thousands of lives.

Although this article concerns itself with the HIV/AIDS problem in the United States, that problem is common to all nations; and it is only through a united international effort that we can hope to control the disease and prevent further transmission. Basic control actions—including professional and public education, risk-behavior reduction in the high-risk groups, and screening of blood supplies—can be implemented, but the obstacles to complete control remain pervasive in our political societies. Further information about the magnitude of HIV infection and HIV incidence rates within many populations, and updating of projections of infection, disease, and mortality by the use of updated mathematical models should help convince political and medical authorities, as well as the general public, about the ove impact of this disease on our society.

References

1. Quinn, T. C., J. M. Mann, J. W. Curran, and P. Piot. AIDS in Africa: an epidemiologic paradigm. *Science* 234:955–963, 1986.

2. Piot, P., F. A. Plummer, F. S. Mhalu, J. L. Chin, and J. M. Mann. AIDS: an international perspective. *Science* 239:573–579, 1988.

3. World Health Organization. Acquired immunodeficiency syndrome (AIDS): CDC/WHO case definition for AIDS. *Weekly Epidemiol Rec* 61:69–73, 1986.

4. United States Centers for Disease Control. Table V: estimated years of potential life lost (YPLL) before age 65 and cause-specific mortality, by cause of death—United States, 1986. *MMWR* 37:163, 1988.

5. Morgan, W. M., and J. W. Curran. Acquired immunodeficiency syndrome: current and future trends. *Public Health Rep* 101:459–465, 1986.

6. Curran, J. W., H. W. Jaffe, A. M. Hardy, W. M. Morgan, R. M. Selik, and T. J. Dondero. Epidemiology of HIV infection and AIDS in the United States. *Science* 239:610–616, 1988.

7. Medley, G. F., R. M. Anderson, D. R. Cox, and L. Billard. Incubation period of AIDS in patients infected via blood transfusion. *Nature* 328:719–721, 1987.

8. Jaffe, H. W., W. W. Darrow, D. F. Echenberg, P. M. O'Malley, J. P. Getchell, V. S. Kalyanaraman, R. H. Byers, D. P. Drennan, E. H. Braff, and J. W. Curran. The acquired immunodeficiency syndrome in a cohort of homosexual men: a six-year follow-up study. *Ann Intern Med* 103:210–214, 1985.

9. United States Centers for Disease Control. Human immunodeficiency virus infection in the United States: a review of current knowledge. *MMWR* 36:1–48, 1987.

10. Chamberland, M. E., and T. J. Dondero. Heterosexually acquired infection with human immunodeficiency virus (HIV) (editorial). *Ann Intern Med* 107:763–768, 1987.

11. Peterman, T. A., R. L. Stoneburner, J. R. Allen, H. W. Jaffe, and J. W. Curran. Risk of HIV transmission from heterosexual adults with transfusion-associated infections. *JAMA* 259:55–58, 1988.

12. Burke, D. S., J. F. Brundage, J. R. Herbold, W. Bemer, L. I. Gardner, J. D. Guzenhauser, J. Voskovitch, and R. R. Redfield. Human immunodeficiency virus (HIV) infections among civilian applicants for United States military service, October 1985 to March 1986: demographic factors associated with seropositivity. *N Engl J Med* 317:131–136, 1987.

13. Quinn, T. C., D. Glasser, R. O. Cannon, O. L. Matuszak, R. W. Dunning, R. L. Kline, C. H. Campbell, E. Israel, A. S. Fauci, and E. W. Hooks. Human immunodeficiency virus infection among patients attending clinics for sexually transmitted diseases. *N Engl J Med* 318:197–203, 1988.

14. Kelen, G. D., S. Fritz, B. Qadish, R. Brookmeyer, J. L. Baker, R. L. Kline, R. M. Cuddy, T. K. Goessel, D. J. Floccare, K. T. Sivertson, S. Altman, and T. C. Quinn. Unrecognized human immunodeficiency virus infection in emergency department patients. *N Engl J Med* 318:1645–1650, 1988.

15. Marwick, C. HIV antibody prevalence data derived from study of Massachusetts infants. *JAMA* 258:171–172, 1987.
16. Brookmeyer, R., and M. H. Gail. A method for obtaining short-term projections and lower bounds on the size of the AIDS epidemic. *J Am Stat Assoc* 83:301–308, 1988.

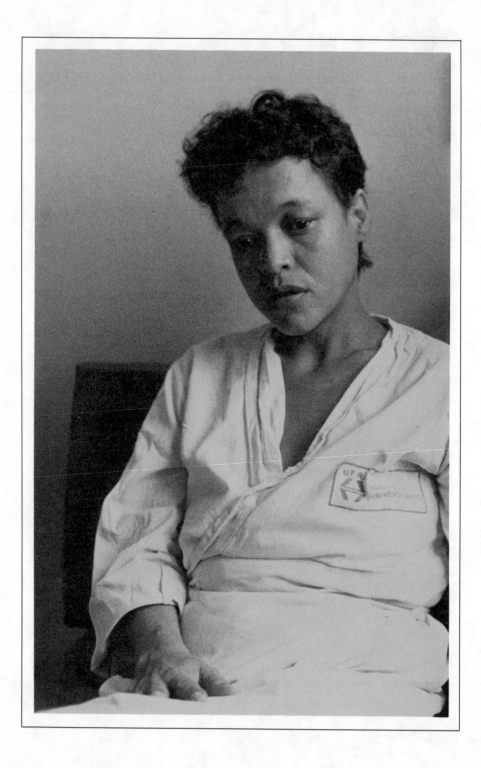

AIDS IN MEXICO: TRENDS AND PROJECTIONS

JOSE LUIS VALDESPINO G., JOSE ANTONIO IZAZOLA L., & BLANCA RICO G.

Broadly speaking, AIDS epidemiology around the world can be regarded as involving four transmission patterns found in distinct geographic regions, as follows:

- In some parts of Africa and the Caribbean, transmission began before the 1970s. High levels of HIV infection have been found, the agent being transmitted predominantly through heterosexual contact, perinatal contact, and blood transfusions (1).

- In the United States and Western Europe, transmission typically began toward the end of the 1970s and has produced high levels of HIV infection among homosexual and bisexual males and intravenous drug abusers. HIV transmission through blood transfusions has been limited. In general, persistent but low levels of heterosexual transmission have occurred, and perinatal transmission has been occurring in hyperendemic areas (2).

- In Latin America outside the Caribbean, transmission began in the early 1980s and has produced moderate prevalences of infection among groups engaging in high-risk practices, chiefly homosexual and especially bisexual males. Blood transfusions have played an important role in HIV transmission, one that has not been completely eliminated; but the proportions of cases occurring as a result of intravenous drug abuse and perinatal contact have been low (3, 4).

31

- In Asia and Oceania, transmission of HIV began in the mid-1980s among groups engaging in high-risk practices. However, there is as yet no evidence of transmission through blood products, and levels of perinatal transmission are low (4).

Analysis of these different epidemiologic patterns suggests that HIV transmission first involves homosexuals with many partners; but then, as the epidemic progresses, the agent comes to spread mainly between heterosexuals with fewer partners. Perinatal transmission reflects HIV transmission to women, both sexually and through blood transfusions. The experiences of some countries to date have indicated that transmission via blood transfusion can be controlled by energetic measures designed to detect HIV infections in blood donors (5).

AIDS Epidemiology in Mexico

As of June 1988 a cumulative total of 1,502 AIDS cases had been reported in Mexico, the number having grown exponentially and having doubled, on the average, once every 7.7 months. Besides age distribution, the dynamics of past HIV transmission in Mexico is reflected in the sex ratio, there having been 11 male AIDS cases for every female case.

Among adult males, 92.7% of those afflicted acquired the infection through sexual contact. Of this 92.7%, most (58.6%) was accounted for by people identified as homosexuals, a smaller share (26.3%) by ones identified as bisexuals, and the remaining 7.8% by ones identified as heterosexuals. Also, 5.7% of the adult males with AIDS were infected via contaminated blood or blood products, with 4.3% being transfusion recipients, 1.1% hemophiliacs, and 0.3% having been infected through intravenous drug abuse. Regarding the relatively small number of adult females with AIDS, some two-thirds appear to have acquired their infections through blood transfusions and the remainder through heterosexual contact.

Overall, the most frequent mode of HIV transmission in the adults with AIDS was sexual contact, which accounted for 87.6% of the reported cases, while transfusion with contaminated blood or blood products accounted for 10.8% and intravenous drug abuse for 0.3%. In addition, 56 pediatric AIDS cases were reported, of which transmission through contaminated blood accounted for 67.9%, sexual contact for 5.4%, and perinatal transmission for 19.6% (6). The modes of transmission of the remaining 1.3% of adult cases and 7.1% of pediatric cases are unknown.

Current Trends and Projections

Trends in the numbers of AIDS cases in Mexico indicate that the disease is spreading from the large cities to the suburbs and country-side. Also, the incidence of AIDS is rising faster among women and children than among young men, even though the latter still account

Table 1. Reported AIDS cases in Mexico by time of onset, 1981–June 1988, and exponential projections of case numbers based on the 1983–1986 and 1983–June 1987 data.

Year and first or second half		Reported AIDS cases		Estimated AIDS cases (cumulative total)	
		No.	Cumulative total	1983–1986	1983–1987 (first half)
1981	1	1	1	5	5
	2	1	2	7	8
1982	1	3	5	12	12
	2	8	13	19	20
1983	1	18	31	30	31
	2	18	49	47	48
1984	1	18	67	75	76
	2	54	121	119	118
1985	1	79	200	189	186
	2	141	341	301	291
1986	1	156	497	477	456
	2	296	793	757	716
1987	1	369	1,162	1,201	1,122
	2	253	1,415	1,905	1,760
1988	1	87	1,502	3,024	2,759
	2			4,798	4,327
1989	1			7,614	6,784
	2			12,081	10,638
1990	1			19,171	16,680
	2			30,421	26,154
1991	1			48,274	41,010
	2			76,602	64,304

for the largest number of cases. It appears that the disease is spreading faster among heterosexual males than among homosexual and bisexual males.

If one directly applies the curves derived from 1983–1986 and 1983–1987 (first half) AIDS case data, the resulting projections indicate that the cumulative number of AIDS cases occurring in Mexico by the end of 1991 could range from 64,304 to 76,602. As Table 1 shows, the higher projection was derived from the 1983–1986 data, while the lower projection was obtained by including data from the first half of 1987. Later data have not been used in the projections because not all cases beginning in the second half of 1987 and the first half of 1988 have been diagnosed.

It should also be noted that exponential growth curves do not accurately describe the AIDS case growth rates observed in all countries. In the United States, for example, no exponential growth of AIDS cases has been seen since 1983. Hence, a number of possible adjusted curves have been proposed, among them a dampened exponential curve. (A principal problem involved in applying this latter curve is accurately determining in advance the point where the exponential growth starts decelerating.) Another alternative is to project various estimates based on changes in the incidence growth rate and doubling interval.

In this regard it appears relevant that growth in the incidence of AIDS cases in Mexico City appears less rapid than it was, and that the doubling intervals observed there are longer than those found in other jurisdictions. It thus appears that the phase of rapid growth in Mexico City may be giving way to slower exponential growth.

Nationwide, by estimating the number of cases associated with different doubling rates, we can project various possible behavior patterns for the epidemic. Table 2 indicates two such possible patterns.

Conclusions

Overall, the number of AIDS cases in Mexico to date has continued to grow at an exponential rate, despite the decelerating growth rate observed in Mexico City. Projections of anticipated AIDS cases based on observed growth rates lead to anticipation of continued exponential growth. However, projections of this growth must be reduced in order to incorporate the observations for Mexico City, where about

Table 2. Estimates of the cumulative AIDS cases that would be expected in Mexico during 1988-1994, by year of origin, if the incidence rate's doubling time were prolonged as shown.

	Intermediate reduced rate of increase			Low reduced rate of increase		
Year	Cumulative cases	Monthly rate of increase (%)	Doubling time (months)	Cumulative cases	Monthly rate of increase (%)	Doubling time (months)
1988	2,427	8	8.6	2,427	8	8.6
1989	6,339	8	8.6	5,622	7	9.9
1990	14,683	7	9.9	13,022	7	9.9
1991	34,011	7	9.9	26,752	6	11.6
1992	69,873	6	11.6	54,960	6	11.6
1993	143,549	6	11.6	100,144	5	13.8
1994	261,563	5	13.8	182,474	5	13.8

20% of the population and one-third of the AIDS cases in the country are concentrated.

AIDS case projections must also consider relevant transmission patterns and sociodemographic factors. For example, HIV is expected to spread most extensively in marginal urban and rural settings, most commonly afflicting people with low socioeconomic status. Increased transmission of the disease among women and children presages a wider age distribution of AIDS cases, even though most cases are still expected to occur among young men.

In this same vein, although the upward trend in HIV transmission among homosexual males is expected to persist, the proportion of AIDS cases among exclusively homosexual males is expected to decline because of increased HIV transmission among bisexuals and heterosexuals. It also seems probable that AIDS cases associated with receipt of blood and blood products will decline over the next four years or so as a result of HIV detection in blood donors.

References

1. Quinn, T. C., J. M. Mann, J. W. Curran, and P. Piot. AIDS in Africa: an epidemiologic paradigm. *Science* 234:955–963, 1986.
2. Curran, J. W., H. W. Jaffe, A. M. Hardy, W. M. Morgan, R. M. Selik, and T. J. Dondero. Epidemiology of HIV infection and AIDS in the United States. *Science* 239:610–616, 1988.

3. St. John, R. K., and F. Zacarías. Status of AIDS in the Americas. Paper presented at the III International Conference on Acquired Immunodeficiency Syndrome held in Washington, D.C., 1-5 June 1987.

4. Valdespino, J. L., J. Sepúlveda, J. A. Izazola, et al. Patrones y predicciones epidemiológicas del SIDA en México. *Salud Pública Mex* 30(4):567-592, 1988.

5. Piot, P., F. A. Plummer, F. S. Mhalu, J. L. Chin, and J. M. Mann. AIDS: an international perspective. *Science* 239:573-579, 1988.

6. Dirección General de Epidemiología. Situación del SIDA en México hasta el primero de junio de 1988. *Bol Mens SIDA (México)* 2 (6):322-330, 1988.

AIDS IN COLOMBIA

JORGE BOSHELL S., MANUEL G. GACHARNA, MARCELA GARCIA, LUZ SOCORRO JARAMILLO, GLADYS MARQUEZ, MARIA MERCEDES FERGUSSON, STELLA GONZALEZ, ELSA Y. PRADA, ROSANA DE RANGEL, & ROSALBA DE CABAS

In 1983, after the first case of acquired immunodeficiency syndrome (AIDS) was diagnosed in Colombia, the Ministry of Health established a national program against AIDS (Programa Nacional de Lucha contra el SIDA) and made a commitment to control the spread of human immunodeficiency virus (HIV) throughout the country. As a result of this program, starting in 1984 AIDS was made a notifiable disease and screening of blood donors became compulsory in blood banks nationwide. At the same time, Colombia's National Institute of Health in Bogotá began seroepidemiologic studies designed to provide the Ministry of Health with current information on the prevalence of HIV infection in the country.

Materials and Methods

Since 1983 the Health Ministry's Directorate of Epidemiology (Dirección de Epidemiología) has collected nationwide data on reported

AIDS cases. Clinical AIDS cases have been diagnosed following the criteria established by the United States Centers for Disease Control (CDC) in Atlanta, Georgia (1).

HIV seroprevalence surveys have examined sera collected from voluntary blood specimen donors in the following groups:

- Female prostitutes and male homosexuals attending State Health Service clinics for sexually transmitted disease (STD).
- High-risk individuals coming to the National Institute of Health in Bogotá for free AIDS testing.
- A total of 762 Amerindians living on reservations located within the Orinoco and Amazon river basins.
- Voluntary blood donors to the Colombian Red Cross in Bogotá.
- A total of 753 individuals from both high-risk and low-risk groups in the city of Villavicencio, Meta, Colombia.

All of the survey specimens were initially screened for HIV antibodies using the Abbott enzyme-linked immunosorbent assay (ELISA) HIV-recombinant kit. Sera found repeatedly positive by ELISA were submitted to the Virus Laboratory at the National Institute of Health (Bogotá) for confirmation by indirect immunofluorescence assay (IIFA) and Western blot analysis.

The IIFA was performed as described by Gallo et al. (2) using HT and H9 continuous cell lines (3) kindly provided in 1987 by Dr. Paul Feorino, Chief of the Virus Laboratory, AIDS Program, at the CDC in Atlanta. Sera were tested at both 1:10 and 1:50 dilutions.

Western blot antigen was kindly provided in 1987 by Dr. Charles Schable, Chief of the AIDS Diagnostic Laboratory at the CDC in Atlanta, and Western blot antigen strips were prepared at the Virus Laboratory (National Institute of Health, Bogotá) following CDC procedures (4). Test sera were incubated with the strips at a 1:100 dilution, and antigen-antibody reactions were detected with commercial enzyme-conjugated anti-human globulins reacted with appropriate chemical substrates. We considered a serum positive if it reacted with one of the core proteins (p15, p18, p24) and one of the envelope glycoproteins (gp41, gp120). Sera reacting only with core or envelope proteins were considered equivocal (following CDC criteria), and therefore the test was not considered confirmatory.

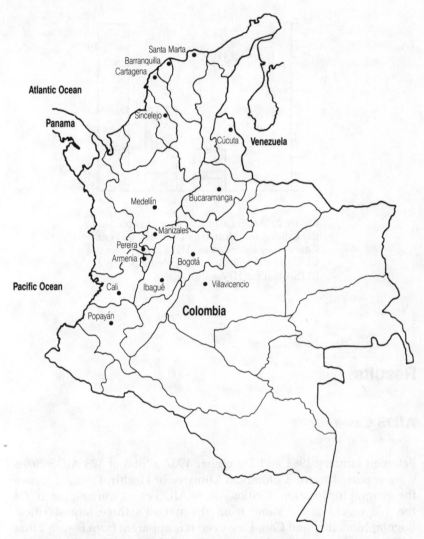

Figure 1. A map of Colombia showing cities where AIDS cases were reported in 1983–1987.

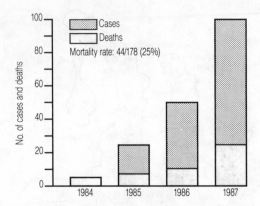

Figure 2. AIDS cases and deaths reported to the Colombian Ministry of Health, by year. Cases were recorded as AIDS if they met the CDC clinical criteria and yielded a positive ELISA test for HIV antibodies.

Results

AIDS Cases

Between January 1984 and December 1987 a total of 178 AIDS cases were reported to the Colombian Ministry of Health. Figure 1 shows the geographic location of cities where AIDS cases were reported. Of the 178 cases, 57.3% came from the nation's three largest cities: Bogotá, Medellín, and Cali. However, it is apparent from Figure 1 that AIDS cases have occurred in most major Colombian cities, suggesting that HIV-1 is already widely distributed in the Republic.

Figure 2 shows the total number of AIDS cases and deaths recorded each year since reporting began. Four cases were reported in 1984, 25 in 1985, 50 in 1986, and 99 in 1987. Most (97%) of these cases have occurred in males, yielding a male:female ratio of 32:1. The five reported female AIDS patients were all prostitutes.

An attempt was made to determine the sexual preferences of patients with the 99 AIDS cases reported during 1987. This study

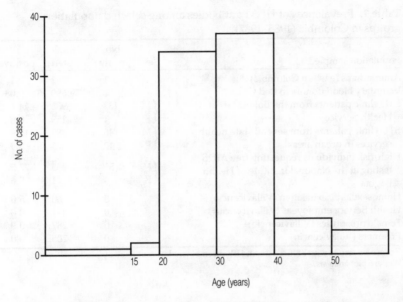

Figure 3. Distribution by age group of 84 Colombian AIDS patients whose cases occurred between January 1984 and December 1987.

showed that 67% of the cases afflicted homosexual males and two cases afflicted heterosexual females (both prostitutes). The sexual preferences of the remaining 31 patients could not be determined.

Figure 3 shows the age distribution of 84 Colombian AIDS patients. The exact ages of the remaining 95 AIDS patients are unknown. Most of the 84 cases afflicted people between 20 and 39 years of age. However, one case of pediatric AIDS occurred in a three-month-old child secondary to blood transfusion.

HIV-1 Seroprevalence

Table 1 shows the prevalence of HIV-1 antibodies among selected population groups in Colombia. The sera used in these studies were collected between 1985 and 1987. The highest antibody prevalence was found among high-risk individuals who participated in a free AIDS testing program offered by the National Institute of Health in

Table 1. Prevalences of HIV-1 antibodies among selected population groups in Colombia (1985–1987).

Population sampled	Sex	No. positive[a]	Total tested	% positive
Amerindians (eastern Colombia)		1	762	0.1
Voluntary blood donors to Red Cross		32	39,690	0.08
STD clinic patients from the Bogotá	M	137	936	14.6
Health Service	F	1	159	0.6
STD clinic patients from several state health	M	46	289	15.9
services in urban areas	F	12	305	3.9
High-risk individuals requesting free AIDS testing at the National Institute of Health,	M	53	235	22.5
Bogotá	F	4	71	5.6
Homosexual/bisexual men (Villavicencio)		3	60	5.0
Health Service employees (Villavicencio)		0	201	0.0
Female prostitutes (Villavicencio)		0	287	0.0
Prisoners (Villavicencio)		0	205	0.0

[a]Positive results with ELISA (Abbott HIV recombinant kit) confirmed by positive IIFA and Western blot analysis.

Bogotá. A relatively high HIV-1 antibody prevalence was also found among patients attending STD clinics in Bogotá and several other urban areas. Most of the patients attending these clinics were female prostitutes or male homosexuals. In each of the three groups classified by sex that are shown in Table 1, the HIV-1 infection rate was significantly higher in males than in females.

For comparison with the results obtained among these high-risk groups in Bogotá and other major urban areas, we examined sera from 753 persons living in Villavicencio, Meta Department. This is a medium-sized commercial city with 174,000 inhabitants that is located in the eastern plains (Llanos Orientales) region. Three out of 60 (5%) of the tested homosexual/bisexual men in Villavicencio had HIV-1

Table 2. Prevalences of HIV-1 antibodies found among volunteers donating blood to the Colombian Red Cross in 1985, 1986, and 1987.

Year	Sex	No. positive[c]	No. tested	% positive
1985[a]		0	804	0
1986[b]		0	809	0
1987[a]	M	32	24,673	0.13
	F	0	13,404	0

[a]Data based on ELISA results from seven major cities.
[b]Data based on ELISA results from Bogotá only.
[c]According to ELISA results obtained with commercial kits.

antibodies, but no member of the other groups tested (female prostitutes, prisoners, and health service employees) was found to be infected. Likewise, only one of 762 Amerindians living in the remote eastern regions of the country was found to have HIV-1 antibodies.

Table 2 shows the prevalence of HIV-1 antibodies among volunteer blood donors in Colombia during 1985, 1986, and 1987. Relatively few donors were tested by the Red Cross in 1985 and 1986, but all were negative. During 1987, 32 of 38,077 donors tested (0.08%) were found to have HIV-1 antibodies. All of the positive donors were males.

Discussion

The results of our studies indicate that HIV-1 infection and AIDS are widely distributed in Colombia and probably occur in most urban areas of the country. To date, the pattern of infection seems similar to that observed in Europe and North America, with most of the AIDS cases occurring among males in the 20–39 year age range.

Infection of these men has probably resulted mainly from homosexual activity. However, there is also evidence of heterosexual transmission of HIV-1 in Colombia, since AIDS cases and HIV-1 antibodies have also been found among prostitutes and intravenous drug abuse has not been reported in the country. Aside from these two high-risk groups, the prevalence of HIV-1 infection in the general population is still quite low, as shown by the antibody rates among blood donors and other low-risk population groups (Table 1).

The total number of reported AIDS cases in Colombia has doubled or tripled every year since reporting began in 1984 (Figure 2). This pattern, essentially the same as that observed worldwide, points up the urgency of developing control measures to halt the spread of HIV-1 infection. In Colombia, these control measures have included public education about AIDS, mandatory testing of blood donors, establishment of HIV-1 diagnostic laboratories, and provision of free AIDS testing services for high-risk persons.

■ ■ ■

Acknowledgments: We are greatly indebted to Dr. Robert B. Tesh for his valuable suggestions and review of the manuscript, to Alcira Díaz for her assistance in preparation of the manuscript, and to Dr. Marcela Salazar, Hector Anaya, and Hilda Guzmán for collecting blood samples from Amerindians on the plains of Vichada and Catatumbo in Guajira, Colombia. Dr. David Saavedra supported us in obtaining sera from the Bogotá STD clinic, Alba Sofía Rojas kindly provided us with the epidemiologic data on the AIDS cases, and Olga Parada collaborated with us at the beginning of the study in Villavicencio. We also wish to acknowledge Faye Cowart from the Laboratory Branch—AIDS Program, CDC, Atlanta, Georgia, USA, for introducing us to the Western blot assay.

References

1. United States Centers for Disease Control. Human immunodeficiency virus (HIV) infection codes: Official authorized addendum ICD-9-CM. *MMWR* 36:507, 1987.
2. Gallo, D., J. L. Diggs, G. R. Shell, P. J. Dailey, M. B. Hoffman, and J. L. Riggs. Comparison of detection of antibody to the acquired immune deficiency syndrome virus by enzyme immunoassay, immunofluorescence, and Western blot methods. *J Clin Microbiol* 23:1049–1051, 1986.
3. Popovic, M., M. G. Sarngadharan, E. Read, and R. C. Gallo. Detection, isolation and continuous production of cytopathic retroviruses (HTLV-III) from patients with AIDS and pre-AIDS. *Science* 224:497–500, 1984.
4. Tsang, V. C. W., K. Hancock, M. Wilson, D. F. Palmer, S. D. Whaley, J. S. McDougal, and S. Kennedy. *Enzyme-linked Immunoelectrotransfer Blot Technique (Western Blot) for HTLV-III/LAV Antibodies.* Immunology Series No. 15, Procedural Guide. Centers for Disease Control, Atlanta, Georgia, United States, December 1986.

AIDS IN BRAZIL, 1982-1988

LAIR GUERRA DE MACEDO RODRIGUES & PEDRO CHEQUER

Brazil has the fourth highest number of reported AIDS cases in the world, surpassed only by the United States, France, and Uganda. In terms of incidence relative to size of population, however, it ranks below fortieth.

The first cases of AIDS in Brazil were identified in 1982 in the states of Rio de Janeiro and São Paulo, where one and four cases were recorded, respectively. In 1983, 31 more cases were recognized; in 1986, 867 were reported; and in 1988, through 30 July, 914 new cases had been diagnosed (Table 1). As the number of cases has grown, the annual incidence of the disease per one million population has increased from 0.05 in 1982 to 6.5 in 1988.

The following report reviews some aspects of the epidemiologic profile of AIDS in Brazil.

Spatial Distribution of Cases

Since the first cases were recognized, southern and central Brazil, and specifically the Southeast region, have had the largest concentration of cases. As of 30 July 1988, this region accounted for 81.1% of the

Source: Ministério de Saúde, Brazil. *Boletim Epidemiológico AIDS* Ano I, No. 6, 1987, and Ano II, No. 1, 1988.

Table 1. Number of AIDS cases, percentages, and case rate per million population by place of residence (region and political unit), Brazil, 1988 (through 30 July) and cumulative 1982–1988.

Region/political unit	1988 (through 30 July)			1982–1988[a]		
	No.	%	Cases/ million pop.	No.	%	Cases/ million pop.
North	8	0.9	1.0	29	0.7	4.1
Rondônia	1	0.1	1.2	5	0.1	7.2
Acre	—	—	—	3	0.1	8.6
Amazonas	3	0.3	1.6	6	0.2	3.6
Roraima	—	—	—	—	—	—
Pará	3	0.3	0.7	14	0.4	3.4
Amapá	1	0.1	4.4	1	0.0	4.8
Northeast	97	10.6	2.4	326	8.2	8.5
Fernando de Noronha	—	—	—	—	—	—
Maranhão	4	0.4	0.8	13	0.3	2.9
Piauí	2	0.2	0.8	7	0.2	2.9
Ceará	16	1.8	2.6	42	1.1	7.3
Rio Grande do Norte	11	1.2	5.0	29	0.7	13.9
Paraíba	5	0.5	1.6	21	0.5	7.0
Pernambuco	20	2.2	2.9	99	2.5	14.8
Alagoas	9	1.0	3.9	22	0.6	10.0
Sergipe	6	0.7	4.4	13	0.3	10.0
Bahia	24	2.6	2.2	80	2.0	7.6
Southeast	697	76.3	11.2	3,204	81.1	55.1
Minas Gerais	17	1.9	1.1	110	2.8	7.6
Espírito Santo	12	1.3	5.0	32	0.8	14.2
Rio de Janeiro	91	10.0	6.8	661	16.7	52.7
São Paulo	577	63.1	18.4	2,401	60.8	82.9
South	86	9.4	4.0	265	6.7	13.0
Paraná	14	1.5	1.7	58	1.5	7.2
Santa Catarina	8	0.9	1.9	28	0.7	7.0
Rio Grande do Sul	64	7.0	7.3	179	4.5	21.4
Central-West	26	2.8	2.7	128	3.2	14.4
Goiás	6	0.7	1.3	36	0.9	8.3
Mato Grosso	8	0.9	5.0	29	0.7	20.3
Mato Grosso do Sul	2	0.2	1.2	18	0.5	11.5
Distrito Federal	10	1.1	5.8	45	1.1	29.5
Total	914	100.0	6.5	3,952	100.0	29.7

Source: National Division for the Control of Sexually Transmitted Diseases/AIDS, Epidemiology Service.

[a]Preliminary data for 1988, through 30 July. Numbers subject to revision.

total of notified cases in the country; 96% of the cases in that region had occurred in the states of São Paulo (2,401 cases, 60.8% of the national total) and Rio de Janeiro (661 cases, 16.7% of the national total). The Southeast region also presents the highest cumulative case rate, at 55.1 cases per million population; for São Paulo and Rio de

Janeiro states, the rates are 82.9 and 52.7, respectively. The Federal District is the political division with the third highest rate, and next, in descending order, are the states of Rio Grande do Sul, Mato Grosso, and Pernambuco.

Case Distribution by Age

The age profile of AIDS cases resembles that observed in the other countries of the Western Hemisphere and in general has not altered much from year to year during the seven years of the epidemic. In the past three years, however, there has been a significant increase in the number of pediatric cases, which now account for 3.1% of total recorded cases. Perinatal transmission and transfusion of contaminated blood or blood products are responsible for these cases.

Since the primary mode of transmission is sexual, it is not surprising that persons 25 to 40 years old constitute the age group most affected, in terms of both absolute number of cases (with 58.2% of the total) and statistical risk (the highest prevalence rates). Within this larger group, the 30-to-34-year-old age group has experienced 22.6% of total reported cases and has the highest case rate of any age group, at 102.9 per million (Table 2).

Case Distribution by Sex

In Brazil, only 295 (7.5%) of reported AIDS cases have occurred in women. This pattern is similar to the distribution by sex in most other countries of the Americas outside the Caribbean, but it differs substantially from the approximately 1:1 sex ratio observed for cases in Central Africa and the ratio of about 4:1 male to female cases observed in Haiti and the Dominican Republic.

Transmission Categories

Sexual transmission has been responsible for 72.8% (2,879) of recorded cases; of those, 91% (2,621) have occurred in homosexual

Table 2. Number of AIDS cases, percentages, and specific case rates per million population, by age group, Brazil, 1988 (through 30 July) and cumulative 1982–1988.

Age group (years)	1988 (through 30 July)			1982–1988[a]		
	No.	%	Cases/ million pop.	No.	%	Cases/ million pop.
Under 1	10	1.1	2.4	29	0.7	7.3
1 to 4	14	1.5	0.9	37	0.9	2.6
5 to 9	6	0.7	0.3	32	0.8	1.9
10 to 14	4	0.4	0.2	28	0.7	1.8
15 to 19	26	2.8	1.6	97	2.5	6.4
20 to 24	105	11.5	7.6	398	10.1	30.7
25 to 29	196	21.4	17.3	717	18.1	67.1
30 to 34	196	21.4	21.1	893	22.6	102.9
35 to 39	142	15.5	18.7	692	17.5	97.0
40 to 44	85	9.3	12.5	435	11.0	67.9
45 to 49	61	6.7	11.1	254	6.4	48.9
50 to 54	15	1.6	3.1	113	2.9	24.7
55 to 59	19	2.1	5.1	81	2.0	23.2
60 and over	12	1.3	1.4	66	1.7	8.3
Unknown	23	2.5	—	80	2.0	—
Total	914	100.0	6.5	3,952	100.0	29.7

Source: National Division for the Control of Sexually Transmitted Diseases/AIDS, Epidemiology Service.

[a]Preliminary data for 1988, through 30 July. Numbers subject to revision.

and bisexual men, and 9% (258) were contracted through heterosexual contact (Table 3).

Next in order of importance is transmission by contact with contaminated blood or blood products, which has been responsible for 743 cases. Most prevalent in this category have been cases among intravenous drug users, followed by cases in transfusion recipients and hemophiliacs. This mode of transmission is highly susceptible to control, and safe, sensitive, and very effective techniques exist that can practically eliminate the risk of infection for hemophiliacs and transfusion recipients. The Federal Government is making a concerted effort to universally control the quality of blood and blood products by screening of donors with the ELISA method. In the public sector, advances have been made in this regard, although unevenly, following the decision of the Ministries of Health and of Social Security and Welfare to institute a new blood quality control policy. Regrettably, even though a highly effective strategy has been defined, cases of AIDS are still occurring among hemophiliacs and recipients of multiple transfusions because the prevalence of HIV infection was already

Table 3. Numbers and percentages of AIDS cases by transmission category and sex, and male to female case ratios, Brazil, 1982–1988.

Transmission category	Male		Female		M/F ratio	Total[a]	
	No.	%	No.	%		No.	%
Sexual transmission	2,801	76.6	78	26.4	36/1	2,879	72.8
Homosexuals	1,793	49.0	—	—	—		
Bisexuals	828	22.6	—	—	—		
Heterosexuals	180	4.9	78	26.4	2/1		
Transmission via blood	558	15.3	185	62.7	3/1	743	18.8
Hemophiliacs	145	4.0	—	—	—		
I.V. drug users	265	7.2	91	30.8	3/1		
Recipients of blood/ blood products	148	4.0	94	31.9	2/1		
Perinatal transmission	22	0.6	17	5.8	1/1	39	1.0
Undetermined/other[b]	276	7.5	15	5.1	18/1	291	7.4
Total	3,657	92.5	295	7.5	12/1	3,952	100.0

Source: National Division for the Control of Sexually Transmitted Diseases/AIDS, Epidemiology Service.
[a]Preliminary data for 1988, through 30 July. Numbers subject to revision.
[b]Case/category not investigated, or investigated but undetermined, or category other than those listed.

significant before the existence of appropriate technology for screening blood. Health promotion activities are being developed for users of intravenous drugs in order to reduce their risk of infection.

Perinatal transmission is third in order of importance and is responsible for 1.0% of total recorded cases. No cases in this category have been linked to breast-feeding, infection having taken place in utero or during birth.

In 291 (7.4%) of the AIDS cases in Brazil, the mode of transmission was undetermined (either investigated but not characterized, or not investigated).

Temporal Distribution

As described above, the number of new cases has been increasing substantially from year to year. The average of notified cases rose from 10 per month in 1984 to 89 per month—or three new cases per day—in 1987. The variety of modes of transmission and the variable incubation period do not allow any classification of cases with respect to this statistic.

Infection Prevalence and Trends

Two bases for estimating the prevalence of HIV infection should be taken into account. The first is serologic surveys carried out in certain population groups by means of diverse methodologies; and the second is projection of the prevalence of infection based on the number of actual cases, using as a parameter the ratio of 50–100 HIV-infected persons for every AIDS case. The percentages of HIV-positive results found in some serologic surveys are listed below.

- Rio de Janeiro, January–May 1987, 17,224 blood donors: 0.34%[1]
- Recife, 3,085 blood donors: 0.16%[2]
- Rio de Janeiro, sample survey of 611 convicts: 1.8%[3]
- Rio de Janeiro, 1987, 100 prostitutes: 6%[4]
- Rio de Janeiro, 1987, 100 transvestites: 37%[4]
- Rio de Janeiro, hemophiliacs (300 tested, 228 positive): 76.0%[5]

It can be seen that the circulation of the virus varies greatly in different groups, which makes it possible to delineate major risk groups based on behaviors or pre-existing conditions.

Using the above-mentioned 1:50 to 1:100 case:infection ratio as the basis for projections, and assuming an underreporting of 1,500 cases through the end of 1987 (which would bring the case total to about 4,000 at that time), the number of asymptomatic infected persons would be between 200,000 and 400,000. These are the epidemiologically significant numbers with regard to circulation of the virus and the appearance of new cases.

The situation calls for the public health entities and society as a whole to unite in intensified prevention and control efforts in order to reduce the risk of infection. Moreover, only a united effort will assure that persons afflicted by this disease are treated humanely, with dignity, and without discrimination.

[1]National Cancer Institute blood blank, Rio de Janeiro.
[2]Hemocentro de Pernambuco, Recife.
[3]Department of Health, Rio de Janeiro.
[4]Fundação Instituto Oswaldo Cruz, Rio de Janeiro.
[5]Instituto Santa Catarina, Rio de Janeiro.

HIV-1 INFECTION IN INTRAVENOUS DRUG ABUSERS WITH CLINICAL MANIFESTATIONS OF HEPATITIS IN THE CITY OF BUENOS AIRES

MARCELO DIAZ LESTREM, HUGO FAINBOIM, NORA MENDEZ, MARTHA BOXACA, OSVALDO LIBONATTI, MIGUEL ANGEL CALELLO, LAURA ASTARLOA, & MERCEDES WEISSENBACHER

Worldwide, the group with the highest prevalence of human immunodeficiency virus (HIV) infection, following promiscuous homosexuals, is intravenous (I.V.) drug abusers (1). Part of this group's epidemiologic significance resides in the fact that once HIV infection establishes itself in local I.V. drug abusers, those people can become the primary source for heterosexual transmission of the virus in their area. In addition, I.V. drug abusers are also exposed by the same intravenous route to various other infections—including those caused by hepatitis viruses B, delta, and non-A non-B (2).

Among I.V. drug abusers, notably those in Europe and the United States, the numbers of AIDS cases occurring and the results of HIV seroprevalence studies point to HIV infection as a growing problem. However, the prevalence of HIV infection among I.V. drug abusers in these two areas varies from place to place—exceeding 50% in some parts of Spain and Italy, for example (2–6), while being lower in other geographic areas of these two countries (7–9) and lower still in other countries, descending to levels such as 6.5% in Scotland (10) and 2.1% in Greece (11).

In Argentina, up to July 1988 a total of 197 AIDS cases had been reported, 12% occurring in people with histories of I.V. drug abuse (12). Overall, the seroprevalence of HIV infection among different groups of Argentine I.V. drug abusers studied has been found somewhat variable but generally high. Specifically, HIV was detected in 22% of a group of I.V. drug abusers enrolled in rehabilitation programs in the city of Buenos Aires (13), in 35% of a group of convicts with histories of I.V. drug abuse in a federal prison (14), and in 39% of a group of I.V. drug abusers who spontaneously came forward for HIV consultation in Buenos Aires (15).

Argentine serologic surveys conducted to determine prevalences of infection by HIV and by viruses for B, delta, and non-A non-B hepatitis have approached the problem from different standpoints. At present there are many reports of hepatitis B virus, non-A non-B hepatitis, and asymptomatic HIV infection in groups of drug addicts, and also reports of hepatitis B virus markers in patients infected with HIV. However, few studies have been done of HIV infections among patients with clinical pictures of acute or chronic hepatitis B or non-A non-B hepatitis. Indeed, within Argentina we know of no such published study.

It is also noteworthy that drug abuse has increased substantially in Buenos Aires and its environs, as well as in other urban Argentine communities, in recent years. The result has been an increased incidence of hepatitis types B and non-A non-B within the context of the nation's hepatitis etiology—an increase that has been especially evident among hospitalized patients.

With regard to one particular group of patients, between December 1986 and September 1987 the Hospital de Enfermedades Infecciosas "Francisco J. Muñiz" of Buenos Aires provided medical care to 99 intravenous cocaine abusers with hepatitis. Since intravenous drug addiction alone was known to entail a high risk of HIV transmission, it was decided to study the incidence of HIV infection in this group of I.V. drug abusers who had presented with hepatitis.

Materials and Methods

All of the 99 patients involved presented clinical and humoral pictures consistent with a diagnosis of hepatitis and exhibited transaminase levels 10 times higher than normal. These subjects were selected from among outpatients and inpatients at the Francisco J. Muñiz Hospital during the aforementioned study period.

Information about each subject—including his or her age, sex, sexual orientation, alcohol intake, type and duration of drug addiction, and previous episodes of hepatitis—was entered on a card designed for this purpose.

The determinations provided for each subject included total and differential bilirubin, erythrosedimentation, Quick's test, a complete hemogram, glutamic-oxaloacetic transaminase (GOT), glutamic-pyruvic transaminase (GPT), and alkaline phosphatase (AP). The presence or absence of certain immunologic markers—hepatitis B surface antigen (HBsAg), antibody to hepatitis B core antigen (anti-HBc), anti-HBc IgM, IgM antibody to hepatitis A (anti-HA IgM), and total anti-delta antibody—was determined by means of enzyme-linked immunosorbent assay (ELISA) testing that employed the Auszyme, Corzyme, Corzyme-M, anti-delta, and HAVAB-M kits commercially available from Abbott Laboratories. Subjects with hepatitis A IgM antibody (anti-HA IgM+) were classified as having hepatitis A. Those with HBsAg and anti-HBc were classified as having hepatitis B—acute hepatitis B if anti-HBc IgM was present, chronic hepatitis B if it was absent (16). Subjects serologically negative for hepatitis A virus, hepatitis B virus, cytomegalovirus, and Epstein-Barr virus were classified as having non-A non-B hepatitis.

The presence of HIV-1 was determined using three tests for screening and one for confirmation. More specifically, test sera were screened using commercial enzyme immunoassay kits from two manufacturers (Virgo HTLV-III ELISA produced by Electronucleonics Inc., Fairfield, NJ, USA, and Vironostika anti-HTLV-III Microelisa System made by Organon Teknika, Turnhout, Belgium) together with one gelatin particle agglutination kit (Serodia HIV produced by Fuji Rebio Inc., Tokyo, Japan).

Sera yielding negative results with all three screening methods were classified as negative for HIV. Those yielding positive results by one or more methods were confirmed by the Western blot test (Biotech/Dupont HIV). This latter test was considered positive if at least two of the three major bands—gp 160/120, gp 41, and p 24—were seen (17).

Results

The average age of the study population was 21 years, within a range of 14 to 32 years. As Table 1 indicates, males comprised 90% of the population—there being 89 males, including four homosexual/bisexual patients. All 99 of the patients were intravenous cocaine

Table 1. Sex, average age, and sexual orientation of the 99 intravenous drug abusers with clinical hepatitis constituting the study population.

Sex	No.	Average age (years)	Sexual orientation	
			Heterosexual	Homosexual/bisexual
Male	89	21	85	4
Female	10	20	10	0
Total	99	21	95	4

abusers, and 10% were also intravenous abusers of morphine, heroin, or other drugs (Table 2).

The subjects' serologic markers related to hepatitis A and B indicated that 62 had acute hepatitis B, 25 had chronic hepatitis B, 10 had hepatitis non-A non-B, and two had hepatitis A (Table 3). Antibodies against the delta agent were detected in five (8%) of the acute cases with hepatitis B and in four (16%) of the chronic cases with hepatitis B (Table 4).

The overall prevalence of HIV-1 antibodies found in the study patients was 47%. More specifically, 47% of the patients with acute hepatitis B tested positive for HIV-1, as did 56% of those with chronic hepatitis B and 40% of those with non-A non-B hepatitis. No HIV-1 antibodies were detected in the two subjects with hepatitis A (Table 5). Likewise, no HIV-1 antibodies were detected in the four subjects with chronic hepatitis B and anti-delta antibodies, but they were found in four of the five subjects with acute hepatitis B and anti-delta antibodies (see Table 4).

The prevalence of HIV-1 did not differ greatly with sex, HIV-1 antibodies being found in 47% of the males and 50% of the females. Two of the four male homosexual/bisexual patients yielded positive serologic results for the virus.

Table 2. Intravenous drugs used by the 99 study subjects.

Drugs	Study subjects	
	No.	(%)
Cocaine alone	89	(90)
Cocaine + morphine	4	(4)
Cocaine + heroin	1	(1)
Cocaine + 2 or more drugs	5	(5)
Total	99	(100)

Table 3. Types of hepatitis associated with particular serologic markers and the numbers of study subjects classified as having those various types.

Type of hepatitis infection and status	Serologic markers	Study subjects No.	(%)
B, acute[a]	HBsAg (+) and anti-HBc IgM (+)	62[a]	(63)
B, chronic[b]	HBsAg (+) and anti-HBc (+)	25[b]	(25)
A, acute	anti-HA IgM (+)	2	(2)
Non-A non-B	HBsAg (−), anti-HBc (−), and anti-HA IgM (−)	10	(10)
Total		99	(100)

[a] Including five cases of delta hepatitis (see Table 4).
[b] Including four cases of delta hepatitis (see Table 4).

The duration of drug addiction could only be established with reasonable certainty for 41 of the 99 study subjects. No correlation was found between their length of addiction and the prevalence of HIV-1 antibodies (Table 6).

At least 37 of the 47 patients seropositive for HIV had never traveled abroad and so must have acquired the infection in Argentina. Eight subjects could have acquired the infection in Brazil and two in Bolivia.

Thirty-five percent of the patients studied said they drank alcoholic beverages and indicated that they consumed over 80 g of ethanol daily. However, no correlation was found between this level of drinking and the prevalence of HIV-1 infection (Table 7).

Discussion and Conclusions

The prevalence of HIV-1 infection (47%) found among the study subjects was higher than the 22% prevalence detected between July and October 1987 among I.V. drug abusers attending two Buenos Aires

Table 4. Cases of delta hepatitis among the study subjects, with and without accompanying HIV infection.

Type of case	No. with HDV / No. with HBV	% HBV-positive subjects with delta antibody	Study subjects with HIV-1 and delta antibodies No. with both / No. with delta antibody
Chronic	4 / 25	16	0 / 4
Acute	5 / 62	8	4 / 5
Total	9 / 87	10	4 / 9

Table 5. The prevalence of HIV-1 antibodies observed among the 99 study subjects, grouped according to the type of hepatitis diagnosed.

Type of hepatitis infection and status	No. of study subjects	Study subjects with antibodies to HIV-1 No.	(%)
B, acute	62[a]	29	(47)
B, chronic	25[b]	14	(56)
A, acute	2	0	(0)
Non-A non-B	10	4	(40)
Total	99	47	(47)

[a]Including five cases of delta hepatitis.
[b]Including four cases of delta hepatitis.

rehabilitation clinics (*13*). However, the latter prevalence increased to 38% when only those I.V. drug abusers carrying hepatitis B markers were included.

Despite the preponderance of males among the 99 patients in our study, no marked variation in the seroprevalence of HIV-1 was observed between the sexes.

The youth of our hepatitis-positive study subjects was noteworthy, the subjects' average age being 21 years. However, this situation is comparable to that found in other groups of Argentine I.V. drug abusers, which have typically been comprised mainly of youths around 20 years of age (*13*). A third of the patients admitted daily alcohol consumption exceeding 80 g of ethanol per day, which is why a transaminase level 10 times higher than normal was required for clinical assignment to that group of patients with some type of viral hepatitis (*11*). However, no difference was found between the seroprevalences of HIV-1 antibodies among study subjects who consumed over 80 g of ethanol per day and those who did not.

Table 6. HIV-1 seroprevalences in 41 study subjects experiencing drug addiction for different lengths of time.

Length of addiction (years)	No. of study subjects	% HIV-1 seropositive
<1	19	47
1–2	9	55
>2	13	53
Total	41	

Table 7. HIV-1 seroprevalences found among study subjects said to consume over 80 g of ethanol per day and other study subjects.

| | Study subjects with daily alcohol consumptions of: | | | | Total | |
| | ≤ 80 g ethanol | | > 80 g ethanol | | | |
	No.	(%)	No.	(%)	No.	(%)
HIV-1 (+)	29	(62)	18	(38)	47	(100)
HIV-1 (−)	35	(67)	17	(33)	52	(100)
Total	64	(65)	35	(35)	99	(100)

The high percentage of study subjects with hepatitis B (88%) appears reasonable for hepatitis-afflicted I.V. drug abusers in Argentina, as does the low percentage (2%) with hepatitis A (18–20).

There was not any great variation in the seroprevalences of HIV-1 antibodies among study subjects with different hepatitis markers. Specifically, HIV-1 infection was detected in 47% of the 62 subjects with acute hepatitis B infections (including five with the delta marker), in 56% of the 25 subjects with chronic hepatitis B infections (including four with the delta marker), and in 40% of the 10 subjects with non-A non-B hepatitis. These findings are consistent with those of Muñoz Domínguez and colleagues (21), who found a significantly lower seroprevalence of HIV-1 in subjects with non-A non-B hepatitis than in those with hepatitis B.

Overall, however, it seems clear that the high prevalence of HIV-1 is related not to the presence of hepatitis B (whether acute or chronic) or non-A non-B hepatitis, but to the route of transmission that their agents share with HIV-1. This is corroborated by a low incidence of HIV antibodies found among nonaddicts and nonintravenous drug addicts positive for HBsAg (22).

Previous studies have reported a direct correlation between HIV prevalence and the length of drug addiction. In our case no correlation was found, perhaps because of the sample's small size (the duration of addiction being known in only 41 cases) and because very few of our subjects had been drug addicts for more than 5 years. However, some investigators have maintained that acquisition of hepatitis B virus and HIV generally takes place early, during the first two years of drug addiction, and that the prevalences of their markers do not rise notably thereafter (23).

The 10% prevalence of anti-delta antibodies among the 87 study subjects with hepatitis B infections deserves comment, because

Argentina is regarded as nonendemic for the delta virus. For example, Fay and colleagues found anti-delta antibodies in only 1.8% of 340 Argentine subjects with hepatitis B infections who were not I.V. drug addicts (24). Delta hepatitis was also found to be uncommon in a population of HIV-seropositive I.V. drug abusers in the United States (25). On the other hand, it has been postulated that HIV infection could reactivate both hepatitis B virus and the delta agent (26). (It is known that HIV affects the immune response to hepatitis B virus, and it may prolong productive replication of this virus—27).

HIV-1 antibodies were detected in four of the five subjects with acute hepatitis who were coinfected with hepatitis B virus and the delta agent; but there was no evidence of HIV-1 infection in the four similarly coinfected study subjects with chronic hepatitis B. With I.V. drug addiction being on the increase in Argentina, the results of this research presage a significant increase in the delta agent's prevalence in our country in the immediate future.

Overall, the results of this study are noteworthy because they serve to affirm a high incidence of hepatitis B among I.V. drug abusers with hepatitis, to indicate a prevalence of associated delta agent infection significantly higher than that found by previous studies in Argentina, and to demonstrate a high prevalence (47%) of concomitant HIV-1 infection within the study population.

References

1. Organización Panamericana de la Salud. Programa Especial de la Organización Mundial de la Salud sobre el Síndrome de Inmunodeficiencia Adquirida. *Boletín Epidemiológico* 8(1–2):1–5, 1987.

2. Conte, D., P. Ferroni, G. P. Lorini, G. P. Aimo, C. Mandelli, M. Casana, L. Brunelli, G. C. Bignotti, P. A. Bianchi, and A. R. Zanetti. HIV and HBV infection in intravenous drug addicts from northeastern Italy. *J Med Virol* 22:299–306, 1987.

3. Migneco, G., R. Attianess, and C. La Cascio. Infezione da HBV, HDV, e HTLV-III in tossicodipendienti, in cirratici ed in emodializzati. *Boll Soc Ital Biol Sper* 62(10):1905–1910, 1986.

4. Cunco Crovazi, P., G. Icardi, and A. Ponzio. Prevalenza dell'Infezione da HTLV-I e III in Tossicodipendienti: Studio Retrospetivo di 6 Anni. Paper presented at the Congress on AIDS and Related Syndromes held in Rome, Italy, 12–25 May 1987.

5. Gelosa, L., B. Borroni, and A. Panuccio. Sulla Prevalenza di Anticorpi Anti HIV in Soggetti Carcelati. Paper presented at the Congress on AIDS and Related Syndromes held in Rome, Italy, 12–25 May 1987.

6. Bertaggia, A., G. Francarilla, and L. Salmaso. Prevalenza e Tipo di Presentazione dell' Infezione da HIV in Omosessuali e Tossicodipendienti nel Veneto. Paper presented at the Congress on AIDS and Related Syndromes held in Rome, Italy, 12–25 May 1987.

7. De Carolis, M., V. Profeta, and F. Leone. Andamento dell'Infezione da HIV in una Popolazione de Tossicodipendienti nella Provinzia di Terano. Paper presented at the Congress on AIDS and Related Syndromes held in Rome, Italy, 12–25 May 1987.

8. Niutta, R. Raconto della Difusione dell'Infezione da HIV em Basilicata. Paper presented at the Congress on AIDS and Related Syndromes held in Rome, Italy, 12–25 May 1987.

9. Titti, F., G. Rezza, and P. Verani. HIV, HTLV-I, e HBV in Tossicodipendienti: Follow Up e Possibile Correlazione tra le Varie Infezione. Paper presented at the Congress on AIDS and Related Syndromes held in Rome, Italy, 12–25 May 1987.

10. Follet, E., L. Wallace, and E. McCruden. HIV and HBV infection in drug abusers in Glasgow (letter). *Lancet,* April 1987, p. 920.

11. Roumeliotou-Karayanis, A., N. Tassopoulos, and E. Karpodini. Prevalence of HBV, HDV, and HIV infections among intravenous drug addicts in Greece. *Eur J Epidemiol* 3:143–146, 1987.

12. Argentina, Secretaria de Salud, Programa Nacional de Control de Enfermedades de Transmisión Sexual y SIDA. Informe de casos acumulados hasta el 20/6/88. Buenos Aires, 1988.

13. Weissenbacher, M., O. Libonatti, R. Gertiser, E. Muzzio, R. Hosokawa, L. Chamo, J. Naveira, L. Astarloa, and M. Boxaca. Prevalence of HIV and HBV Markers in a Group of Drug Addicts in Argentina. Paper presented at the IV International Conference on AIDS, held in Stockholm, 12–16 June 1988.

14. Benetucci, J., L. Astarloa, S. Multare, S. Zarate, E. Massio, J. Rubens, M. Boxaca, and M. Weissenbacher. Prevalence of Infection among a Closed Population of Prisoners in Argentina. Paper presented at the IV International Conference on AIDS, held in Stockholm, 12–16 June 1988.

15. Muchinik, G., O. Fay, P. Cahn, M. B. Bouzas, G. Picchio, E. Richard, J. Biglione, M. Taborda, E. Bianco, A. Anselmo, M. de Tezanos Pintos, and A. Miroli. HIV Seropositivity in High-Risk Groups in Argentina: Future Impact on Heterosexual Transmission. Paper presented at the IV International Conference on AIDS, held in Stockholm, 12–16 June 1988.

16. Fagan, E., and R. Williams. Serological responses to HBV infection. *Gut* 27:858–867, 1986.

17. Committee on HIV, Association of State and Territorial Public Health Laboratory Directors. Third Consensus Conference on HIV Testing: Report and Recommendations, 8–10 March 1988, Kansas City. Department of Health and Human Services, 1988.

18. Buti, M., R. Estebán, and R. Jardi. Etiología de las hepatitis agudas en toxicómanos. *Gastroenterol Hepatol* 9:11–14, 1986.

19. Pérez, R., I. Pastrana, and L. Rodrigo. Enfermedad hepática en 325 drogadictos asturianos: papel de los virus de la hepatitis. *Gastroenterol Hepatol* 9:37–44, 1986.

20. Kunches, L., D. Craven, and B. Werner. Seroprevalence of hepatitis B virus and delta agent in parenteral drug abusers. *Am J Med* 81:591–595, 1986.

21. Muñoz Domínguez, F., M. Lago, A. Sánchez, F. G. Escandón, J. A. Iniguez, M. Alcazar, and C. Navarro. Anti-HIV, Low Prevalence in Intravenous Drug Abusers in Madrid Area with Non A Non B Hepatitis vs. B Hepatitis. Paper presented at the IV International Conference on AIDS, held in Stockholm, 12–16 June 1988.

22. González, J., S. Rivas, and R. Hosokawa. Detection of HIV Antibodies in HBsAG Positive Sera. In: *Libro de resúmenes de la Segunda Conferencia Internacional sobre el Impacto de las Enfermedades Virales en el Desarrollo de Países de Latinoamérica y de la Región del Caribe.* Mar del Plata, Argentina, 1988.

23. Espinoza, P., I. Bouchard, and C. Buffer. Forte prevalence de l'infection par le virus de l'hépatite B et le virus HIV chez les toxicomanes français incarcérés. *Gastroenterol Clin Biol* 11:286–292, 1987.

24. Fay, O., G. H. Tamme, J. A. Basualdo, M. Ciocca, H. Fainboim, J. Astuo, A. Motta, M. Narac, J. Polazzi, M. Rammer, J. Rev, J. Rojman, L. Schjman, J. Clones, R. Tery, and F. Villamina. Antidelta antibody in various HBsAg positive Argentine populations. *J Med Virol* 22:257–268, 1987.

25. Nyanjom, D., W. Greaves, S. Barves, R. Delapenha, C. Saxinger, C. Callender, and W. Frederick. Unusual Hepatitis B Markers in HIV Seropositive Patients. Paper presented at the IV International Conference on AIDS, held in Stockholm, 12–16 June 1988.

26. Shattock, A. G., I. B. Hillary, F. Mulearhy, G. Kelly, and J. O. O'Connor. Reactivation of Hepatitis B and Hepatitis D by Human Immunodeficiency. Paper presented at the IV International Conference on AIDS, held in Stockholm, 12–16 June 1988.

27. Gilson, R. J. C., I. V. D. Weller, A. Hawkins, J. Waite, C. A. Carne, A. J. Robinson, G. Kelly, M. Briggs, and R. S. Tedder. Interactions between Hepatitis B Virus (HBV) and HIV in Homosexual Men. Paper presented at the IV International Conference on AIDS, held in Stockholm, 12–16 June 1988.

EPIDEMIOLOGY OF AIDS AND HIV INFECTION IN THE CARIBBEAN

JAI P. NARAIN, B. HULL, C. J. HOSPEDALES,
S. MAHABIR, & D. C. BASSETT

Since the first case was reported in the United States in 1981, cases of acquired immunodeficiency syndrome (AIDS) have been reported in increasing numbers from almost all parts of the world, including the Caribbean countries. An estimated 5–10 million persons worldwide are likely to be infected with human immunodeficiency virus (HIV), the causative agent of AIDS (1). In the Americas, which reports the majority of the world's AIDS cases, five countries—the United States of America, Brazil, Canada, Haiti, and Mexico—account for 95% of all reported cases (2). The data also demonstrate that the entire Caribbean area has exceptionally high rates of AIDS. This paper describes the magnitude of AIDS and HIV infection in 18 English-speaking Caribbean countries and Suriname, and discusses the implications of the changing epidemiologic pattern of the disease in this area.

Background

Since its inception in 1975, the Caribbean Epidemiology Center (CAREC) has collected and analyzed communicable-disease surveillance data from its 19 member countries: Anguilla, Antigua and Barbuda, Bahamas, Barbados, Belize, Bermuda, the British Virgin Islands, the Cayman Islands, Dominica, Grenada, Guyana, Jamaica, Montserrat, St. Kitts and Nevis, Saint Lucia, St. Vincent and the

61

Grenadines, Suriname, Trinidad and Tobago, and the Turks and Caicos Islands. These countries have a combined population of 6.3 million people and share a similar colonial history and similar problems, especially in health.

AIDS surveillance in the area began in 1982; since 1985, the countries routinely have reported AIDS cases to CAREC, using a standard PAHO/WHO form. HIV antibody testing began in the Caribbean in 1985, first in Trinidad and Tobago and subsequently in many other countries. As of August 1988, almost all the 19 countries and territories had already acquired HIV antibody testing equipment and supplies, and their technicians had been trained with CAREC assistance.

Methods

We reviewed and analyzed data on AIDS cases from the 19 Caribbean countries which have been reporting cases on a quarterly basis to CAREC in Port of Spain, Trinidad. A standard reporting form is used, and it provides information on distribution of cases according to age, sex, and transmission category.

The countries also report the number of HIV tests performed on donated blood and the number of tests performed for diagnostic purposes. Information on HIV infection in specific population groups was gathered through various surveys and studies conducted in different countries, most of which are still unpublished.

For the purpose of surveillance and for reporting to CAREC, a positive serologic test is defined as a repeatedly reactive antibody test with ELISA, followed by a positive confirmation test with Western blot assay. The WHO/PAHO AIDS case definition is used by all the reporting countries.

Results

The first confirmed case of AIDS in the Caribbean occurred in Jamaica in 1982. In Trinidad and Tobago, eight cases were reported in 1983—all in homosexual or bisexual males.

As of 30 June 1988, the CAREC member countries had reported 827 cases, 80% of which were reported since January 1986 (Table 1). The number of reported cases was 187 for 1986 and 306 for 1987, repre-

Table 1. Reported cases by year and country as of 30 June 1988.

Country	Year							Total
	1982	1983	1984	1985	1986	1987	1988[a]	
Anguilla	—	—	—	—	2	—	1	3
Antigua	—	—	—	—	2	1	0	3
Bahamas	—	—	—	36	50	90	38	214
Barbados	—	—	2	9	20	24	8	63
Belize	—	—	—	—	1	7	0	8
Bermuda	—	—	—	30	21	21	3	75
British Virgin Is.	—	—	—	—	—	—	—	0
Cayman Is.	—	—	—	1	1	1	1	4
Dominica	—	—	—	—	—	5	1	6
Grenada	—	—	—	2	1	5	3	11
Guyana	—	—	—	—	—	12	20	32
Jamaica	1	0	1	4	6	33	17	62
Montserrat	—	—	—	—	—	—	—	0
St. Kitts and Nevis	—	—	—	—	—	1	—	1
Saint Lucia	—	—	—	4	0	7	0	11
St. Vincent and the Grenadines	—	—	1	0	2	6	3	12
Suriname	—	—	—	—	2	5	1	8
Trinidad and Tobago	—	8	19	45	77	86	75	310
Turks and Caicos Is.	—	—	—	—	2	2	—	4
Total	1	8	23	131	187	306	171	827

[a] Data for six months only.

senting an increase of 63%. Of the 827 total cases, 492 had died, giving an overall case fatality ratio of 59.4%.

Nearly 90% of the cases were reported from five countries— Trinidad and Tobago, Bahamas, Bermuda, Barbados, and Jamaica; 75% were from the first three countries (Figure 1).

The distribution of cumulative cases and of deaths in selected countries were as follows: Trinidad and Tobago, 310 cases and 200 deaths; Bahamas, 214 and 104; Bermuda, 75 and 58; Barbados, 63 and 43; and Jamaica, 62 and 38. In Guyana, the first 12 cases were reported in 1987; up to June in 1988, 20 additional cases had been reported. Similarly, Jamaica reported six cases in 1986 and 33 in 1987. Montserrat and the British Virgin Islands are the only two territories in the Americas that have not reported any AIDS cases to date. The annual incidence rates of reported cases in some Caribbean countries are among the highest in the world. During 1987, the rates per 100,000 population varied from 0 to 38.3, median 4.27. Countries with high rates were Bahamas (38.3), Bermuda (35.3), Barbados (9.4), and Trinidad and Tobago (7.0) (Table 2). Of the five countries with the majority of reported cases, only Bermuda did not report an increase in case

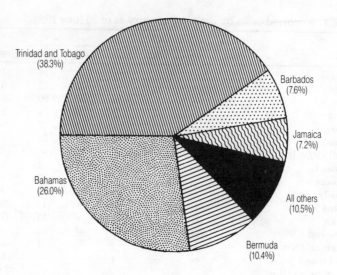

Figure 1. Distribution by country of reported AIDS cases among CAREC member countries, as of 30 June 1988.

rates from 1986 to 1987. Overall, the 20–44-year age group had the most cases; the number of reported cases peaked among 25–34-year-olds (Table 3).

Of 737 adult cases (≥ 15 years old) reported up to June 1988, 564 (76.5%) were among males and 173 (23.5%) among females; the male to female ratio was 3.3:1. The proportion of AIDS reported in females has increased from year to year. While none of the 31 persons with AIDS reported up to 1984 were females, the proportion increased to 18.3%, 23.0%, 25.5%, and 28.9% in 1985, 1986, 1987, and 1988 (up to June), respectively.

Table 4 shows the distribution of reported adult cases by transmission categories: homosexual or bisexual males (45.0%), heterosexual males and females (44.1%), intravenous drug users (7.8%), blood transfusion recipients (1.9%), and hemophiliacs (0.3%). Overall, sexual HIV transmission was responsible for 89% of the total cases reported up to June 1988. Of 45 intravenous drug users with AIDS, 44 (98%) were reported from Bermuda.

The first pediatric AIDS cases reported in the Caribbean were 11 cases in 1985, followed by 14 and 30 cases in 1986 and 1987, respectively. The male to female ratio of cumulative AIDS cases in children is 1.4:1. Of children under 5 years of age who have AIDS, all were born to HIV-positive mothers. The Bahamas reported the highest

Table 2. Number of reported AIDS cases and case rate per 100,000 population in selected CAREC member countries[a] in 1987, and cumulative case rate per 100,000 as of 30 June 1988.

Country	Mid-year population in 1987	No. of cases reported in 1987	1987 case rate per 100,000	Cumulative case rate per 100,000
Bahamas	235,000	90	38.3	91.1
Barbados	256,000	24	9.4	24.6
Bermuda	59,400	21	35.3	126.3
Guyana	988,000	12	1.2	3.2
Jamaica	2,400,000	33	1.4	2.6
Trinidad and Tobago	1,230,000	86	7.0	25.2

[a]Countries reporting fewer than 10 new cases in 1987 are not included.

Table 3. Age and sex distribution of cases reported as of 30 June 1988.

Age (years)	Male	Female	Total	%[a]
<1	22	12	34	5.3
1–4	15	13	28	4.4
5–14	2	2	4	0.6
15–19	9	2	11	1.7
20–24	53	28	81	12.6
25–34	187	77	264	41.2
35–44	98	24	122	19.1
45–54	47	15	62	9.7
>55	27	7	34	5.3
Unknown	143	20	163	—
Total	603	200	803[b]	100.0

[a]Percentages based on total cases for whom age information was available.
[b]For 24 cases, information on the sex was not available.

Table 4. Distribution of adult AIDS cases by major transmission categories, in CAREC member countries, 1982–June 1988.

Transmission categories	Male	Female	Unknown	Total	%[a]
Homosexual	170	—	—	170	29.5
Bisexual	89	—	—	89	15.5
Heterosexual	121	102	31	254	44.1
I.V. drug abuse	40	5	0	45	7.8
Transfusion	5	2	4	11	1.9
Hemophiliac	2	0	0	2	0.3
Other risk factors	0	0	0	0	0
No risk factor	4	1	0	5	0.9
Unknown	108	32	36	176	—
Total	539	142	71	752	100.0

[a]Percentages were calculated with a denominator of 576, excluding cases with unknown risk factors.

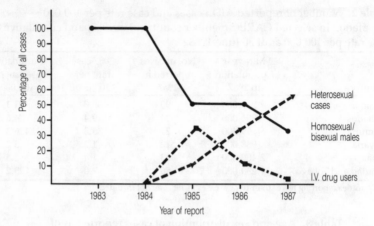

Figure 2. Proportion of reported cases by major risk categories in the Caribbean, 1983–1987.

proportion of perinatally transmitted AIDS; 19% of reported cases were in children, compared to an overall Caribbean percentage of 10.3.

Comparison of risk behavior data over the last five years demonstrates a shift from the predominantly homosexual spread seen earlier in the epidemic toward the present pattern of predominantly heterosexual transmission (Figure 2). The number of homosexuals and bisexuals with AIDS continues to increase, but the relative increase of those who appear to have acquired AIDS heterosexually has been far greater.

As a result, the proportion of heterosexual persons with AIDS has steadily increased, while that among homosexuals and bisexuals has declined over the years. Of cases reported in 1986, 27% were heterosexual contact cases. This proportion increased to 56.2% in 1987 and to 61.1% of cases reported in 1988 up to June. In all countries reporting more than 60 cumulative cases, those cases associated with heterosexual contact have been increasing.

In Trinidad and Tobago, among persons with AIDS resulting from sexual transmission, the proportion attributable to heterosexual contact increased from none in 1983 and 1984, to 13%, 25%, and 47% during the middle of 1985, 1986, and 1987, respectively. Data from Bermuda from 1985 to 1987 show an increase in heterosexual contact cases (from 6% to 24% of the total) and a decrease in reported cases among intravenous drug users. In Guyana, which started reporting cases in 1987, all but two of the 34 cases have been among males, predominantly among homosexuals or bisexuals.

Table 5. Seroprevalence in several population groups, 1985–1988.

Population groups	Country	Year	No. tested	% positive
1. Homosexual/bisexual males	Trinidad and Tobago	1983	100	40.0
	Jamaica	1985–86	125	15.0
2. Prison inmates	Trinidad and Tobago	1987–88		
	—Males		59	10.2
	—Females		217	3.7
	Jamaica	1988	12	8.3
3. Prostitutes	Antigua	1986–88	470	1.7
	Guyana	1987	77	0
	Trinidad and Tobago	1988	223	13.0
4. Cocaine abusers	Trinidad and Tobago	1987	150	2.0
5. STD patients	Guyana	1986	26	0
	Jamaica	1985–86	2,400	0.1
	Trinidad and Tobago	1987–88	1,700	2.5
6. Migrant farm workers	Dominica	1985–87	202	0
	Grenada	1985–87	133	0
	Jamaica	1985–86	7,470	0.6
	Saint Lucia	1985–86	1,086	1.6
	St. Vincent and the Grenadines	1985–87	1,038	1.1
7. Healthy adults, as part of viral hepatitis survey	Trinidad and Tobago	1983	983	0.2
8. Prenatal clinic attendees	Trinidad and Tobago	1988	203	0
9. Food handlers	Jamaica	1985–86	4,000	0
10. Hospital patients other than those with STD or cancer	Trinidad and Tobago	1985–86	370	0.5

HIV Infection

Some seroprevalence studies have been conducted in the Caribbean to assess the extent of HIV infection in specific population groups (Table 5).

One of the first serologic studies was conducted among homosexuals in Trinidad and Tobago (3); subsequent serosurveys and screenings have been conducted in persons from other identified high-risk groups, specifically prostitutes and persons seeking treatment at sexually transmitted disease clinics. In sexually active populations not at high risk, surveys have been conducted on women attending prenatal clinics and also on persons without known risk factors, such as blood donors. HIV seroprevalences range from 15–40% among homosexual and bisexual males, 4–10% among prisoners, 0–13% among prostitutes, 2% among cocaine users, and 0–2.5% among individuals attending STD clinics.

As of July 1988, 15 Caribbean countries were testing donated blood for HIV antibodies. The prevalence of HIV infection in nine countries reporting data has ranged from 0.04% to 1.55%, with a median of 0.26% (Table 6).

A 1982 outbreak of hepatitis B in Trinidad and Tobago provided an opportunity to obtain serum samples from a representative sample of 983 adults from the general population. Two of these persons (0.2%) had antibodies to HIV and both were from known risk groups. Among 4,000 food handlers tested in Jamaica during 1985–1986, none were found to have antibodies to HIV (4).

Discussion

Our analysis of the cases reported to CAREC reveals that AIDS in the Caribbean occurs primarily among young to middle-aged adults and, although males are still more likely than females to have AIDS, the gap is narrowing. The proportion of new cases attributable to heterosexual transmission is increasing. Given the prevailing pattern of sexual behavior, the rapid spread of HIV from bisexuals (and possibly from intravenous drug abusers in some countries) to heterosexual persons, and the size of the heterosexual population, it is inevitable that sexual transmission will continue to occur and to increase in the Caribbean. This will, in turn, directly and significantly affect perinatal transmission of HIV, which is already a substantial problem in many countries of the area.

The World Health Organization's Global Program on AIDS has described three distinct epidemiologic patterns of AIDS in the world. In general, the epidemiology in the Caribbean does not fit easily into any pattern. In large countries, the epidemic began among homosexuals (Pattern I) and then shifted rapidly towards Pattern II, in which heterosexual transmission is the predominant mode of spread. The

Table 6. HIV seroprevalence (%) among blood donors.[a]

Country	1986	1987
Bahamas	—	0.50
Barbados	—	0.11
Bermuda	0.04	0.09
Cayman Islands[b]	—	0.49
Grenada[b]	—	0.26
Jamaica	0.27	0.23
St. Vincent and the Grenadines[b]	—	0.45
Suriname	—	0.04
Trinidad and Tobago	1.5	1.55

[a] Based on quarterly reporting system.
[b] Based on fewer than 500 donors tested.

male to female ratio up to 1985 was 5.9:1, but has declined steadily since then.

The Caribbean countries have a serious AIDS problem with one of the highest annual incidence rates in the world. Since the virus was introduced in the late 1970s, primarily among the homosexual population by gay and bisexual men traveling between the Caribbean and North America, and considering that AIDS often has a 7–8 year or longer incubation period, the yearly increase in heterosexual contact cases has been extremely rapid. In part, this could be explained by factors related to the sexual behavior of the population, such as a higher ratio of bisexual to homosexual males than in North America, the nature of sexual/marital relationships, and perhaps the increasing level of STDs. It is generally believed that most Caribbean homosexuals, unlike those in the United States, tend to be bisexual because homosexuality is not well tolerated in the area. Strong social and religious disapproval makes it difficult to follow a homosexual lifestyle openly—many homosexuals are married, have children, and perhaps continue to engage in both homosexual and heterosexual activity. HIV probably was introduced into the heterosexual population when bisexual males had sexual contact with women. This hypothesis is supported further by data from Trinidad and Tobago which show that, while initial cases resulting from heterosexual contact were women with bisexual partners, 72% of the heterosexual cases reported in 1987 were among males whose only risk activity was frequent sexual contact with females (5), indicating female-to-male transmission of HIV.

Further spread of HIV in the community may have been facilitated by the fact that men and women tend to have multiple sexual partners (6). In many communities, it seems, sex is not often linked to monogamous relationships: serial consensual unions are common, and uninterrupted and civilly sanctioned monogamous marriages are in the minority (S. Mintz, as quoted in 5). The fluidity of sexual relationships and the custom for men to have multiple partners have been documented in several anthropological studies (7, 8). In addition, risk factors such as teenagers engaging in unprotected sex (9) and the increasing levels of sexually transmitted diseases, particularly syphilis, have further contributed to rapid spread of HIV in the Caribbean.

This increase in heterosexual transmission in the Caribbean has inevitably resulted in more HIV infection. Pediatric AIDS is already a substantial problem in many countries, where the proportion of children among reported AIDS cases is 10%. This figure is far greater than that from North America and Europe, where the proportion is less than 3% (10, 11). However, some Caribbean countries are still at the initial stages of the epidemic; in Guyana, for example, where the first cases were reported as recently as 1987, AIDS cases are at present exclusively among males. Given the general trend seen in most other Caribbean countries, this is expected to change.

Faced with the increasing problem of AIDS and HIV infection, the governments of all Caribbean countries have taken the problem very seriously: national AIDS committees have been established, education of health care workers and the general public has been started, and almost all countries now screen donated blood. The majority of countries have started implementing short-term programs (one year) for AIDS prevention and control, and most have developed medium-term plans (three years) with assistance from the Pan American Health Organization, the World Health Organization's Global Program on AIDS, and CAREC.

Priorities and strategies for the medium-term programs for AIDS control in the Caribbean are based on available epidemiologic evidence. These priorities include strengthening of epidemiologic surveillance through HIV serosurveys and serosurveillance studies, and prevention of sexual transmission and of perinatal transmission through information and education strategies aimed both at those engaged in high-risk behaviors and at the general population. To this end, it is important to conduct knowledge, attitude, and practice surveys, especially of specific target groups, and to follow these studies with interventions. Such surveys have been carried out in some countries, including Grenada and Jamaica. It is also important to take steps to reduce the social and economic impact of HIV on individuals, groups, and societies. In the absence of a vaccine or an effective therapy, the development and strengthening of AIDS education and information campaigns and of counselling services in all countries of the Caribbean remain the most important strategies for containing the spread of the virus.

References

1. World Health Organization, Global Program on AIDS. Update on AIDS, July 1988.
2. St. John, R., M. Clifford, and F. Zacarías. Epidemiology of AIDS in the Americas. Paper presented at the IV International Conference on AIDS, Stockholm, 12–16 June 1988.
3. Bartholomew, C., C. Saxinger, J. W. Clard, M. Gail, A. Dudgeen, B. Mahabir, B. Hull-Drysdale, F. Cleghorn, R. C. Gallo, and W. A. Blattner. Transmission of HTLV-1 and HIV among homosexual men in Trinidad. *JAMA* 257(19):2604–2608, 1987.
4. Murphy, E., P. Figueroa, W. N. Gibb, et al. Retroviral epidemiology in Jamaica, West Indies: Introduction of HIV into an HTLV-1 endemic island. Paper presented at the III International Conference on AIDS, Washington, D.C., 1–5 June 1987.
5. Cleghorn, F., et al. In: *Proceedings of the London Conference on Global Impact of AIDS*, March 1988, p. 55.
6. Bishop, J. Family life in the Caribbean—Sociocultural issues which affect AIDS prevention strategies. Presented at the CAREC Workshop on Prevention Counselling, July 1988.
7. Kerr, M. *Personality and Conflict in Jamaica*. Collins, London, 1963.
8. Hodge, M. Young women and the development of stable family life in the Caribbean. *A Journal of the Caribbean Artists Movement*, 1977.
9. Jagdeo, T. P. Myths, misconceptions and mistakes: a study of Trinidad adolescents. The Family Planning Association of Trinidad & Tobago, 1986.
10. Centers for Disease Control. Reports on selected racial/ethnic groups. *MMWR* 37:1–3, 1988.
11. Health Education Authority and Public Health Laboratory Service AIDS Centre, United Kingdom. A quarterly epidemiological briefing on AIDS/HIV in the United Kingdom. Issue 1, March 1988.

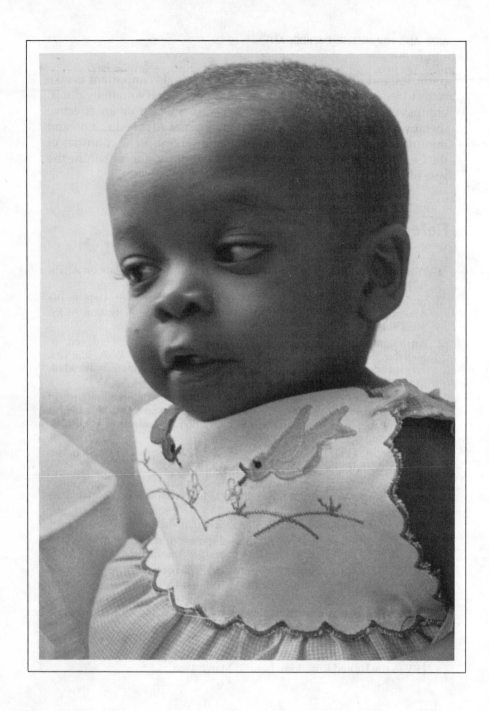

PERINATAL TRANSMISSION OF THE HUMAN IMMUNODEFICIENCY VIRUS

JEAN W. PAPE & WARREN JOHNSON, JR.

Two years after the first adult patients with the acquired immunodeficiency syndrome (AIDS) were reported, cases of a similar syndrome in infants and children were described (1–6). Since these early reports, the number of cases of pediatric AIDS has continued to increase worldwide at the same rate as that of AIDS cases in adults (7, 8). However, underreporting of AIDS cases probably occurs more frequently among infants and children than among adults because the clinical presentation of human immunodeficiency virus (HIV) infection is more subtle and serologic tests are less reliable in this population.

Like adults, children can acquire AIDS by transfusion of infected blood or blood products (9–11); as indicated in Table 1, up to 30% of the infected children may acquire their infections by this route (7, 8, 12). Another potential mode of HIV transmission in developing countries is by "medical" injections with contaminated syringes or needles (12, 13). However, by far the most important risk factor for AIDS in children is vertical transmission from an infected mother to her fetus or infant (13–19). Casual transmission of HIV between adults and children has not been documented, even in crowded housing with unsanitary conditions where there have been two or more infected people per family (14, 15).

Table 1. Known and suspected routes of pediatric HIV transmission, showing reported percentages of transmission by those routes in developed and developing countries.

Route of transmission	Developed countries	Developing countries
Vertical (perinatal) transmission[a]	70–80%	80–100%
Transfusions	20–30%	0–20%
"Medical" injections	Not reported	Suspected
Casual transmission	Not reported	Not reported

[a]Including transmission of HIV during delivery and by infected breast milk.

Vertical HIV Transmission

Vertical transmission of HIV occurs transplacentally during pregnancy and probably during labor and delivery as a result of contact with contaminated blood or body fluids. In addition, postpartum transmission via infected breast milk has been documented.

Because the transmission mechanisms have not been fully elucidated and serologic methods commonly used to diagnose HIV infection in infants are unreliable, it is difficult to determine the precise rate of transmission. Mothers infected with HIV produce IgG antibodies that are transferred to the fetus transplacentally, resulting in cord blood being positive for antibody when tested by enzyme-linked immunosorbent assay (ELISA) or the Western blot (WB) technique.

As many as 25% of the infants seropositive at birth will continue to have maternal antibody beyond one year of age, while a similar percentage of those infected may not be identified by ELISA anti-HIV screening alone (20). Because neonates are not fully immunocompetent, they produce a less vigorous antibody response to HIV infection (21). Indeed, fetal synthesis of specific IgM antibody is not a useful marker of infection in utero because it is short-lived and because of nonspecific binding of IgM (22).

Demonstration of virus by the method of in situ hybridization is promising but is technically difficult and not always successful (16). Viral culture is the definitive method for confirming infection in the neonate. For these reasons, there is a wide range in the apparent rate of transmission from an infected mother to her fetus or infant, available studies having reported transmission rates that range from 0% to 70% (4–6, 23–37). The true transmission rate is probably between 20% and 60%, depending on the health status of the mother. In general, the transmission rate appears higher among women with more advanced disease (6, 20, 32).

Intrauterine Transmission

A substantial number of reports support the occurrence of intrauterine transmission (1-3, 38, 39). Intrauterine HIV infection selectively affecting one monozygotic twin and not the other has also been reported (40). The exact period at which HIV infection of the fetus occurs is not yet known. However, HIV has been detected in fetal tissues at 15 and 20 weeks of gestation (41, 42). In addition, studies of AIDS patients' sex partners have shown that seropositive women have twice as many miscarriages as seronegative ones, with most of these miscarriages occurring during the first trimester of pregnancy (43). In utero HIV infection could also account for the rare occurrence of a dysmorphic syndrome in children born to seropositive mothers (44).

Transmission during Labor and Delivery

HIV has been isolated from cervical secretions (45, 46), which suggests that they could be a source of infection. Transmission by this route is commonly seen in other diseases caused by vertically transmitted agents such as cytomegalovirus and herpes simplex. To reduce this risk, it has been suggested that seropositive women should be delivered by cesarean section (26). However, there is no convincing evidence that cesarean section reduces the risk of HIV transmission to newborns.

Transmission via Breast Milk

HIV is present at high titers in cell-free breast milk and in the cellular fraction of colostrum (47). Transmission of another retrovirus, human T-cell leukemia virus type I (HTLV-I) via breast milk has been reported (48). In addition, five cases of HIV transmission by infected breast milk have recently been documented (49–52). In all cases the nursing mother was either symptomatic or recently infected by transfusion with HIV-contaminated blood.

Breast-feeding during the period of maternal seroconversion may carry more risk of transmission (50). However, in the usual situation of an infected mother breast-feeding her infant, the risk of transmission appears to be low (53). Forty-eight infants less than one year of age became HIV-seronegative or remained seronegative while being breast-fed by HIV-seropositive mothers. These children who remained seronegative or became seronegative were breast–fed for at least as long a period as those who remained seropositive.

In industrialized countries it may be appropriate to follow U.S. Centers for Disease Control guidelines that recommend that infected women stop breast-feeding their infants. However, in developing countries a major cause of infant death is diarrheal disease, which can be directly linked to artificial feeding. Until more information is available, infected women from impoverished areas of the world are better advised to continue breast-feeding.

The Importance of Perinatal Infections

The actual numbers of pediatric AIDS cases and of HIV-infected children is unknown. However, an indirect way to determine the importance of pediatric AIDS is to analyze the pattern of transmission of HIV in heterosexual adults and particularly in women of childbearing age. In general, the situation in most countries corresponds to one of two recognized patterns.

Pattern I

In North America, Western Europe, parts of South America, Australia, and New Zealand, AIDS is primarily a disease of young homosexual and bisexual men. This is reflected by a large difference in the sex ratio (the male to female ratio is approximately 8:1 in Western Europe and 11.5:1 in the United States). These regions exhibit the "Pattern I" type of HIV distribution (54).

Under these circumstances, children are less likely to be infected. In the United States and Western Europe, respectively, only 1.5% and 2.5% of all AIDS cases occur among children under 13 years of age (7, 8). Underscoring this point, 70% of the children with AIDS in the United States and 68% of those with AIDS in Western Europe come from families in which the mother has AIDS or is infected with HIV.

It is also true that in the industrialized countries perinatal transmission usually occurs among women who belong to one of the following high-risk groups: intravenous drug abusers, women originally

Table 2. HIV seroprevalence rates found among selected U.S. populations.

Group	Place	% seropositive	Year(s)	Source
I.V. drug abusers	Dallas, Texas	1	1987	57
	New York City	61	1986	57
Prostitutes	Las Vegas, Nevada	0	1986–1987	56
	New Jersey	45	1986–1987	56
Women of childbearing age	Inner-city hospitals, Massachusetts	0.8	1988	58
	Inner-city hospitals, New York	1.6–3	1988	58
Newborns	New York State	0.8	1988	59
	Bronx, New York City	2.3	1987	59

from regions where heterosexual transmission of HIV is common (Central Africa, the Caribbean), and women who have received a blood transfusion or who have an infected sex partner.

Actually, in Pattern I countries intravenous drug abuse has been the source of most AIDS cases contracted through heterosexual contact and the indirect source of most perinatally acquired AIDS cases. In the United States, women account for notably high percentages of the patients infected through intravenous drug abuse and heterosexual contact. Specifically, while they account for only 8% of all AIDS cases in the United States, 19% of all cases acquired through intravenous drug abuse and 52% of those acquired by heterosexual contact have occurred in women. HIV transmission by these two routes is particularly important among black and Hispanic women, who account for 71% of all female AIDS cases. As a result of the large number of AIDS cases acquired in this manner by women in these minorities, 75% of all children with AIDS, 80% of those under five years of age, and 85% of all those infected perinatally are black or Hispanic youngsters.

HIV seroprevalence rates in the sexually active heterosexual population have direct consequences for perinatal infections. As could be expected, HIV seropositivity rates tend to be highest among risk groups living in geographic locations with the largest numbers of reported AIDS cases. As Table 2 indicates, seroprevalence rates among intravenous drug abusers have been found to range from 1% in Dallas, Texas, to 61% in New York City. Similarly, HIV seropositivity rates for female prostitutes in the United States have been found to vary from 0% to over 45%, with the highest rates occurring among prostitutes who are also intravenous drug abusers (55).

HIV seropositivity rates among women of childbearing age tend to be highest in populations served by inner-city hospitals located in places reporting large numbers of AIDS cases. Hence, rates found among women of childbearing age served by inner-city hospitals in Massachusetts and New York were respectively 0.8% and 1.6%; rates were lower and comparable in both states (0.13%) among women using hospitals in nonmetropolitan areas (56, 57).

HIV seropositivity rates over 3% have been found among parturients in New York City. It is estimated that 1,620 to 4,800 HIV-infected infants are born each year in the United States (57), 900 in New York State alone. The seropositivity rate among newborns in New York State is 0.83%, while rates as high as 2.29% have been recorded in the Bronx, New York City (58).

Pattern II

In Pattern II regions, heterosexual contact with an infected person is the predominant mode of HIV transmission. Such regions include Central, East, and West Africa, as well as the Caribbean. The overall male to female ratio of AIDS cases in these regions is 1.5 to 1.

Women in Pattern II countries usually acquire the infection from infected heterosexual or bisexual men. However, rapid risk-factor changes from bisexual contact to heterosexual contact have occurred in Haiti and other Caribbean countries, resulting in a doubling of the percentage of female AIDS patients within a five-year period (59–61). Indeed, while the roles of risk factors in Haiti such as bisexuality and receipt of blood transfusions have progressively decreased, the percentages of patients having a spouse with AIDS or admitting to prostitution have tripled within the same period.

This shift from a primarily bisexual mode of transmission to a heterosexual mode of transmission could occur in countries that now fit Pattern I, resulting in more women and children being infected. In Pattern II countries, blood transfusion is the second most important risk factor, particularly among women (59, 62).

In contrast to the picture in Pattern I countries, intravenous drug abuse is rarely reported in Africa and is only found among 1% of the Caribbean AIDS patients outside Bermuda and Puerto Rico, where intravenous drug abuse is important. The possible role of "medical" injections in the transmission of HIV by contaminated needles or syringes has been raised in Pattern II countries but is difficult to assess (12, 13).

As a result of the important role of heterosexual transmission in Pattern II countries, prostitutes are both the victims and the prime

Table 3. HIV seroprevalence rates among prostitutes of four Pattern II countries, as determined by ELISA with Western blot or radioimmunoassay confirmation.

Country and region	% seropositive	Year
Rwanda (Butare), East Africa	88	1984
Kenya (Nairobi), East Africa	67	1985
Zaire (Kinshasa), Central Africa	27	1985
Haiti (Port-au-Prince), Caribbean	66	1987

Table 4. Seroprevalence of HIV among women of childbearing age in certain African, Caribbean, and North American localities, as indicated by ELISA with Western blot or radioimmunoassay confirmation.

City/country and region	% seropositive	Year
Africa:		
Kinshasa, Zaire (Central Africa)	5	1980
Dar es Salaam, United Republic of Tanzania (East Africa)	3.6	1986
Malawi (Southern Africa)	4	1986
North America:		
Bronx, New York, USA	2.6	1986
New York, New York, USA	3	1987
Jacksonville, Florida, USA	0.7	1986
Caribbean:		
Port-au-Prince, Haiti	8	1987
San Juan, Puerto Rico	1.7	1986

reservoir of HIV. However, the seropositivity rate among prostitutes varies according to their geographic location, socioeconomic status, and associated sexually transmitted diseases (59, 62–66). In Africa, HIV seropositivity among prostitutes is much higher in Central and East African countries (27–88%) than in West and North Africa (1–20%) (see Table 3).

Though prostitution plays a significant role in the spread of HIV (67–69), the seroprevalence rate among apparently healthy women of childbearing age reveals that a surprisingly large proportion of those living in urban areas are infected with the virus (Table 4). Overall, 3% to 7% of the apparently healthy women in some parts of Africa and the Caribbean may be seropositive (59, 62, 70–74). These rates are much higher than those generally reported in the United States (25, 55, 57). Rates are usually higher in urban than in rural areas.

Perinatal transmission is a significant problem in Pattern II countries. Up to 35% of all AIDS cases occur among children (75, 76), with more than 80% and up to 100% of all pediatric subjects with AIDS being born to seropositive mothers (12, 15, 17, 77). However, even the large number of pediatric AIDS cases reported in Pattern II countries underrepresents the real problem.

Among other things, because of the high infant mortality from diarrheal and respiratory infections, the full impact of HIV in the pediatric population is not well-defined. Seropositive women in Haiti and parts of Africa have reported having lost at least twice as many infants prior to their current pregnancy as had seronegative women (6, 43). One-third of the children with diarrhea who died after discharge from a rehydration unit in Port-au-Prince had antibody to HIV (78). Therefore, it appears that a majority of the children in the developing countries who are infected with HIV may not live long enough to develop clinical AIDS. It has been found that the mortality rate among children 0–5 years old born to HIV seropositive mothers is 99 deaths per thousand person-months, as compared to one death per thousand person-months among seronegative children (15).

Severe malnutrition is also common among seropositive children (15, 78), and may be a presenting manifestation of HIV infection (79). Forty-five percent of children 2 to 29 months old who were hospitalized consecutively for severe malnutrition in pediatric wards in Bujumbura, Burundi, were HIV seropositive (80). Most of these children were expected to die, since severe malnutrition is a major determinant of death among children in developing countries.

Problems Associated with Control of Perinatal Infections

Control of perinatal infection depends on effective measures to prevent HIV transmission in women.

Transfusion of infected blood and blood products is an important mode of HIV transmission in countries where mandatory screening procedures are not in effect. Although present blood screening procedures for HIV appear simple, they are prohibitive in most developing countries. The present cost of the ELISA test used by most blood banks for screening blood and blood products may be the equivalent of three to ten times the amount many developing countries are spending for health care per person annually. In addition, the necessary infrastructure for adequately performing the test is not available in remote villages. The best approach at present may be to use rapid and simple methods for HIV testing that do not require complicated equipment (81–83). Some of these tests appear to have good specificity but more variable sensitivity (84).

Even more important than blood screening are control measures designed to prevent HIV transmission involving women who are I.V. drug abusers or who have acquired the infection by heterosexual contact. This target population can be more readily identified in Pattern I countries, where a significant proportion of infected women are I.V. drug abusers or sex partners of I.V. drug abusers. In countries where such drug abuse is important, information campaigns directed at adolescents should pay particular attention to education on drug abuse.

In contrast to the situation in Pattern I countries, most women in Pattern II countries may not belong to any high-risk group or recall any high-risk exposure to HIV. One possible approach for identifying potentially infected men and women in Pattern II countries would be to screen the following groups:

1. Those with symptoms, signs, or infections associated with the presence of HIV;[1]
2. Sex partners of seropositive individuals and of patients with AIDS or suspected AIDS;
3. Those with other sexually transmitted diseases;
4. Those having children with AIDS or suspected AIDS;
5. Those who have received a blood transfusion within the last 10 years;
6. Pregnant women early in the course of pregnancy;
7. Women with previous miscarriage or death of a child 0–5 years old within the last 10 years;
8. All male and female prostitutes (85).

Like blood screening for HIV, identification of potentially infected individuals is a continuing process that will require funds not readily available in countries where it would be most appropriate.

[1]Common signs and symptoms or infections associated with HIV in Pattern II countries include the following: (1) chronic diarrhea with severe weight loss ($\geq 10\%$ of body weight in three months), (2) prurigo, (3) persistent or intermittent fever, (4) unexplained lymphadenopathy, (5) oral thrush, (6) herpes zoster, (7) genital herpes, and (8) nontyphoid salmonellosis.

Once seropositive women are identified, information and counseling to prevent heterosexual spread and perinatal transmission should be initiated. Also, women should be informed about their risk of sexually acquiring HIV and should be encouraged to have only one lifetime sexual partner. In addition, women who have more than one regular sexual partner and those who have sexual contact with HIV-infected men should be told to reduce their risk by insisting that their partners always use condoms during intercourse.

It is also true, however, that in many developing countries where women depend on men for support, they may have no choice regarding whether or not their sexual partners use condoms. In addition, the target population in both developed and developing countries may not be very responsive to health education strategies. The high illiteracy rates prevailing in Pattern II countries and the lack of motivation of I.V. drug abusers in Pattern I countries are not conducive to health interventions. Contraceptive methods including condoms are available and often free in many developing countries, and yet less than 5–10% of the women of childbearing age actually use them.

Infected women already pregnant should be made aware of the high rate of vertical transmission and the likelihood of manifest disease in their offspring. In addition, infected pregnant women should be informed of the high probability that they may develop AIDS and die before their child is five years old. If possible, termination of pregnancy should be offered to women who desire it; however, in many countries elective abortion is illegal.

Serosurveys in almost all countries have shown a higher HIV seropositivity rate in urban than in rural areas. This difference is probably related to the greater sexual promiscuity, particularly sexual contact with prostitutes, existing in large cities.

Health education should be directed at all sexually active individuals. Ongoing educational interventions have been successful in convincing prostitutes to use condoms (86, 87). In male-dominant societies, another approach is to convince men to use condoms when practicing "risky sex." In Haiti, women who become infected usually have one male sex partner who in turn has had many other sex partners and contact with prostitutes. Hence, the control of the infection in women and children in Haiti is dependent upon control of the infection in men. Within this context, it should be noted that a limitation on the number of sex partners may not be easily accepted in societies where polygamy is common.

Once health education interventions are developed, the most pressing need is to monitor their efficacy in leading to fewer sexual partners, reduced contact with prostitutes, and increased utilization of condoms. A multisectoral approach should be used in every community to mobilize all members in an open crusade against what has become a challenge for society, a challenge for the world.

References

1. Oleske, J., A. Minnefor, R. Cooper, Jr., et al. Immune deficiency syndrome in children. *JAMA* 249:2345–2349, 1983.
2. Scott, G. B., B. L. Buch, J. G. Leterman, et al. Acquired immunodeficiency syndrome in infants. *N Engl J Med* 310:76–81, 1984.
3. Rubinstein, A., M. Sicklick, A. Yupta, et al. Acquired immunodeficiency syndrome with reversed T4/T8 ratio in infants born to promiscuous and drug-addicted mothers. *JAMA* 249:2350–2356, 1983.
4. Blanche, S., C. Rouzioux, F. Veber, et al. Prospective Study on Newborns of HIV Seropositive Women. Paper presented at the III International Conference on Acquired Immunodeficiency Syndrome, held in Washington, D.C., on 1–5 June 1987. Book of Abstracts, Abstract TH.7.4, p. 158.
5. Braddick, M., J. K. Kreiss, T. Quinn, et al. Congenital Transmission of HIV in Nairobi, Kenya. Paper presented at the III International Conference on Acquired Immunodeficiency Syndrome, held in Washington, D.C., on 1–5 June 1987. Book of Abstracts, Abstract TH.7.5, p. 158.
6. Nzilambi, N., R. W. Ryder, F. Behets, et al. Perinatal HIV Transmission in Two African Hospitals. Paper presented at the III International Conference on Acquired Immunodeficiency Syndrome, held in Washington, D.C., on 1–5 June 1987. Book of Abstracts, Abstract TH.7.6, p. 158.
7. Centers for Disease Control. Update: AIDS worldwide. *MMWR* 37 (18):286–295, 1988.
8. Centers for Disease Control. *AIDS Weekly Surveillance Report*. United States AIDS Program, Center for Infectious Diseases, June 20, 1988, pp. 1–5.
9. Curran, J. W., D. N. Lawrence, H. J. Jaffe, et al. Acquired immunodeficiency syndrome (AIDS) associated with transfusions. *N Engl J Med* 310:69–75, 1984.
10. O'Duffy, J. F., and A. F. Isles. Transfusion-induced AIDS in four premature babies. *Lancet* 2:1346, 1984.
11. Wykoff, R. F., E. R. Pearl, and F. T. Saulsbury. Immunologic dysfunction in infants infected through transfusion with HTLV-III. *N Engl J Med* 312:294–296, 1985.
12. Mann, J. M., H. Francis, F. Davachi, et al. Risk factors for human immunodeficiency virus seropositivity among children 1–24 months old in Kinshasa, Zaire. *Lancet* 2:654–657, 1986.
13. Pape, J. W., B. Liautaud, F. Thomas, et al. The acquired immunodeficiency syndrome in Haiti. *Ann Intern Med* 103(5):674–678, 1985.

14. Friedland, O. H., H. R. Saltzman, M. F. Rogers, et al. Lack of transmission of HTLV-III/LAV infection to household contacts of patients with AIDS or AIDS-related complex with oral candidiasis. *N Engl J Med* 314:344–345, 1986.

15. Pape, J. W., R. I. Verdier, S. Jean, et al. Transmission and Mortality of HIV Infection in Haitian Children. Paper presented at the IV International Conference on AIDS, held in Stockholm on 12–16 June 1988. Book of Abstracts 2, Abstract 6581, p. 292.

16. Pyun, K. H., H. D. Ochs, M. T. Dufford, and R. J. Wedgwood. Perinatal transmission with HIV virus. *N Engl J Med* 317(10):611–614, 1987.

17. Lesbordes, J. L., S. Chassignol, E. Ray, et al. Malnutrition and HIV infection in children in the Central African Republic. *Lancet* 2:337–338, 1986.

18. Centers for Disease Control. Update, acquired immunodeficiency syndrome Europe. *MMWR* 35:35–46, 1986.

19. Centers for Disease Control. Recommendations for assisting in the prevention of perinatal transmission of human T-lymphotropic virus type III/lymphadenopathy associated virus and acquired immunodeficiency syndrome. *MMWR* 34:721–732, 1985.

20. Mok, J. G., A. De Rossia, A. E. Ades, et al. Infants born to mothers seropositive to HIV. *Lancet* 1:1164–1168, 1987.

21. Harnish, D. G., O. Hammerberg, J. R. Walken, and K. L. Rosenthal. Early detection of HIV in a newborn. *N Engl J Med* 316:272–273, 1987.

22. Johnson, J. P., P. Nain, and S. Alexander. Early diagnosis of human immunodeficiency virus infection in the neonate. *N Engl J Med* 316:273–274, 1987.

23. Semprini, E. A., A. Vucetian, G. Pandi, and M. M. Cossu. HIV infection and AIDS in newborn babies of mothers positive for HIV antibody. *Br Med J* 294:610, 1987.

24. Scott, G. B., M. T. Mastrucci, S. C. Hutto, and W. P. Parks. Mothers of Infants with HIV Infection: Outcome of Subsequent Pregnancies. Paper presented at the III International Conference on Acquired Immunodeficiency Syndrome, held in Washington, D.C., on 1–5 June 1987. Book of Abstracts, Abstract THP.91, p. 178.

25. Luizi, G., B. Ensoli, G. Turbessi, et al. Transmission of HTLV-III infection by heterosexual contact. *Lancet* 2:1018, 1985.

26. Chiodo, F., E. Ricchi, P. Costogliola, et al. Vertical transmission of HTLV-III. *Lancet* 1:739, 1986.

27. Thomas, P. A., M. J. Lubink, J. Milberg, et al. Cohort comparison study of children whose mothers have AIDS. *Pediatr Infect Dis* 6:247–251, 1987.

28. Scott, G. B., M. A. Fischl, N. Klimar, et al. Mothers of infants with acquired immunodeficiency syndrome: Evidence for both symptomatic and asymptomatic carriers. *JAMA* 253:363, 1985.

29. Rubinstein, A. Pediatric AIDS. *Curr Probl Pediatr* 16:365–409, 1986.

30. Andiman, W. A., J. Simpson, L. Dember, et al. Prospective Studies of a Cohort of 50 Infants Born to Human Immunodeficiency Virus Seropositive Mothers. Paper presented at the IV International Conference on

AIDS, held in Stockholm on 12–16 June 1988. Book of Abstracts 2, Abstract 6590, p. 294.

31. Weintrub, P. S., C. Rumsey, D. Wara, et al. Prospective Evaluation of Infants of HIV Antibody Positive Women. Paper presented at the IV International Conference on AIDS, held in Stockholm on 12–16 June 1988. Book of Abstracts 2, Abstract 6593, p. 295.

32. Mok, J., R. Hague, L. MacCallum, et al. Perinatal Transmission of HIV: Prospective Study. Paper presented at the IV International Conference on AIDS, held in Stockholm on 12–16 June 1988. Book of Abstracts 2, Abstract 6580, p. 291.

33. Levy, J., F. Puissant, G. Soumenkoff, et al. Prospective Study of Vertical Transmission of HIV. Paper presented at the IV International Conference on AIDS, held in Stockholm on 12–16 June 1988. Book of Abstracts 2, Abstract 6582, p. 292.

34. Willoughby, A., H. Méndez, J. Hittelman, et al. Epidemiology of Perinatal Transmission of Human Immunodeficiency Virus. Paper presented at the IV International Conference on AIDS, held in Stockholm on 12–16 June 1988. Book of Abstracts 2, Abstract 6588, p. 293.

35. Ryder, R. W., W. Nsa, F. Behets, et al. Perinatal HIV Transmission in Two African Hospitals: One-year Follow-up. Paper presented at the IV International Conference on AIDS, held in Stockholm on 12–16 June 1988. Book of Abstracts 1, Abstract 4128, p. 291.

36. Terragna, A., A. De Maria, F. Sampietro, et al. Perinatal HIV Infection: Evaluation of the Risk for the Mother and Child. Paper presented at the IV International Conference on AIDS, held in Stockholm on 12–16 June 1988. Book of Abstracts 1, Abstract 4028, p. 266.

37. Grosch-Wörner, I., S. Koch, M. Vocks, et al. Newborns of HIV-positive Mothers: Berlin Follow-up Experience. Paper presented at the IV International Conference on AIDS, held in Stockholm on 12–16 June 1988. Book of Abstracts 1, Abstract 7255, p. 441.

38. Cowan, M. J., D. Hellmann, D. Chudwin, et al. Maternal transmission of AIDS. *Pediatrics* 73:382–386, 1984.

39. Wilmer, E., A. Fischer, C. Griscelli, et al. Possible transmission of human lymphotropic retrovirus (LAV) from mother to infant with AIDS. *Lancet* 2:229–230, 1988.

40. Menez, B. R., S. M. Kikrig, and S. Pahwa. Monozygotic twins discordant for the acquired immunodeficiency syndrome. *Am J Dis Child* 140:678–679, 1986.

41. Lapointe, N., J. Michaud, D. Pekovic, et al. Transplacental transmission of HTLV-III. *N Engl J Med* 312:1325–1326, 1985.

42. Jovaisas, E., M. A. Koch, A. Schaefer, et al. LAV/HTLV-III in 20-week foetus. *Lancet* 2:1129, 1985.

43. Pape, J. W. Outcome of Offspring of HIV Infected Pregnant Women in Haiti. In: R. F. Schinazi and A. J. Nahmias (eds.). *AIDS in Children, Adolescents and Heterosexual Adults.* New York, Elsevier Science Publishing Co., Inc., 1987, pp. 216–219.

44. Marion, R. W., A. A. Wiznia, R. G. Hutcheon, et al. Human T-cell lym-

photropic virus type III (HTLV-III) embryopathy: A new dysmorphic syndrome associated with intrauterine HTLV-III. *Am J Dis Child* 140:638–640, 1986.

45. Vogt, M. W., D. J. Witt, D. E. Craven, et al. Isolation of HTLV-III/LAV from cervical secretion of women at risk for AIDS. *Lancet* 1:525–527, 1986.

46. Wofsy, C. B., J. B. Cohen, L. B. Haver, et al. Isolation of AIDS-associated retrovirus from genital secretions of women with antibodies to the virus. *Lancet* 1:527–529, 1986.

47. Thiry, L., S. Sprecher-Goldenberger, T. Jonckheer, et al. Isolation of AIDS virus from cell-free breast milk of three healthy virus carriers. *Lancet* 1:891–892, 1985.

48. Hino, S., K. Yamaguchi, S. Katamine, et al. Mother to child transmission of human T-cell leukemia virus type I. *Jpn J Cancer Res* 76:474–480, 1985.

49. Ziegler, J. B., D. A. Cooper, R. O. Johnson, and J. Gold. Postnatal transmission of AIDS-associated retrovirus from mother to infant. *Lancet* 1:896–898, 1985.

50. Ziegler, J. B., G. J. Stewart, R. Penny, et al. Breastfeeding and Transmission of HIV from Mother to Infant. Paper presented at the IV International Conference on AIDS, held in Stockholm on 12–16 June 1988. Book of Abstracts 1, Abstract 5100, p. 339.

51. Weinbreck, P., V. Loustaud, F. Denis, and F. Liozon. Breastfeeding and HIV-1 Transmission. Paper presented at the IV International Conference on AIDS, held in Stockholm on 12–16 June 1988. Book of Abstracts 1, Abstract 5102, p. 340.

52. Colebunders, R. L., B. Kapita, W. Nekwei, et al. Breastfeeding and Transmission of HIV. Paper presented at the IV International Conference on AIDS, held in Stockholm on 12–16 June 1988. Book of Abstracts 1, Abstract 5103, p. 340.

53. Stanback, M., J. W. Pape, R. I. Verdier, et al. Breastfeeding and HIV Transmission in Haitian Children. Paper presented at the IV International Conference on AIDS, held in Stockholm on 12–16 June 1988. Book of Abstracts 1, Abstract 5101, p. 340.

54. Piot, P., F. Plummer, S. Mhalu, et al. AIDS: an international perspective. *Science* 239:573–579, 1988.

55. Centers for Disease Control. Supplement, human immunodeficiency virus infection in the United States: a review of current knowledge. *MMWR* 36(Suppl. 5,6):1–48, 1987.

56. Hoff, R., V. P. Berardi, B. J. Weiblen, et al. Seroprevalence of human immunodeficiency virus among childbearing women. *N Engl J Med* 318(9):525–530, 1988.

57. Sperling, R., H. S. Sacks, L. Mayer, and R. Berkowitz. Serosurvey of an Obstetrical Population in a Voluntary Hospital in New York City. Paper presented at the IV International Conference on AIDS, held in Stockholm on 12–16 June 1988. Book of Abstracts 1, Abstract 4030, p. 267.

58. Novick, L. F., D. Berns, R. Stricof, and R. Stevens. HIV Seroprevalence in Newborn Infants in New York State. Paper presented at the IV International Conference on AIDS, held in Stockholm on 12–16 June 1988. Book of Abstracts 1, Abstract 7221, p. 433.

59. Pape, J. W., and W. D. Johnson, Jr. Epidemiology of AIDS in the Caribbean. In: P. Piot and J. Mann (eds.). *Bailliere's Clinical Tropical Medicine and Communicable Diseases, AIDS and HIV Infection in the Tropics, 1988* (in press).

60. Hospedales, C. J. The Epidemiology of AIDS in the Caribbean and Action to Date. Paper presented at the First International Conference on the Global Impact of AIDS, held in London, 1988. Book of Abstracts, Abstract 529.

61. Guerrero, E., E. A. De Moya, I. Garris, et al. Predominance of Heterosexual Transmission of HIV Infection in the Dominican Republic. Paper presented at the IV International Conference on AIDS, held in Stockholm on 12–16 June 1988. Book of Abstracts 2, Abstract 5502, p. 239.

62. Quinn, T. C., J. M. Mann, J. W. Curran, and P. Piot. AIDS in Africa: an epidemiologic paradigm. *Science* 234:955–963, 1986.

63. Neequarye, A. R., J. Neequarye, J. A. Mingle, and A. D. Ofari. Preponderance of females with AIDS in Ghana. *Lancet* 2:978, 1986.

64. Mann, J. M., T. C. Quinn, H. Francis, et al. Sexual Practices Associated with LAV/HTLV-III Seropositivity among Female Prostitutes in Kinshasa, Zaire. Paper presented at the II International Conference on AIDS, held in Paris, France, on 23–25 June 1986.

65. Van de Perre, P., and M. Carael. HIV Infection in Prostitutes in Africa. In: R. F. Schinazi and A. J. Nahmias (eds.). *AIDS in Children, Adolescents and Heterosexual Adults*. New York, Elsevier Science Publishing Co., Inc., 1987, pp. 166–167.

66. Van de Perre, P., N. Clumeck, M. Carael, et al. Female prostitutes, a risk group for infection with human T-cell lymphotropic virus type III. *Lancet* 2:524–527, 1985.

67. Simonsen, N., P. Plummer, N. Gakinya, et al. Longitudinal Study of a Cohort of HTLV-III/LAV Infected Prostitutes in Nairobi. Paper presented at the II International Conference on AIDS held in Paris, France, on 23–25 June 1986.

68. Van de Perre, P., D. Rouvroy, P. Lepage, et al. Acquired immunodeficiency syndrome in Rwanda. *Lancet* 2:62–65, 1984.

69. Kreiss, J. K., D. Koech, F. A. Plummer, et al. AIDS virus in Nairobi prostitutes: spread of the epidemic to East Africa. *N Engl J Med* 314(7):414–418, 1986.

70. Clumeck, N., M. R. Guroff, P. Van de Perre, et al. Seroepidemiological studies of HTLV-III antibody prevalence among selected groups of heterosexual Africans. *JAMA* 254:2592–2602, 1985.

71. Koenig, E. R., J. Pittaluga, M. Bogart, et al. Prevalence of antibodies to the human immunodeficiency virus in Dominicans and Haitians in the Dominican Republic. *JAMA* 257(5):631–634, 1987.

72. Gürtler, L. G., G. Zoulek, G. Frösner, et al. Prevalences of HIV-1 and HIV-2 Antibodies in a Selected Malawian Population. Paper presented at the III International Conference on Acquired Immunodeficiency Syndrome, held in Washington, D.C., on 1–5 June 1987. Book of Abstracts, Abstract THP. 93, p. 179.

73. Mhalu, F., E. Mbena, U. Bredberg-Raden, et al. Prevalence of HIV Anti-

bodies in Healthy Subjects and Groups of Patients in Some Parts of Tanzania. Paper presented at the III International Conference on Acquired Immunodeficiency Syndrome, held in Washington, D.C., on 1–5 June 1987. Book of Abstracts, Abstract TP.86, p. 76.

74. Boulos, R., N. Halsey, J. R. Brutus, et al. Risk Factors for HIV-1 Infection in Pregnant Haitian Women. Paper presented at the IV International Conference on AIDS, held in Stockholm on 12–16 June 1988. Book of Abstracts 1, Abstract 5119, p. 344.

75. Ndinuyeze, A., G. Bugingo, and A. Ntilivamundo. Adult and Pediatric AIDS and AIDS Related Syndrome in Rwanda. Paper presented at the Second International Symposium on AIDS and Associated Cancers in Africa. Naples, 1987. Book of Abstracts, Abstract 5-2-2.

76. Bartholomew, C., F. Cleghorn, B. Hull, et al. Transition from Homosexual to Heterosexual AIDS in Trinidad. Paper presented at the IV International Conference on AIDS, held in Stockholm on 12–16 June 1988. Book of Abstracts 2, Abstract 5505, p. 240.

77. Lepage, P., and P. Van de Perre. Strategies in the Identification and Control of HIV-infected Women in Africa. In: R. F. Schinazi and A. J. Nahmias (eds.). *AIDS in Children, Adolescents and Heterosexual Adults.* New York, Elsevier Science Publishing Co., Inc., 1987, pp. 214–215.

78. Oriol, L., J. W. Pape, J. Clarke, et al. Factors Associated with Mortality Post-discharge from a Rehydration Unit in Port-au-Prince, Haiti. (Manuscript in preparation.)

79. Scott, B. G., W. Park, and M. Jonas. Protein-calorie Malnutrition as a Presenting Manifestation of Human Retrovirus (HTLV-III) Infection in Infants and Children. Paper presented at the First International Conference on AIDS, held in Atlanta, 1985.

80. Excler, J. L., B. Standaert, E. Ngendandumwe, and P. Piot. Malnutrition et infection à HIV chez l'enfant en milieu hospitalier au Burundi. *Pediatrie* 42(9):715–718, 1987.

81. Weisner, D., D. Taylor, A. Suarez, et al. Passive Hemagglutination Assay for HIV Antibody Screening. Paper presented at the IV International Conference on AIDS, held in Stockholm on 12–16 June 1988. Book of Abstracts 2, Abstract 5593, p. 262.

82. Said, O. I., J. A. Hinda, S. Bygdeman, and L. Grillner. Evaluation of a Particle Agglutination Test for Detection of HIV Antibodies. Paper presented at the IV International Conference on AIDS, held in Stockholm on 12–16 June 1988. Book of Abstracts 2, Abstract 5596, p. 262.

83. Rosenheim, M., M. Ritterband, F. Fish, et al. A Method for Anti-HIV Antibodies Testing in Developing Countries. Paper presented at the IV International Conference on AIDS, held in Stockholm on 12–16 June 1988. Book of Abstracts 2, Abstract 5600, p. 263.

84. Kabeya, C. M., F. Spielberg, N. K. Kifuani, et al. Comparison of Rapid HIV Antibody Screening Assays, Mama Yemo Hosp. Kinshasa, Zaire. Paper presented at the IV International Conference on AIDS, held in Stockholm on 12–16 June 1988. Book of Abstracts 2, Abstract 5595, p. 262.

85. Pape, J. W. Identification and Control of HIV Infected Pregnant Women. In: R. H. Schinazi and A. J. Nahmias (eds.). *AIDS in Children, Adolescents*

and Heterosexual Adults. New York, Elsevier Science Publishing Co., Inc., 1987, pp. 257–260.

86. Plummer, F., M. Braddick, W. Cameron, et al. Durability of Changed Sexual Behavior in Nairobi Prostitutes: Increasing Use of Condom. Paper presented at the IV International Conference on AIDS, held in Stockholm on 12–16 June 1988. Book of Abstracts 1, Abstract 5141, p. 350.

87. Lamptey, P., A. Neequays, S. Weir, and M. Potts. A Model Program to Reduce HIV Infection among Prostitutes in Africa. Paper presented at the IV International Conference on AIDS, held in Stockholm on 12–16 June 1988. Book of Abstracts 1, Abstract 5149, p. 352.

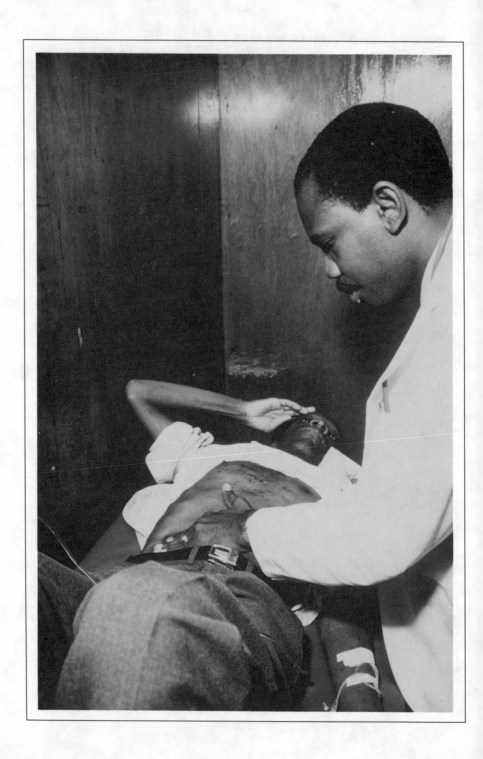

PREVALENCE OF INFECTION WITH HUMAN IMMUNODEFICIENCY VIRUS IN CUBA

HECTOR TERRY MOLINERT, ENRIQUE GALBAN GARCIA, & RODOLFO RODRIGUEZ CRUZ

Actions for the prevention and control of acquired immunodeficiency syndrome (AIDS) in Cuba go back to the beginning of 1983, when a National Multidisciplinary Commission was created and given the fundamental objective of advising the Ministry of Public Health on the measures that needed to be adopted to prevent the disease. This occurred long before the first case was reported in Cuba in mid-1986.

Subsequently, the first measures taken were to suspend imports of blood products from countries that had reported AIDS cases and to implement a system for special epidemiologic surveillance of patients with Kaposi's sarcoma and opportunistic infections.

At the end of 1985, when tests were available to detect antibodies to the human immunodeficiency virus (HIV) that causes AIDS, a much more complete and efficient control program was designed. The general purpose of this program, initiated in January 1986, was to use scientific grounds to guide the efforts aimed at preventing the spread of AIDS, a spread that was occurring in numerous countries on several continents.

The principal immediate objectives of the Cuban program have been as follows:

1. to design and employ a system for epidemiologic surveillance of HIV infection and disease;
2. to determine groups at risk;

3. to establish quality control of all blood and blood products utilized in the country;

4. to make early diagnoses and to treat patients and carriers of the
   virus;

5. to carry out an epidemiologic study and trace the contacts of all
   seropositive individuals identified;

6. to minimize the possibility of perinatal transmission by conducting serologic tests on all pregnant women during the first trimester of pregnancy and terminating the pregnancies of seropositive
   women; and

7. to carry out publicity and educational activities directed at reducing the risk of sexual transmission of HIV.

In addition, insofar as it was possible to develop an appropriate
diagnostic technology that would reduce the high cost of importing
equipment and reagents, a strategy was developed for screening
large groups in the general population. So far, this strategy has been
implemented without great difficulty.

The Current Situation

As of 30 May 1988 a total of 2,224,748 serologic tests to detect HIV
antibodies had been performed. This total represents approximately a
third of the country's sexually active population and somewhat more
than a fifth of the entire population. Overall, 227 of the resident
Cubans tested (0.01 per 100 tested) were identified as seropositive
(Table 1).

The total tested population of 2,224,748 included blood donors,
members of groups at risk (international travelers, homosexuals, people with sexually transmitted diseases, AIDS case contacts, etc.),
adult patients admitted to clinical/surgical and gynecological/obstetric
hospitals, women in the first trimester of pregnancy, and other
groups from the general Cuban population. Also included were some
32,000 foreign students who came to reside in our country for
extended periods, among whom an additional 131 seropositives were
detected.

Table 1 shows the prevalence of seropositivity in each of the principal groups investigated. The highest seropositivity (4.5 seropositives
per 100 tested) was found among the contacts of seropositive individuals. Within the group of international travelers, merchant seamen

Table 1. HIV seropositivity among the various Cuban population g
tested, January 1986–May 1988.

Population group	1986	1987	1988 (January– May)	Total	HIV prev (No. serop per 100 test
Specific groups at risk:					
Blood donors	304,856	491,884	238,942	1,035,682	0.0018
Pregnant women		79,063	83,949	163,012	0.002
Hospital inpatients		99,348	199,937	299,285	0.003
Patients with other sexually transmitted diseases (syphilis or gonorrhea)		9,552	33,753	43,305	0.016
Contacts of HIV seropositive people	766	350	242	1,358	4.5
Other groups at risk	280,487	144,856	48,547	473,890	0.03
General population of:					
Cabaiguán		37,744		37,744	0.019
Varadero		11,359	11,502	22,861	0.004
Old Havana			103,583	103,583	0.0019
Guantánamo			6,277	6,277	0.00
Isle of Youth			5,001	5,001	0.00
Subtotal (Cubans)	586,109	874,156	731,733	2,191,998	0.01
Foreigners	17,652	6,452	8,646	32,750	0.4
Total	603,761	880,608	740,379	2,224,748	

Source: Cuba, Ministerio de Salud Pública, Dirección Nacional de Epidemiología.

(not shown in the table) exhibited the highest seroprevalence (0.6 seropositives per 100 tested). People with other sexually transmitted diseases (syphilis or gonorrhea) showed a prevalence of 0.016 seropositives per 100 tested, nearly 10 times higher than that observed among blood donors but relatively low compared to seroprevalences found by similar studies published in the international literature.

Tables 2 and 3 show the clinical classification of the 227 seropositive individuals up through the last evaluation performed at the end of May 1988. The 33 cases in Group IV (see Table 3) were distributed among all five recognized subgroups and categories, though cases of secondary (opportunistic) infections predominated. These 33 cases included those of eight patients who had already died.

More than 97% of the seropositives identified acquired the infection sexually, with heterosexual transmission predominating in absolute terms. However, male homosexuals and bisexuals experienced a higher relative risk. Heterosexual transmission in both directions (man to woman and woman to man) has been confirmed, as have

Table 2. Distribution of individuals seropositive for HIV according to the classification for HIV infection of the U.S. Centers for Disease Control (CDC).

Group	Seropositive individuals No.	(%)
I (acute infection)	—	(0.0)
II (asymptomatic infection)	148	(65.2)
III (persistent generalized lymphadenopathy)	46	(20.3)
IV (other illness)	33	(14.5)
Total	227	(100)

Source: Cuba, Ministerio de Salud Pública, Dirección Nacional de Epidemiología.

both directions of male homosexual transmission (active to passive and passive to active). The male:female ratio was 3:1 among the infected subjects and very similar among those who were ill.

Epidemiologic investigation and contact tracing have made it possible to conclude that sexual relations with foreigners, both within and outside the country, were the source of contagion for almost three-fourths of the total infected population. Secondary cases resulting from sexual contact with these latter people were less important as a source of detected seropositivity.

Only five of the seropositives (2.2%) acquired the infection through a nonsexual mechanism of HIV transmission, one perinatally and four via blood transfusions received before blood quality control had been established in the country (Table 4).

Table 3. Distribution of the 33 HIV seropositive individuals in CDC Group IV (other diseases).

Group IV subgroup	Subgroup category	Cases No.	(%)
A (systemic disease)	—	3	(9.1)
B (neurologic disease)	—	3	(9.1)
C (secondary infections)	1[a]	15	(45.5)
C (secondary infections)	2[b]	10	(30.3)
D (secondary cancers)	—	1	(3.0)
E (other disorders)	—	1	(3.0)
Total		33	(100)

Source: Cuba, Ministerio de Salud Pública, Dirección Nacional de Epidemiología.
[a]Secondary infections specified in the CDC surveillance definition for AIDS.
[b]Other specified secondary infections.

Table 4. Modes of HIV transmission to the 227 seropositive Cubans whose cases were detected from January 1986 through May 1988.

Mode of transmission	Seropositive individuals	
	No.	(%)
Sexual relations with foreigners	161	(70.9)
Sexual relations with known seropositives	61	(26.8)
Blood transfusions (before 1986)	4	(1.8)
Perinatal transmission	1	(0.4)
Total	227	(100)

Source: Cuba, Ministerio de Salud Pública, Dirección Nacional de Epidemiología.

It is noteworthy that only one of the four seropositives infected by transfusion was a hemophiliac. This illustrates the low index of HIV circulation in Cuba as compared to other countries (in the United States, for example, the prevalence of HIV infection among hemophiliacs is around 70%, and in many countries of Western Europe it exceeds 50%).

Table 5 shows the chronologic evolution of the prevalence of seropositivity among blood donors in our country. These data indicate a progressive decline in the overall number of seropositive blood donors, even though the requirements for donating blood have not been modified and the number of donations has increased. This circumstance, together with the fact that almost all the seropositive individuals detected were from one of the principal high-risk groups, suggests that this virus has not extended into the population of young sexually active males who constitute our main source of blood donors.

The tests performed on pregnant women have revealed a seroprevalence similar to that found in other young people. Specifically, four seropositives were detected among 163,012 pregnant women tested, yielding a seroprevalence (0.002 per 100) similar to that found in blood donors (see Table 1). Three of the four seropositive women were contacts of seropositive individuals, and the remaining one was a promiscuous young woman who had frequent sexual relations with foreigners.

A prospective analysis of the prevalence of seropositivity among pregnant women reveals a declining trend similar to that observed among blood donors. In 1987 (when this investigation began) three seropositive pregnant women were detected from among the 79,063

Table 5. Changes of HIV seroprevalence among blood donors in Cuba, based on data for 1986, 1987, and early 1988.

Year	No. tested	No. seropositive	HIV prevalence (No. seropositive per 100 tested)
1986	304,856	14	0.0046
1987	491,884	5	0.0012
1988 (Jan.–May)	238,942	—	0.0000
Total	1,035,682	19	0.0018

Source: Cuba, Ministerio de Salud Pública, Dirección Nacional de Epidemiología.

tested, yielding a seroprevalence of 0.0038 per 100 tested, while in 1988 only one seropositive pregnant woman was found among the 83,949 tested, yielding a prevalence of 0.0012 per 100 tested.

Screening of the General Population

Once a test to detect HIV antibodies became available, studies were begun on the sexually active groups in the general population with a view to making a relatively quick determination of the magnitude of HIV spread.

To date, five population groups have been investigated in this manner. The testing has been carried out on volunteers from the selected populations, and in all cases has been preceded by an information campaign explaining the objectives and nature of the screening. The level of acceptance by the inhabitants has been high, and the information activities and taking of samples have been carried out by the regular primary health care services, reinforced by the educational facilities of the schools of medicine and nursing and supported by local citizens' organizations. Processing of the samples has been accomplished quickly and has not interfered with the program's other activities.

In all cases, the screening has tested over 90% of the estimated population, and a subsequent evaluation of the quality of the work carried out has been conducted. The following accounts provide more detailed descriptions of the studies performed.

Cabaiguán

This municipality, in the province of Sancti Spíritus, has a population of about 40,000 inhabitants over 15 years of age. In 1987 large-scale screening was carried out here because of Cabaiguán's relatively high prevalence of seropositive inhabitants (with respect to other municipalities in the country) belonging to various high-risk groups.

A total of 37,744 inhabitants were tested, of whom seven were found to be seropositive (0.019 seropositives per 100). It was confirmed that all seven (mainly male homosexuals/bisexuals) were associated with a focus of infection located in this municipality.

Varadero

This locality was selected for screening because every year it receives tens of thousands of foreign tourists, most of them from countries where HIV infection has reached significant endemic levels.

The first study carried out in this community of approximately 12,000 adult inhabitants, concluded at the beginning of 1987, only detected one seropositive individual among the 11,359 people tested, indicating a prevalence of 0.009 per 100. Subsequent epidemiologic investigation showed that the infected person was a male homosexual who had frequent sexual relations with foreigners.

In March of 1988 (one year later), the screening was repeated; on this occasion 11,502 people were tested and all were shown to be serologically negative.

Old Havana

In February 1988 a testing program began screening a population of about 111,000 residents over age 15 in the capital city area of Old Havana. This region, located around the Port of Havana, was known to have a high incidence of sexually transmitted diseases (mainly syphilis and gonorrhea). Since HIV is commonly transmitted the same way as these diseases and since people exposed to these diseases may also be exposed to HIV, it was logical to suppose that screening this population would lead to detection of the virus in the capital.

In a little over two months 103,583 persons were tested. However, only two of them showed antibodies to HIV. This prevalence (0.002

seropositives per 100 tested) was almost the same as the seropreva-lences found among blood donors and pregnant women. Once again, epidemiologic investigation of the seropositive subjects made it clear that the sources of infection were seropositive individuals who had had contact with foreigners.

Guantánamo

The epidemiologic importance of this municipality derives from its having the highest prevalence of leprosy patients in the country. For this reason, mass screening was being conducted in Guantánamo to detect anti-leprosy antibodies by means of an innovative ELISA tech-nique developed in our setting that makes it possible to identify lep-rosy patients early.

It was decided to expand this program in order to assess the sero-prevalence of HIV. To date, more than 6,000 Guantánamo residents have been tested serologically for HIV, and all the results have been negative.

Other Studies

Our program has envisioned systematic screening of the special population groups considered to be at risk for HIV infection. Despite this assumption of risk, the fact is that the prevalences found among these groups, although higher than those found in the general popu-lation, appear very low compared to prevalences reported for similar groups in other countries.

For example, the seroprevalence of HIV infection (0.016 per 100) found among sexually transmitted disease patients is very low, con-sidering that prevalences reported for such patients in the United States, Western Europe, and certain African countries have exceeded 10%.

Similarly, the seroprevalence found among hospitalized patients (0.003 per 100) is between a hundred and a thousand times lower than that found in some sentinel hospitals in the United States. The same is true of Cuban prisoners, who show a prevalence of 0.01 seropositives per hundred tested.

Conclusions

The results of these serologic and epidemiologic investigations of HIV's prevalence and spread in one-third of the Cuban population of sexually active age, together with contact tracing and implementation of the other prevention and control measures envisioned in our program, make it possible for us to suggest that the extent of the spread of the causative agent of AIDS in our setting is very limited and that, far from showing the increases evident in many countries, HIV circulation is tending to decline.

Bibliography

Centers for Disease Control. Revision of the CDC surveillance case definition for acquired immunodeficiency syndrome. *MMWR* 36(Suppl 1):1S–15S, 1987.

Centers for Disease Control. Human immunodeficiency virus infection in the United States. *MMWR* 36(Suppl 6):1S–48S, 1987.

Cuba, Ministerio de Salud Pública. *Programa Nacional de Prevención y Control del SIDA.* January 1986.

Pan American Health Organization. PAHO Guidelines for the Acquired Immunodeficiency Syndrome (AIDS). Mimeographed document. Washington, D.C., 22 October 1987.

World Health Organization. Special Programme on AIDS: Strategies and Structures, Projected Needs. Document WHO/SPA/GEN/87.1. Geneva, 1987.

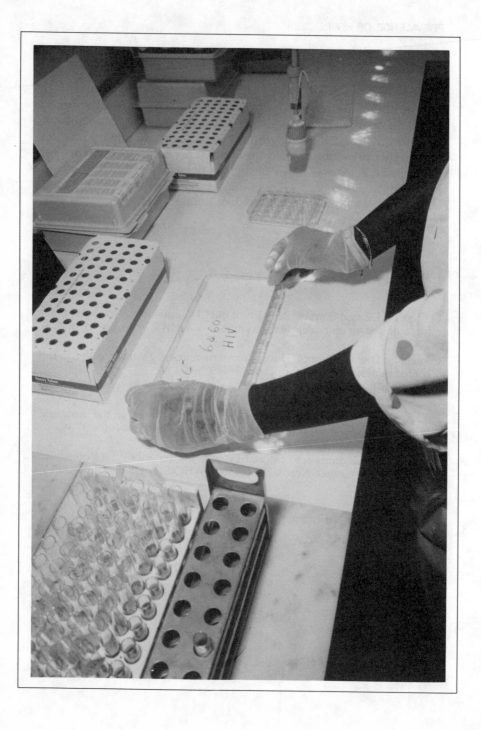

IMMUNOPATHOGENIC ASPECTS OF INFECTION BY THE HUMAN IMMUNODEFICIENCY VIRUS IN VENEZUELA

GLORIA ECHEVERRIA DE PEREZ, LEOPOLDO DEIBIS, CARMEN SILVIA GARCIA, TANIA OLARIA, MERLY MARQUEZ, ISAAC BLANCA, & NICOLAS E. BIANCO

The physiopathogenesis of human immunodeficiency virus (HIV) infection is largely due to profound changes of the lymphocytic sub-populations. Since acquired immunodeficiency syndrome (AIDS) was first described by Gottleib et al. (1), studies have established that the lymphocytes of the infected host are victims of a specific tropism of HIV for those cells and particularly for subpopulations of T lymphocytes that express the CD4 antigen (2–4). The immunopathogenesis of HIV generally compromises not only CD4 lymphocytes but also the large granular lymphocytes (LGL), which have the CD3-, CD16+ phenotype surface marker and whose principal function is natural cytotoxicity (5).

In the last two years, the availability of kits for detecting circulating HIV antigens and anti-HIV antibodies has made possible immunologic and clinical research on the virus-host relationships and their implications for the natural history of HIV infection. A prospective study of 240 patients with HIV infection has been carried out at the National Reference Center for Clinical Immunology in an attempt to establish the immunopathogenic characteristics of HIV infection in Venezuela.

Materials and Methods

Since 1984, the immunopathogenesis of HIV infection has been prospectively evaluated in 240 individuals grouped according to the classification recommended by the U.S. Centers for Disease Control (CDC) in Atlanta, Georgia (6), on the basis of their clinical picture when they were first examined at the center.

Ninety-five patients were asymptomatic HIV carriers (Group II), 34 had persistent chronic lymphadenopathy (Group III), 22 had HIV-related symptoms but did not meet the criteria for AIDS (Group IV–without AIDS), and 89 had AIDS (7). Regarding the risk factors for HIV infection, 234 (97.5%) of the patients were homosexual or bisexual males, heterosexual transmission was confirmed in five of the six females (known seropositive partners), and transmission occurred via blood transfusion in the remaining female.

The presence of antibodies for HIV was investigated using enzyme-linked immunosorbent assay (ELISA) (Abbott HTLV III EIA and some samples of Abbott Recombinant HIV-1 EIA, Abbott Laboratories, Diagnostic Division, Chicago, IL, USA), and their specificity against the isolated virus proteins was tested by means of Western blot (Biotech/Dupont HIV Western blot, Dupont Company, Wilmington, DE, USA).

The presence of free circulating antigens was confirmed by ELISA. In 49 patients the lymphocytic subpopulations were studied at the same time.

Peripheral blood mononuclear cells (PBMC) were obtained by centrifuge on Ficoll-Hypaque gradients (8). Identification of T lymphocytes (CD3) and CD4 and CD8 subpopulations was done by first marking the cell surface with monoclonal antibodies against CD3, CD4, and CD8 antigens (OKT-3, 4, 8, Ortho Diagnostic Systems, Inc., and Leu-2, 3, 4 donated by Dr. E. Engleman of Stanford University, USA). In the second phase, a secondary fluorescein-marked antibody was added, and the samples were then examined with a fluorescence microscope (GAMFIT, Ortho Diagnostic Systems, Inc., USA). All assays included two control samples obtained from healthy volunteer blood donors or laboratory personnel, and a total of 100 controls was accumulated.

The number of CD16 cells was determined by indirect immunofluorescence, using the B73.1 monoclonal antibody (Leu11a, donated by Dr. Félix Tapia, Instituto de Biomedicina, Caracas) (9). Natural cytotoxic activity was evaluated against the K562 cell line in a short-

Table 1. Distribution of free HIV serum antigen in patients grouped according to the U.S. Centers for Disease Control classification, Caracas, Venezuela, 1984–1988.

Antigen	Clinical group			AIDS patients	Total
	II[a]	III[b]	IV[c]		
Positive	7	0	2	13	22
Negative	13	10	4	7	34
Total	20	10	6	20	56

[a] Asymptomatic infection.
[b] Persistent generalized lymphadenopathy.
[c] Other illness associated with HIV.

duration (four hours) microcytotoxicity assay by release of radioactive chromium (^{51}Cr) (*10, 11*). In a second set of experiments, the PBMC obtained from patients and controls were treated with recombinant interleukin-2 (rIL-2) before the cytotoxicity assay against K562 cells.

The statistical significance of differences between mean results was analyzed by application of the Student-Fisher t-test for unpaired data, using a Hewlett-Packard model 67 calculator.

Results

All the patients studied had anti-HIV antibodies detected by ELISA and confirmed by Western blot, with visible bands for the proteins of at least two viral genes.

Sera of 56 patients at different clinical stages of the infection were studied; free antigen was detected in 22 cases (39%). Table 1 shows the distribution of the results by CDC clinical group. In cases diagnosed as AIDS, 13 of 20 individuals (65%) had measurable levels of serum antigen, whereas circulating HIV antigen was detected in only one-third (seven of 20) of the asymptomatic carriers (Group II).

The CD4 population was lower in all the clinical groups than in the controls (Figure 1). It is notable that the asymptomatic carriers had absolute values of CD4 below 50% of the values observed in controls ($398/mm^3$ compared to $825/mm^3$), a significant reduction ($p < 0.005$). An increase of the CD8 population was evidenced in all the groups, with the exception of the AIDS patients; the increase was most pronounced in the patients with persistent generalized lymphadenopa-

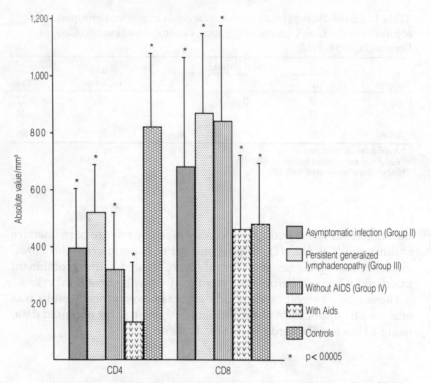

Figure 1. Absolute values ($\bar{x} \pm 1SD$) of CD4 and CD8 antigens in controls and HIV-infected patients grouped according to the U.S. Centers for Disease Control classification, Caracas, Venezuela, 1984–1988.

thy (Group III). A reduced CD4/CD8 ratio in all groups reflects the changes in the CD4 and CD8 populations.

The population of large granular lymphocytes (LGL, natural cytotoxic cells) was evaluated both in terms of variations in the CD3⁻, CD16⁺ subpopulation and in their lytic activity against the K562 cell line. A significant depletion of these LGL was detected in AIDS patients compared to controls, but the reduced values in seropositive patients without AIDS were not statistically significant. While the cytotoxic function against K562 cells was diminished in both groups, in neither case was the reduction significant (Table 2). The response of this subpopulation after stimulation with IL-2 was also investigated in both infected patients and controls. In both groups, a considerable increase of lytic function was observed (Table 3).

Table 2. Functional activity of natural cytotoxic lymphocytes in 22 HIV-infected patients and 11 controls, Caracas, Venezuela, 1984–1988.

Clinical group	CD16+ lymphocytes[a]		
	% (+ SD)	Absolute value per mm^3 ($\bar{x} \pm$ SD)	Lysis[b] (%)
AIDS (n=7)	8 ± 1	139 ± 112[c]	28 ± 13
Without AIDS (n=15)	11 ±3	280 ± 150	28 ± 13
Controls (n=11)	11 ± 2	327 ± 77	36 ± 11

[a] CD3⁻, CD16+ (Leu 11c)
[b] Release of ^{51}Cr, K562 cell line
[c] $p < 0.005$ vs. controls

In 49 patients with HIV infection, the presence or absence of serum antigen was investigated along with the values for subpopulations of T lymphocytes. The number of CD4 cells in HIV-infected patients without AIDS but with detectable levels of serum antigen was significantly less ($p < 0.05$) than in patients in the same clinical group but negative for antigen. However, among patients with AIDS, depletion of the CD4 population was not correlated with the presence or absence of HIV antigen (Table 4).

Table 3. Response of natural cytotoxic lymphocytes to recombinant interleukin-2 (rIL-2) in HIV-infected patients and controls in Caracas, Venezuela, 1984–1988.

	Baseline (% cytotoxicity)	After rIL-2 (500 u/ml)
Patients		
1	20	30
2	8	30
3	74	71
4	34	37
5	33	53
6	14	58
7	32	71
Controls		
1	52	71
2	28	71
3	34	73

Table 4. Absolute values of CD4 and detection of HIV antigen in serum in patients in Caracas, Venezuela, 1984–1988.

Clinical group	CD4 per mm^3	
	Positive for antigen (n) x̄ ± SD	Negative for antigen (n) x̄ ± SD
With AIDS (n=16)	(10) 142 ± 220	(6) 110 ± 102
Without AIDS (n=33)	(8) 219 ± 172	(25) 436 ± 342[a]

[a]Difference significant ($p < 0.05$)

Discussion

One of the most notable findings in the initial report of AIDS (1) was the depletion of CD4 lymphocytes. Since then, the specific tropism of HIV for lymphocytes and glial cells has been confirmed. Recently, alterations of the LGL that carry the phenotype CD3⁻, CD16⁺ have also been found to be among the profound immunopathogenic effects of HIV infection on the immune system (5).

CD4 lymphocytes are particularly susceptible to the cytopathic action of HIV (2–4), as are other cells that have the CD4 molecule on their surface (macrophages, Langerhans cells, and glial cells). CD4 appears to be the receptor molecule for HIV, and the HIV-CD4 interaction is mediated by the gp120 and gp41 proteins of the virus (12). Moreover, monoclonal antibodies directed against epitopes of the CD4 molecule can inhibit the cytopathic effect of HIV in vitro (13).

The CD4 subset is made up of lymphocytic subpopulations that activate CD8 suppressor lymphocytes and of subpopulations of helper cells that cooperate with B lymphocytes in the synthesis of specific antibodies. The phenotype of the first subpopulation is CD4⁺, CD45R⁺, and that of the second is CD4⁺, CDW29⁺ (14, 15, 16). Recent research has yielded preliminary information on the immuno-pathogenic effects of HIV on these subpopulations. Vuillier et al. (17) evaluated 352 patients at different clinical stages of HIV infection, and compared them with 16 high-risk seronegative homosexuals and 61 controls. The findings reveal a decrease in the number of CD4 lymphocytes from the initial stages of the infection, with reduction of the CD4⁺, CDW29⁺ and CD4⁺, CD45R⁺ subpopulations in asymptomatic carriers, persons with AIDS-related complex, and AIDS patients. However, in Group III patients the CD4⁺, CD45R⁺ subpopulation remained intact, while in high-risk seronegatives the CD4$^+$, CDW29$^+$ subpopulation showed a significant increase.

Although the pattern of progressive reduction of CD4 in infected patients found in the study reported here was similar to that described in other studies, the CD4 values in Group II patients (asymptomatic carriers) in the present study showed a greater depletion of that subset than was reported by Vuillier et al. (17) and Andrieu et al. (18).

This finding is important considering that the more depleted CD4 lymphocytes become, the greater the likelihood that AIDS will develop within a shorter time period (18, 19, 20), which could imply a more accentuated cytopathic effect of HIV in the patients studied. The seven (35%) of 20 Group II patients who had circulating HIV antigen experienced a loss of specific immune response to tetanus toxoid-type soluble antigens (results not presented in detail here) similar to that reported by Fauci et al. (12).

In contrast to CD4$^+$ lymphocytes, the numbers of CD3$^+$, CD4$^-$, CD8$^+$ lymphocytes (responsible for suppressor and cytotoxic functions) are generally significantly increased in peripheral blood. The apparent resistance of CD8 lymphocytes to HIV infection was suggested by C. M. Walker et al. (21). Moreover, evidence of the existence of cytotoxic T lymphocytes (CTL) of phenotypes CD3$^+$, CD8$^+$, CD11$^-$ that are specific against components of HIV was found by B. D. Walker et al. (22) using recombinant vaccinia virus transfected with the different HIV genes, which induces the expression of the virus proteins in B lymphocytes previously transformed by the Epstein-Barr virus. Furthermore, in bronchoalveolar washings from patients infected by HIV, Plata et al. (23) found CTL directed against autologous alveolar macrophages previously hybridized with DNA probes that contained the complete HIV genome. It has not yet been determined for certain whether the elevated number of CD8$^+$ lymphocytes observed even in critical stages of HIV infection implies an active state of specific in vitro defense against HIV. Moreover, studies of the CD3$^+$, CD4$^-$, CD8$^+$, CD11$^+$ subpopulation, which is basically formed by suppressor T lymphocytes, have not clarified the situation. This subpopulation does not generally show changes during different clinical stages of the infection, but Vuillier et al. (5) reported a significant increase in these lymphocytes in high-risk seronegative homosexuals. Thus, the immunopathogenic role that might be played by suppressor lymphocytes in patients with HIV infection is unknown.

In the present study, the CD3$^+$, CD4$^-$, CD8$^+$ subpopulation appears to have increased significantly in groups II, III, and IV (without AIDS)

HIV-infected patients; however, the absolute value of this subpopulation in AIDS patients was similar to that in controls.

Initial observations based on the in vitro testing of the LGL cells' activity against tumor cell lines such as the K562 indicated diminished lytic activity in AIDS patients (24–26). Later, Ruscetti et al. (27) reported that LGL with the CD16$^+$, Leu19$^+$ phenotype from healthy donors, activated in vitro with IL-2, had optimal lytic activity against white blood cells infected by HTLV-I or HIV. Studies of CD3$^+$, CD16$^+$ subpopulations (28, 29) found that the LGL were capable of serving as effectors for antibody-dependent cellular cytotoxicity against P-815 cell lines, concomitant with a considerable decrease in natural cytotoxic action against the K562 line. The recent studies of Vuillier et al. (5) have provided more concrete information about the LGL complex (CD3$^-$, CD8$^+$, CD16$^+$, Leu19$^+$) during the course of HIV infection. When this population is analyzed as a whole, a decline of the CD3$^-$, CD16$^+$ lymphocytes is observed, probably associated with lymphopenia induced by HIV. Nonetheless, on investigating the same population using two-color flow cytometry (simultaneous use of two monoclonal antibodies), a significant reduction of the number of CD3$^-$, CD8$^+$, CD16$^+$ lymphocytes was found, particularly those that expressed low-density CD8$^+$ (CD3$^-$, CD8BD$^+$, CD16$^+$), which account for 95% of this population in peripheral blood under normal conditions. Moreover, in high-risk seronegative individuals, a similar but less marked reduction of the CD3$^-$, CD8BD$^+$, CD16$^+$ lymphocytes was demonstrated.

The present study, in contrast to other studies (12, 18), recorded changes in the LGL population (CD3$^-$, CD16$^+$) that confirm the depletion of these natural cytotoxic cells originally reported by Vuillier et al. (5). The decrease was significant ($p < 0.05$) only in patients with AIDS. Furthermore, controverting the idea that the cytotoxic capacity of CD3$^-$, CD16$^+$ cells against K562 lines declines (12, 25, 26, 29), patients in the present study showed an insignificant decline, compared to controls, in the lytic capacity, and unconfirmed results indicate that it can be maintained within the normal range in patients with terminal AIDS, in whom more than 80% of the total volume of LGL is depleted. The increase in lytic action against the K562 cell line after its incubation with recombinant IL-2 was similar to previously reported results (12, 25). The cause of the progressive depletion of the CD3$^-$, CD16$^+$ lymphocytic subpopulation remains obscure. Moreover, reduction of the cell volume of this subset appears to be similar to that observed for the CD4 lymphocytes, which suggests the need to carry out prospective investigations to explain both the depletion mechanism and also its implications for the natural history of HIV infection.

Even though HIV antigens were more commonly detected in the blood of AIDS patients (65%), our results show significant depletion of CD4 lymphocytes in those patients, independent of the presence or absence of circulating antigen. The absolute values of CD4 in the HIV-infected patients without AIDS appear to be lower. Finally, the free antigen was detectable in only 35% of the asymptomatic carriers.

These findings have made it possible to begin to define the immunopathogeny of HIV infection and possible geographic and demographic variations. Nonetheless, many questions have yet to be resolved and will require the application of new immunologic, clinical, and therapeutic approaches.

■ ■ ■

Acknowledgments: The work reported here was financed in part by the Venezuelan Ministry of Health and Social Welfare, the National Commission for the Study of AIDS, CONICIT (Strengthening of Centers), and the National Racetrack Institute.

References

1. Gottlieb, M. S., R. Schroff, H. M. Schanker, *et al. Pneumocystis carinii* pneumonia and mucosal candidiasis in previously healthy homosexual men. *N Engl J Med* 305:1425–1431, 1981.

2. Dalgleish, A. G., P. C. Beverly, P. R. Clapham, *et al.* The CD4 (T4) antigen is an essential component of the receptor for the AIDS retrovirus. *Nature* 312:763, 1984.

3. Klatzmann, D., E. Champagne, S. Chamaret, *et al.* T lymphocyte T4 molecule behaves as the receptor for human retrovirus. *Nature* 312:767, 1984.

4. McDougal, J. S., A. Mawle, S. P. Cort, *et al.* Cellular tropism of the human retrovirus HTLV-III/LAV. I. Role of T cell activation and expression of the T4 antigen. *J Immunol* 135: 3151–3162, 1985.

5. Vuillier, F., N. E. Bianco, L. Montagnier, *et al.* Selective depletion of low density CD8+, CD16+ lymphocytes during HIV infection. *AIDS Research and Human Retroviruses* 4:121–129, 1988.

6. Centers for Disease Control. Classification system for human T-lymphotropic virus type III. Lymphadenopathy-associated virus infection. *MMWR* 35:334, 1986.

7. Centers for Disease Control. Update on acquired immune-deficiency syndrome (AIDS). *MMWR* 31:507–514, 1982.

8. Boyum, A. J. Isolation of mononuclear cells and granulocytes from human blood. *Scand J Clin Lab Invest* 97:1–10, 1968.

9. Rodríguez, M., I. Blanca, M. L. Baroja, et al. Helper activity by human large granular lymphocytes in "in vitro" immunoglobin synthesis. *J Clin Immunol* 7(5):356–364, 1987.

10. Bloom, E. T., and E. L. Korn. Quantification of natural cytotoxicity by human lymphocyte subpopulations isolated by density: heterogeneity of the effector cells. *J Immunol Methods* 58:323–325, 1983.

11. Lozzio, C. B., and B. B. Lozzio. Human chronic myelogenous leukaemia cell line with positive philadelphia chromosome. *Blood* 45:321–334, 1975.

12. Fauci, A. S. The human immunodeficiency virus: infectivity and mechanisms of pathogenesis. *Science* 239:617–622, 1988.

13. Ho, D. D., R. J. Pomerantz, and J. C. Kaplan. Pathogenesis of infection with human immunodeficiency virus. *N Engl J Med* 317:278–286, 1987.

14. Morimoto, C., N. L. Letvin, A. W. Boyd, et al. The isolation and characterization of the human helper inducer T cell subset. *J Immunol* 134:3762–3768, 1985.

15. Morimoto, C., N. L. Letvin, J. A. Distaso, et al. The isolation and characterization of the human suppressor inducer T cell subset. *J Immunol* 134:1508–1515, 1985.

16. Takeuchi, T., M. Dimaggio, H. Levine, et al. CD11 molecule defines the two types of suppressor cells within the T8[+] population. *Cell Immunol* 111:398–409, 1988.

17. Vuillier, F., C. Lapresle, and G. Dighiero. Comparative analysis of CD4-4B4 and CD4-2H4 lymphocyte subpopulations in HIV negative homosexual, HIV seropositive and healthy subjects. *Clin Exp Immunol* 71:8–12, 1988.

18. Andrieu, J. M., D. Eme, A. Venet, et al. Serum HIV antigen and anti-p24 antibodies in 200 HIV seropositive patients: correlation with CD4 and CD8 lymphocyte subsets. *Clin Exp Immunol* 73:1–5, 1988.

19. Polk, B. F., R. Fox, R. Brookmeyer, et al. Predictors of the acquired immunodeficiency syndrome developing in a cohort of seropositive homosexual men. *N Engl J Med* 316:61–67, 1987.

20. Fahey, J. L., J. Giorgi, O. Martinez-Maza, et al. Immune pathogenesis of AIDS and related syndromes. *In: Acquired Immunodeficiency Syndrome* (eds. J. C. Gluckman and E. Vilmer), Paris, Elsevier, 1987, p. 107.

21. Walker, C. M., D. J. Moody, D. P. Stites, and J. A. Levy. CD8[+] lymphocytes can control HIV infection in vitro by suppressing virus replication. *Science* 234:1563–1566, 1986.

22. Walker, B. D., S. Chakrabarti, B. Moss, et al. HIV-specific cytotoxic T lymphocytes in seropositive individuals. *Nature* 328:345–348, 1987.

23. Plata, F., B. Autran, L. Pedroza Martins, et al. AIDS virus-specific cytotoxic T lymphocytes in lung disorders. *Nature* 328:348–351, 1987.

24. Poli, G., M. Introna, F. Zariaboni, et al. Natural killer cells in intravenous drug abusers with lymphadenopathy syndrome. *Clin Exp Immunol* 62:128, 1985.

25. Alcocer-Varela, J., D. Alarcón-Segovia, and C. Abid-Mendoza. Immunoregulatory circuits in the acquired immune deficiency syndrome and related complex. Production of and response to interleukin 1 and 2,

NK function and its enhancement by interleukin 2 and kinetics of the autologous mixed lymphocyte reaction. *Clin Exp Immunol* 60:31:, 1985.

26. Spicuett, G. P., and A. G. Dalgleish. Cellular immunology of HIV infection. *Clin Exp Immunol* 71:1–7, 1988.

27. Ruscetti, F. W., J. A. Mikovits, V. S. Kalyanaraman, *et al.* Analysis of effector mechanisms against HTLV-I and HTLV-III/LAV-infected lymphoid cells. *J Immunol* 136:3619–3624, 1986.

28. Bonavida, B., J. Katz, and M. Gottlieb. Mechanism of defective NK cell activity in patients with acquired immune deficiency syndrome (AIDS) and AIDS-related complex. I. Defective trigger on NK cells for NKCF production by target cells, and partial restoration by IL 2. *J Immunol* 137:1157–1164, 1986.

29. Katz, J. D., R. Mitsuyasu, M. S. Gottlieb, *et al.* Mechanism of defective NK cell activity in patients with acquired immunodeficiency syndrome (AIDS) and AIDS-related complex. II. Normal antibody-dependent cellular cytotoxicity (ADCC) mediated by effector cells defective in natural killer (NK) cytotoxicity. *J Immunol* 139:55–60, 1987.

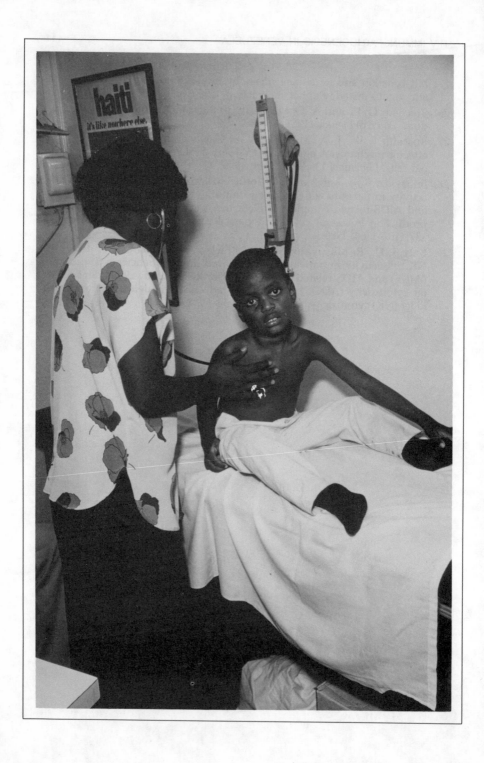

RETROVIRUSES IN THE CARIBBEAN

C. BARTHOLOMEW & F. CLEGHORN

Adult T-cell leukemia was first described as a specific clinical entity by Takatsuki et al. (1) in 1977. In 1980 Poiesz and his colleagues at the National Cancer Institute (2) reported detection and isolation of the first human T-lymphotropic virus, HTLV-I, thereby culminating a long and hitherto fruitless search for a human retrovirus. This work subsequently yielded the first clue to the relationship between HTLV-I and adult T-cell leukemia (ATL)—a clue derived from seropositive responses obtained with ATL case serum samples provided to the researchers by Ito of Kyoto University (3).

After clusters of ATL cases were recognized on the islands of Shikoku and Kyushu in southwestern Japan, Catovsky et al. (4) reported cases among six black West Indians residing in the United Kingdom. The virus-disease relationship was documented by a high seroprevalence of antibodies to HTLV-I in these patients, who were born in Grenada, Guyana, Jamaica, St. Vincent and the Grenadines, and Trinidad and Tobago. Subsequently, Clark et al. (5) did an epidemiologic survey of the seroprevalence of antibodies to HTLV-I on the island of St. Vincent, finding a seroprevalence of 3.3%. More recent studies in Suriname and Barbados have shown respective HTLV-I antibody seroprevalences of 3.0% and 4.25% (6, 7).

Similar surveys in Jamaica have shown an overall seroprevalence of 5.4% in the general population (5) and have found as many as 70% of all cases of non-Hodgkin's lymphoma in Jamaica to exhibit high-titer HTLV-I antibodies, which suggests that HTLV-I has contributed significantly to the occurrence of lymphoreticular neoplasia on that island (8).

In 1982 a random survey of the Trinidad population was conducted to determine the seroprevalence of hepatitis B infection. This survey detected high seroprevalences of hepatitis B antibodies in both major ethnic groups—people of African and Asian (Indian) origin (9).[1] When the stored sera from this survey were tested for HTLV-I antibodies, 37 (2.3%) of 1,578 samples tested by an enzyme-linked immunosorbent assay (ELISA) were found positive for HTLV-I. However, 31 of 802 (3.9%) of the Trinidadians of African ancestry were seropositive, together with five of 208 (2.4%) persons of mixed African ancestry, while only one person out of 448 (0.2%) of Indian descent was seropositive (10). This disparity in ethnic seroprevalence stood in marked contrast to the seroprevalence of hepatitis B antibodies in the two major racial groups.

The almost exclusive restriction of HTLV-I infection to the Afro-Trinidadian population supports the hypothesis of Gallo et al. (11) that HTLV-I came to the Caribbean via the African slave trade. (Although Trinidad is a cosmopolitan island, the people of Indian origin have tended to settle in the rural agricultural lands of central Trinidad, while the Afro-Trinidadians have tended to congregate in the urban areas.) The lone Trinidadian of Indian origin who was seropositive for HTLV-I gave a history of frequent sexual contact with many women of African descent throughout the Caribbean islands.

The modes of transmission of hepatitis B, HTLV-I, and the human immunodeficiency virus (HIV) are very similar—namely, by sexual contact (12); parenterally via blood transfusion (13) or intravenous drug abuse (14); and from mother to child (15), possibly in utero (16), intrapartum (17), or in breast milk (18). It has been found that HTLV-I, like HIV in the Western Hemisphere, is transmitted more readily from male to female than from female to male (19).

A prospective survey of lymphoreticular malignancies in Trinidad and Tobago conducted from 1 October 1985 to 31 March 1988 found that non-Hodgkin's lymphoma accounted for 69 of 176 (39.2%) of all subjects with lymphoreticular malignancies who were enrolled in the study. Of these 69 cases, 35 (50.7%) were positive for HTLV-I antibod-

---

[1]Trinidad and Tobago, the two southernmost islands in the Caribbean Basin, have a 1.2 million population consisting mainly of people of African (41%) and Asian (Indian) origin (41%), people of mixed racial descent (16%), Caucasians (1%), and Chinese (1%). The people of African descent came to Trinidad via the Portuguese slave trade from 1680 onwards, while those of Indian origin came after the abolition of slavery as indentured laborers beginning in 1845.

ies. Not unexpectedly, all the patients with ATL in Trinidad and Tobago to date have been people of African ancestry.

HIV-1–associated AIDS in the Caribbean

The first case report of AIDS in the English-speaking Caribbean was from Trinidad in early 1983 (20). Barbados, Bermuda, Grenada, Jamaica, Saint Lucia, and Suriname reported their first cases in 1984; and Antigua, the Bahamas, Cayman Islands, St. Kitts/Nevis, and St. Vincent and the Grenadines reported cases in 1985. Anguilla's first case was reported in 1987 (21).

Worldwide, three general patterns of HIV-1 transmission have been found (22). The first pattern, involving a spread of the virus that began in the mid-1970s to early 1980s, was one in which transmission occurred primarily through homosexual contact, with intravenous drug abuse playing the next largest role. Regions where this pattern has prevailed include Western Europe, North America, some parts of South America, Australia, and New Zealand.

The second pattern, involving virus introduced into the affected communities in the early to late 1970s, has affected primarily heterosexuals. Where this pattern prevails homosexual transmission has not been a major factor, but transmission via HIV-infected blood has come to pose a major public health problem. Pattern II has been observed increasingly in parts of Latin America, the Caribbean, and in Central Africa. However, as will be discussed later, the pattern typically observed in the individual "English-speaking" Caribbean islands does not conform to this classification or indeed to any of the three principal patterns described.

The third pattern is one in which the virus has been introduced more recently, in the early to mid 1980s; both homosexual and heterosexual transmission are only just being documented, and parenteral transmission is not a significant problem at present. Areas experiencing this pattern include Asia, the Pacific region (apart from Australia and New Zealand), the Middle East, Eastern Europe, and some rural parts of South America.

Regarding the Caribbean, the initial risk groups affected in Antigua, Barbados, Grenada, Guyana, St. Kitts, and Trinidad and Tobago consisted of homosexual/bisexual men. In these places, especially Trinidad and Tobago, the infection has spread slowly into the heterosexual community via bisexual behavior. In contrast, the AIDS epidemic on Saint Lucia was begun by heterosexual contacts of migrant Saint Lucian laborers from Belle Glade, Florida (23).

Intravenous drug abuse is rarely practiced on these islands. On Bermuda, however, 58.0% of the AIDS cases reported up to May 1988 had occurred among intravenous drug abusers, while only 21.0% had afflicted known homosexual or bisexual men (24).

The Bahamas, which reported its first AIDS case in 1985, has provided detailed information on the risk categories of AIDS patients seen during 1987 (25). The mode of transmission in the Bahamas is predominantly sexual, with heterosexual transmission accounting for 59% of AIDS cases, homosexual/bisexual males accounting for 10%, transfusions accounting for 1%, and perinatal transmission accounting for up to 19%. In all, 63% of the heterosexual AIDS cases were found in cocaine abusers (not intravenous drug abusers), who in turn were identified with sexual promiscuity and prostitution as a result of drug abuse. Because of this heterosexual predominance, the high percentage of pediatric AIDS cases is not surprising.

HTLV-I, HIV, and AIDS in Trinidad and Tobago

The first risk group to be affected with AIDS in Trinidad and Tobago was homosexual/bisexual men, among whom the numbers of cases initially doubled about every 12 months. Specifically, there were eight cases in this risk group in 1983, 19 new cases in 1984, 33 in 1985, and 51 in 1986. In 1987 the number of new cases in homosexual/bisexual men fell to 33, but the number of new AIDS cases in heterosexuals kept rising—from five in 1985 and 17 in 1986 to 29 in 1987—so that these almost equalled the number of new homosexual/bisexual cases. Of these 29 heterosexual cases, 15 occurred in males and 14 in females. This trend continued through the first half of 1988, when 33 heterosexual cases and 29 homosexual/bisexual cases were reported. Fourteen of the 33 heterosexual cases occurred in males and 19 in females (Figure 1).

While 173 (56.3%) of all the AIDS cases reported in Trinidad and Tobago occurred among homosexual/bisexual men, bisexual men accounted for a large share (up to 71 cases or 41% of the total). The pattern that emerges is one of heterosexual transmission increasing rapidly in the community, largely as a result of bisexual men becoming infected and transmitting the disease to women.

Regarding patterns of HTLV-I and HIV infection, a study was made

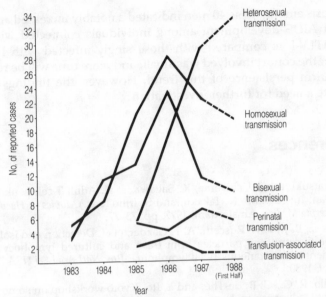

Figure 1. Reported AIDS cases in Trinidad and Tobago, by apparent mode of transmission, through 30 June 1988.

of a cohort of 100 apparently healthy homosexual men who frequently attended a sexually transmitted disease (STD) clinic in Port of Spain, Trinidad. Forty percent of these men were seropositive for HIV in 1984 and 15% were seropositive for HTLV-I. When adjusted for age, this latter figure represented a HTLV-I seroprevalence six times higher than that of the general population. Six percent of the men in the cohort were coinfected with HTLV-I and HIV; none of the cohort members were found to be intravenous drug abusers.

Another more recent study of HTLV-I prevalence in HIV-infected individuals was made in 1987. Of 285 consecutive HIV-positive sera tested for HTLV-I antibodies, 35 (12.3%) were found positive. Of these 35 apparent coinfections, 16 (45.7%) occurred in homosexual/bisexual males and 17 (48.5%) occurred in heterosexual individuals (11 males and 6 females). The other two coinfected individuals, both adult males, were an intravenous drug abuser and a man whose risk category was unknown.

With respect to the first study, after four-and-a-half years of follow-up, five (14.7%) of the 34 homosexual men infected with only HIV had progressed to AIDS, as compared to three (50%) of the six coinfected with HTLV-I and HIV. Trend analysis of the dates of AIDS diagnosis among these 40 men indicated a notably increased apparent risk of AIDS development among individuals coinfected with HIV and HTLV-I as compared with those singly infected with HIV. Of course, the cohort involved was small, and more time will be required to confirm persistence of this trend. However, the findings clearly indicate a need for further investigation.

References

1. Takatsuki, K., T. Uchiyama, K. Sagawa, et al. Adult T-cell Leukaemia in Japan. In: S. Seno, K. Takaku, and S. Irino (eds.). *Topics in Haematology, Excerpta Medica*. Amsterdam, 1977, pp. 73–77.
2. Poiesz, B. J., F. W. Ruscetti, A. F. Gazdar, et al. Detection and isolation of type C retrovirus particles from fresh and cultured lymphocytes of a patient with cutaneous T-cell lymphoma. *Proc Natl Acad Sci USA* 77:7415–7419, 1980.
3. Gallo, R. C., G. B. de-Thé, and Y. Ito. Kyoto workshop on some specific recent advances in human tumour virology. *Cancer Res* 41:4738–4739, 1981.
4. Catovsky, D., M. F. Greaves, M. Rose, et al. Adult T-cell lymphoma/leukaemia in blacks from the West Indies. *Lancet* 1:639, 1982.
5. Clark, J., C. Saxinger, W. N. Gibbs, et al. Seroepidemiologic studies of human T-cell leukaemia/lymphoma virus type 1 in Jamaica. *Int J Cancer* 36:37, 1985.
6. Hull, B. Unpublished data, 1988.
7. Reidel, D. A., A. S. Evans, W. C. Saxinger, and W. A. Blattner. A Retrospective Study of Human T-cell Leukaemia/Lymphoma Virus Type 1 (HTLV-I) Transmission in Barbados. Unpublished data, 1987.
8. Blattner, W. A., W. N. Gibbs, C. Saxinger, et al. Human T-cell leukaemia/lymphoma virus associated neoplasia in Jamaica. *Lancet* 1:61, 1983.
9. Bartholomew, C. Unpublished data, 1983.
10. Bartholomew, C., W. Charles, R. Gallo, and W. Blattner. The Ethnic Distribution of HTLV-I and HTLV-III Associated Diseases in Trinidad, West Indies. In: *International Symposium on African AIDS, Brussels, 1985*.
11. Gallo, R. C., A. Sliski, and F. Wong-Staal. Origin of human T-cell leukaemia/lymphoma virus. *Lancet* 2:962, 1983.
12. Tajima, K., S. Tominaga, T. Suchi, et al. Epidemiological analysis of the distribution of antibody to adult T-cell leukaemia virus associated antigen: Possible horizontal transmission of adult T-cell leukaemia virus. *JAMA* 73:893, 1982.
13. Essex, M., M. F. McLane, T. H. Lee, et al. Antibodies to human T-cell leukemia virus membrane antigens (HTLV-MA) in hemophiliacs. *Science* 221:1061, 1983.

14. Robert-Guroff, M., S. H. Weiss, J. A. Giron, et al. Prevalence of antibodies to HTLV-I, II, and III in intravenous drug abusers from an AIDS-endemic region. *JAMA* 255:3133, 1986.

15. Nakano, S., Y. Ando, M. Ichijo, et al. Search for possible routes of vertical and horizontal transmission of adult T-cell leukaemia virus. *Gann* 75:103, 1984.

16. Kajiyama, W., S. Kashiwagi, H. Ikematsu, et al. Intrafamilial transmission of adult T-cell leukaemia virus. *J Infect Dis* 154(88):51, 1986.

17. Kajiyama, W., S. Kashiwagi, J. Hayashi, et al. Intrafamilial clustering of anti-ATLA-positive persons. *Am J Epidemiol* 124:800–806, 1986.

18. Kinoshita, K., T. Amagasaki, S. Hino, et al. Milk-borne transmission of HTLV-I from carrier mothers to their children. *Gann* 78(7):674, 1987.

19. Tajima, K., and Y. Hinuma. Epidemiological features of adult T-cell leukaemia virus. In: G. Mathe and P. Reizenstein (eds.). *Advances in the Biosciences, Vol. 50: Pathophysiological Aspects of Cancer Epidemiology.* Oxford, Pergamon Press, 1984.

20. Bartholomew, C., C. Raju, and N. Jankey. The acquired immune deficiency syndrome in Trinidad: a report of two cases. *West Indian Med J* 32:177, 1983.

21. Caribbean Epidemiology Center. AIDS in the Caribbean: an update. *CAREC Surveillance Report* 14:5, 1988.

22. Piot, P., F. A. Plummer, F. S. Mhalu, et al. AIDS: an international perspective. *Science* 239:573, 1988.

23. St. Catherine, L. Personal communication, 1988.

24. Surveillance Unit, Department of Health of Bermuda. Acquired Immune Deficiency Syndrome (AIDS) Update. Hamilton, Bermuda, 1988.

25. Ofosu-Barto, K., and R. N. Bain (eds.). *Statistics on AIDS in the Bahamas, 1985–1987.* Nassau, 1988.

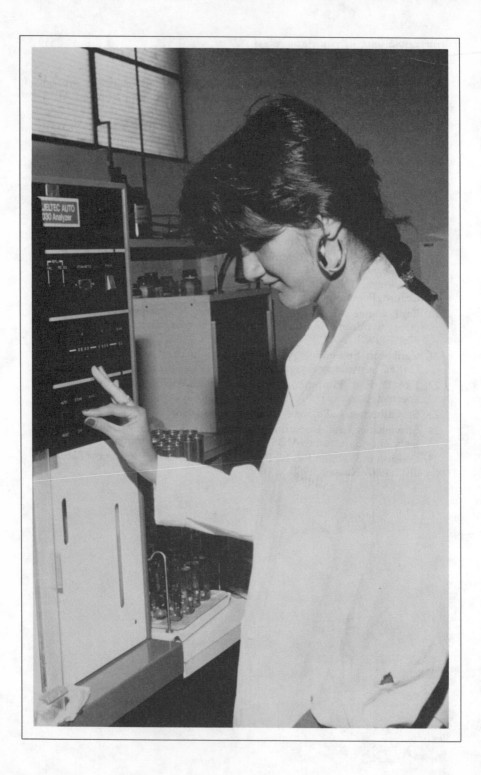

A SIMPLE PROCEDURE FOR OBTAINING LARGE AMOUNTS OF HIV ANTIGENS FOR SERODIAGNOSTIC PURPOSES

JAIRO IVO-DOS-SANTOS & BERNARDO GALVÃO-CASTRO

Several assays for detection of human immunodeficiency virus (HIV) antibodies have been developed. Among these, the enzyme-linked immunosorbent assay (ELISA) (1) and the Western blot test (2, 3) are the methods of choice used respectively for screening sera and confirming seropositivity. Nearly all these tests utilize viral antigens that are either purified by sucrose density gradient centrifugation (4, 5) or obtained by genetic engineering (6, 7). The consequent need for high-cost equipment and reagents such as ultracentrifuges and approved Western blot tests precludes routine use of HIV confirmatory assay in laboratories lacking resources. In this communication we report the results of an effort to devise a simpler, cheaper, and less time-consuming way to obtain viral antigens suitable for serologic confirmation of HIV infection.

Materials and Methods

A lymphoblastoid H9 cell line infected with productively replicating HIV-1, kindly provided by Dr. R. C. Gallo of the U.S. National Cancer Institute in Bethesda, Maryland, USA, was cultured as described elsewhere (8). The culture medium (RPMI 1640 plus 10% fetal calf serum, 2 mM glutamine, 100 units/ml penicillin, and 100 μg/ml streptomycin) was changed every three or four days.

Virus Purification

A differential centrifugation protocol for virus purification was followed. The infected cells (10^6/ml) were initially spun down at low speed (200 times the acceleration of gravity [g] for 10 minutes at 4°C). The supernatant was then centrifuged at 5,000 g for 30 minutes at 4°C to remove cellular debris, and the viruses present in the supernatant were pelleted by centrifuging at 41,000 g for 2 hours at 4°C. The device used was a Beckman J2-21 centrifuge with a JA 21 rotor. The supernatant was carefully removed, and the viral pellet was resuspended at one five-hundredth of the original volume in 0.01 M Tris, 0.15 M NaCl, and 0.25% Triton-X-100 nonionic detergent at a pH of 7.2. The protein concentration was determined by Lowry's technique (9), and the viral suspensions were maintained at −70°C until use.

Western Blot

A sample of semipurified HIV antigen was dissociated in sodium dodecyl sulfate (SDS) and 2-mercaptoethanol, and was subjected to SDS–gel electrophoresis in a 10% acrylamide gel. The resulting protein bands were then transferred to nitrocellulose paper (Schleicher and Schuel, Dassel, Federal Republic of Germany) in a transblot apparatus (BioRad Laboratories, USA) at 40 volts over the course of 14–16 hours. Twenty percent methanol in 0.025 M Tris and 0.192 M glycine was used as a transfer buffer. The nitrocellulose paper was blocked (that is, the remaining protein-binding sites were inactivated) in a 0.3% Tween 20 and phosphate-buffered (pH 7.2) saline solution with 5% non-fat dry milk for 60 minutes. The strips were then incubated with serum samples diluted 1:100 in the same buffer for 60 minutes. All incubations and washings (in PBS/0.3% Tween 20) were carried out at room temperature.

The strips were subsequently incubated with a goat anti-human horseradish peroxidase labeled IgG diluted 1:1,000 in blocking solution for 60 minutes. After washings, the strips were incubated with a chromogenic substrate consisting of diaminobenzidine (0.25 mg per ml), citrate-phosphate buffer (pH 5.0), and 0.001% H_2O_2. The reaction was stopped by immersion of the strips in distilled water.

For comparison, a commercially available Western blot assay (Du Pont Company, Wilmington, Delaware, USA) was carried out according to the manufacturer's instructions.

Serum Samples

Serum samples were obtained from 85 patients. Twenty-one of these patients had the acquired immunodeficiency syndrome (AIDS), 17 had the AIDS-related complex (ARC), 27 had persistent generalized lymphadenopathy (PGL), and 20 had asymptomatic HIV infections. The clinical criteria used to evaluate the clinical status of the AIDS, ARC, and PGL cases were those of the U.S. Centers for Disease Control in Atlanta, Georgia (10). The serum samples were found to be positive by ELISA (1), indirect immunofluorescence (IIF) (11), and Western blot assay (Du Pont Company, Wilmington, Delaware, USA). Sera from six healthy persons without any evidence of HIV infection were included as negative controls.

Results

The usual yield of the semipurification procedure was 100–120 μg of total protein per 50 ml of infected cell supernatant. Although the viral pellets were contaminated with proteins of culture medium and/or cellular origin, as evidenced by Red Ponceau staining of antigens transferred to nitrocellulose paper (data not presented), these contaminants did not interfere with immunostaining of the viral proteins. However, because of their presence we did not determine the actual amount of viral protein in the pellet.

In general, a good correlation was found between the results obtained with our "homemade" Western blot assay and with the commercial assay (Figure 1). However, some differences were observed in the intensity of reactivity to the *gag* p55, *env* gp120, and gp160 antigens. Some AIDS sera that did not react with p55 of the commercial kit did react with the p55 of our Western blot assay (Table 1). On the other hand, the commercial Western blot assay consistently showed a reaction to gp160 in all appropriate sera, while evidence of this reaction was absent when our semipurified antigens were used.

In the course of this work, we verified that it was necessary to maintain the percentage of cells expressing the virus above 90% in order to avoid any appreciable background. At the opposite extreme, when we obtained the virus from a culture where only about 30% of the cells were expressing the virus (as indicated by IIF), the yield was

Table 1. Comparison of the Western blot assay results obtained with our "homemade" method and the commercial (Du Pont) assay. Aside from negative controls (not shown), the sera tested were from patients with AIDS, the AIDS-related complex (ARC), persistent generalized lymphadenopathy (PGL), and asymptomatic HIV infection (HIV). "gp" = glycoprotein, "p" = protein.

| | | Sera testing positive from patients with: | | | | | | | |
| | | AIDS (n=21) | | ARC (n=17) | | PGL (n=27) | | HIV (n=20) | |
Band	Antigen	No.	(%)	No.	(%)	No.	(%)	No.	(%)
gp160	"Homemade"	0	(0)	0	(0)	0	(0)	0	(0)
	Commercial	20	(95)	17	(100)	27	(100)	20	(100)
gp120	"Homemade"	9	(43)	16	(94)	27	(100)	13	(65)
	Commercial	20	(95)	17	(100)	27	(100)	19	(95)
p66	"Homemade"	20	(95)	17	(100)	27	(100)	20	(100)
	Commercial	21	(100)	16	(94)	27	(100)	20	(100)
p55	"Homemade"	17	(81)	15	(88)	25	(93)	20	(100)
	Commercial	4	(19)	10	(59)	11	(41)	13	(65)
p51	"Homemade"	18	(86)	17	(100)	27	(100)	20	(100)
	Commercial	17	(81)	15	(88)	27	(100)	20	(100)
gp41	"Homemade"	21	(100)	15	(88)	27	(100)	18	(90)
	Commercial	20	(95)	15	(88)	27	(100)	16	(80)
p31	"Homemade"	18	(86)	15	(88)	26	(96)	16	(80)
	Commercial	18	(86)	14	(82)	26	(96)	15	(75)
p24	"Homemade"	12	(57)	15	(88)	24	(89)	19	(95)
	Commercial	17	(81)	17	(100)	26	(96)	19	(95)
p18	"Homemade"	9	(43)	13	(76)	22	(81)	13	(65)
	Commercial	15	(71)	8	(47)	22	(81)	16	(80)

so low that we were unable to perform an adequate assay (data not presented).

Discussion

Over the past three years HIV antibody tests have transformed our understanding of the epidemiology of AIDS and HIV infection. The starting point was the finding of cell lines suitable to serve as hosts for the growth of the virus (8). This permitted establishment of serologic procedures for screening and confirmatory diagnosis. However, the costs of confirmatory tests such as the Western blot are so high as to hamper their routine use in countries that have insufficient resources.

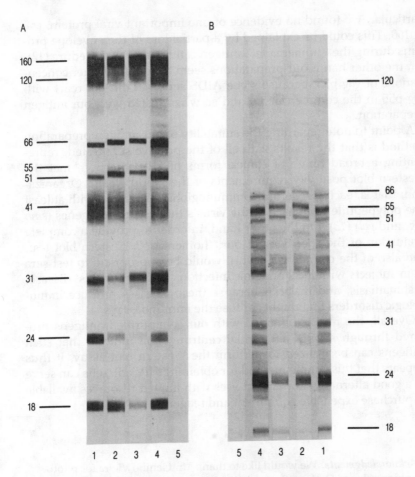

Figure 1. Photographs showing the reactivity of IgG antibodies to HIV-1 antigens electroblotted onto nitrocellulose strips from (A) the commercial Western blot assay and (B) our "homemade" Western blot assay (7 μg of protein per strip). The numbered strips were tested against sera from patients with AIDS (1), the AIDS-related complex (2), persistent generalized lymphadenopathy (3), and asymptomatic HIV infection (4), as well as against normal human sera (5). The numbers at the left and right represent molecular weights (in daltons × 10^{-3}).

The data presented here indicate that a cheaper and simpler methodology could be employed to procure suitable amounts of viral antigens for use in a Western blot confirmatory assay. However, we have observed some differences between the results obtained with our "homemade" Western blot assay and with a commercial product. In particular, we found no evidence of one important viral protein, *env* gp160. This could be explained by a partial loss of the envelope proteins during the "homemade" antigen centrifugation procedure (12). On the other hand, our preparations seem to contain higher concentrations of *gag* p55, because some AIDS sera that did not react with *gag* p55 in the commercial test did so when tested with our antigen preparation.

A point to note regarding the suitability of our antigen preparation method is that the results with all of the positive sera tested, representing a broad range of clinical forms of HIV infection, met the Western blot positivity requirements of the World Health Organization; that is, each test serum's immunoglobulins reacted with at least one polypeptide from each of the virus's three structural genes (*env*, *gag*, and *pol*) (13). On the other hand, in order to provide a complete evaluation of the specificity of our "homemade" Western blot test, and also of the commercial test, it would be appropriate to test sera from subjects with local endemic infections such as Chagas' disease, leishmaniasis, and malaria—because these diseases produce immunologic disorders that might confuse the immunoassays.

Overall, the results obtained with our semipurified antigens procured through simple differential centrifugation indicate that such antigens can be utilized to perform the Western blot assay. It thus appears that this simple method for obtaining HIV antigens can serve as a good alternative for laboratories with limited resources available to purchase expensive equipment and reagents.

■ ■ ■

Acknowledgments: We would like to thank Mr. Genilto Vieira for photographic work and Dr. Vera Bongertz for review of this manuscript.

The work reported here was supported by a grant (No. 10/0212-7) from the Bank of Brazil Foundation (Fundação Banco do Brasil).

References

1. Weiss, S. H., J. J. Goedert, M. G. Sarnaghadaran, and A. J. Bodner. Screening test for HTLV-III (AIDS agent) antibodies: specificity, sensitivity and applications. *JAMA* 253:221–222, 1985.

2. Schupbach, J., M. Popovic, R. V. Gilden, M. A. Gonda, M. G. Sarnaghadaran, and R. C. Gallo. Serological analysis of a subgroup of human T-lymphotropic retroviruses (HTLV-III) in Swiss patients with AIDS. *Science* 224:503–505, 1984.

3. Ulstrup, J. C., K. Skjaug, J. Figenshau, J. Orstavik, N. Bruun, and G. Petersen. Sensitivity of Western blotting compared with ELISA and immunofluorescence during seroconversion after HTLV-III infection. *Lancet* 1:1151–1152, 1986.

4. Sarnaghadaran, M. G., M. Popovic, L. Brush, J. Schupbach, and R. C. Gallo. Antibodies reactive with human T-lymphotropic retroviruses (HTLV-III) in the serum of patients with AIDS. *Science* 224:503–505, 1984.

5. Gallo, D., J. L. Diggs, G. R. Shell, P. J. Dailey, M. N. Hoffman, and J. L. Riggs. Comparison of detection of antibody to the acquired immunodeficiency syndrome virus by enzyme immunoassay, immunofluorescence, and Western blot methods. *J Clin Microbiol* 23:1049–1051, 1986.

6. Steimer, K. S., K. W. Higgins, M. A. Powers, J. C. Stephans, A. Gyenes, C. George-Nascimento, P. A. Luciw, P. J. Barr, R. A. Hallewell, and R. Sanchez-Pescador. Recombinant polypeptide from the endonuclease region of the acquired immunodeficiency syndrome retrovirus polymerase (pol) gene detects serum antibodies in most infected individuals. *J Virol* 58:9–16, 1986.

7. Dawson, G. J., J. S. Heller, C. A. Wood, R. A. Gutiérrez, J. A. Webber, J. C. Hunt, S. A. Hojvat, D. Senn, and S. G. Devare. Reliable detection of individuals seropositive for the human immunodeficiency virus (HIV) by competitive immunoassays using *Escherichia coli*-expressed HIV structural proteins. *J Infect Dis* 157:149–155, 1988.

8. Popovic, M., M. G. Sarnaghadaran, E. Read, and R. C. Gallo. Detection, isolation, and continuous production of cytopathic retroviruses (HTLV-III) from patients with AIDS and pre-AIDS. *Science* 224:497–500, 1984.

9. Lowry, D. H., N. J. Rosebrough, A. L. Faar, and R. J. Randall. Protein measurement with the folin phenol reagent. *J Biol Chem* 193:265–275, 1951.

10. Centers for Disease Control. Classification system for human T-lymphotropic virus type III/lymphoadenopathy-associated virus infection. *MMWR* 35:334–339, 1986.

11. Sandstrom, E. G., R. T. Schooley, D. D. Ho, M. G. Byington, M. G. Sarnaghadaran, M. E. Maclane, M. Essex, R. C. Gallo, and M. S. Hirsh. Detection of human anti-HTLV-III antibodies by indirect immunofluorescence using fixed cells. *Transfusion* 25:308–310, 1985.

12. McGrath, M., O. Witte, T. Pincus, and I. L. Weismann. Retrovirus purification: method that conserves envelope glycoprotein and maximizes infectivity. *J Virol* 25:923–927, 1978.

13. Pan American Health Organization. Report of the Meeting on Guidelines for Evaluation and Standardization of HIV Antibody Kits. Washington, D.C., 2–3 December, 1987.

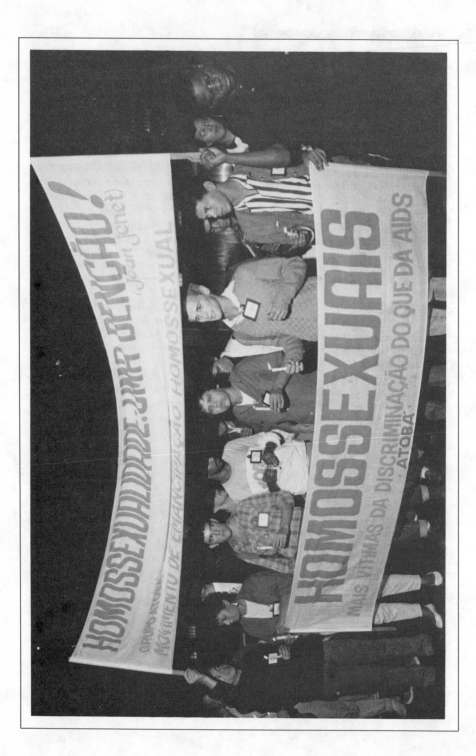

PUBLIC INFORMATION ABOUT AIDS IN BRAZIL, THE DOMINICAN REPUBLIC, HAITI, AND MEXICO

LYDIA S. BOND

Partly because no one can hazard a guess as to when a vaccine against AIDS may be developed or a cure for it discovered, we need to press forward with public health education to help prevent transmission of the human immunodeficiency virus (HIV). Only education can foster the deep individual awareness that leads to self-imposed, willing, meaningful, and sustained changes in behavior and to the recognition that everyone must assume responsibility for his or her own health, because the kind of life chosen today may determine whether one lives tomorrow.

Brandt (1) has found numerous parallels between AIDS and syphilis regarding their associated scientific aspects, public health issues, civil liberties, and social attitudes. In general, he feels that as the search for the "magic bullet against AIDS" continues, it is well to remember that the advent of penicillin did not eradicate syphilis. Similarly, no single treatment or vaccine is likely to free us from AIDS. Therefore, educators and planners working against AIDS need to improve their understanding of relevant relationships between behavior and health—and of relevant biological, cultural, economic, and political influences that affect behavior and sexuality.

In working toward this goal, surveys have been conducted in the four Latin American countries with the largest numbers of reported AIDS cases (Brazil, Haiti, Mexico, and the Dominican Republic) to

Source: From a paper presented at the IV International Conference on AIDS held in Stockholm, Sweden, June 1988.

ascertain public knowledge and attitudes about AIDS transmission and the prevention of HIV infection. The principal aim of these surveys was to provide a basis for developing campaigns and public education programs. In addition, the surveys helped to lay the groundwork for later determination of changes in public knowledge and behavior. The purpose of this article is to report the results of the surveys, results which provide useful insights into public awareness of the problem and available preventive measures.

Materials and Methods Analyzed

The survey findings described here were obtained from published reports and from preliminary information sent to the Pan American Health Organization. Most of the survey instruments included self-assessment by the survey subjects of their knowledge about AIDS and related risk factors, the chances of contracting AIDS, sources of information, modes of transmission and prevention, experience with blood donation, and willingness to be tested.

Since the surveys were not closely comparable in terms of sample size, method of sample selection, questions asked, areas surveyed, or study period, no rigorous comparisons or hemispheric inferences should be made on the basis of the reported data; nor should observed levels of awareness or behavior patterns be attributed to any particular health education effort, since the data reported are the cumulative result of a wide range of circumstances and activities. Finally, it should be noted that the surveys depended on the subjects' recall and other factors prone to bias; however, to the degree that such bias is constant over time, the information reported may be considered reliable in relative terms.

Summary of Results

Brazil

In February 1987 a Brazilian newspaper, Folha de São Paulo, conducted four series of personal interviews with over 5,000 people (2). The first (and by far the largest) series included 4,436 respondents at least 15 years of age in Brasília and seven state capitals;[1] these subjects were grouped in samples representative of the population in terms of sex, age, and socioeconomic status. The other three interview series were conducted only in São Paulo, the nation's largest city, with smaller numbers of respondents chosen at random in public places. The second series included 292 youths of both sexes (people who were 15 to 25 years old); the third included 199 men who identified themselves as homosexuals or bisexuals; and the fourth included 103 street prostitutes.

The four series of interview surveys indicated that 64% of the population sampled in the eight capitals (as compared to 50% in a similar 1985 survey) considered themselves well-informed or reasonably well-informed about AIDS and feared infection. Homosexual and bisexual men (88%), as well as São Paulo youths (65%), were the groups best informed on the nature of AIDS, whereas prostitutes (49%) were the least informed.

Overall, it appears that the Ministry of Health and the news media had made nearly two-thirds of the interview subjects aware of the HIV transmission routes—sexual relations, transfusions, and contaminated needles. However, a considerable share of the prostitutes (49%) and some of the general survey population (23%) believed incorrectly that the disease could also be spread by such acts as kissing, hugging, and shaking hands.

Regarding behavior modification, as Table 1 shows, 20% of the respondents (as compared to 14% in December 1985) said they had changed their lifestyles or sexual practices in a manner that decreased their chances of exposure to HIV infection. Such modifications were reported by a higher proportion of males (27% in 1987, 17% in 1985) than of females (13% in 1987, 12% in 1985). The main modifications reported were in the choice of sexual partners (by 45% of the males and 32% of the females in 1987), in hygienic practices[2] or places frequented[3] (by 7% of the males and 27% of the females), and a reduction or termination of sexual relations with prostitutes (by 12% of the males). Eleven percent of the females said they feared any sexual relations. The fact that lower percentages of respondents reported overall behavior change than reported specific behavior changes

---

[1]Belo Horizonte, in Minas Gerais; Curitiba, in Paraná; Pôrto Alegre, in Rio Grande do Sul; Recife, in Pernambuco; Rio de Janeiro, in Rio de Janeiro; Salvador, in Bahia; and São Paulo, in São Paulo.

[2]Such as bathing before and after intercourse.

[3]Such as bars or brothels.

Table 1. Changes in lifestyles and sexual practices indicated by 1987 interview surveys in eight Brazilian cities (2), as reported by the respondents.

	February 1987 interviews
Modifications of lifestyle or sexual practices to reduce HIV exposure	20% (14% in 1985)
Among males	27% (17% in 1985)
Among females	13% (12% in 1985)
Changes in selection of sexual partners to reduce HIV exposure	
Among males	45%
Among females	32%
Improved hygiene or change in places frequented to reduce HIV exposure	
Among males	7%
Among females	27%
Reported termination or reduction of sexual relations with prostitutes	
(males only)	12%
Reported fear of any sexual relations	
(females only)	11%
Reported use of condoms because of AIDS:	
São Paulo youths of both sexes (people 15–25 years old)	27% (6% in 1985)
Homosexual and bisexual males	49% (17% in 1985)

could conceivably be attributed to the phrasing of the questions or to some respondents not answering particular questions.

The most marked difference between the 1985 and 1987 survey results was in the reported use of condoms. Specifically, in December 1985 6% of the São Paulo young people surveyed and 17% of the homosexual and bisexual males said they used condoms because of AIDS, while in 1987 the respective figures were 27% and 49%.

It also seems clear that information about AIDS had caused changes affecting prostitutes. In particular, 68% of those surveyed who had been practicing their trade for more than a year said the number of customers had decreased. Also, 49% of the prostitutes interviewed in 1987 associated condoms with safe sex. However, few actually insisted on use of condoms, and fatalistic attitudes ("If AIDS is going to happen, it's going to happen") prevailed.

Mexico

Concurrent with the launching of a national AIDS education campaign in 1987, Mexico's Secretariat of Health conducted a survey of 1,961 people at least 15 years of age in Mexico City (3). This survey

Table 2. A summary of data gathered in Mexico City on public awareness of AIDS, HIV transmission routes, and preventive measures through a survey of 1,961 people conducted by the Secretariat of Health in 1987 (3).

	Respondents' answers		
	Yes (%)	No (%)	Do not know (%)
Queries on awareness of AIDS:			
Is AIDS a form of cancer?	50	40	10
Is AIDS an infectious disease caused by a germ?	86	10	4
Is AIDS curable?	36	49	13
Transmission routes (correct):			
Sex with an infected person	92	5	3
Contaminated blood transfusions	96	2	2
Contaminated syringes, needles	93	4	3
Perinatal transmission	89	5	6
Transmission routes (incorrect):			
Through blood donation	75	22	3
Casually, at work	43	47	10
Casually, from a neighbor	25	67	8
Knowledge of preventive measures:			
No vaccine as yet	66	16	18
Celibacy and monogamy with uninfected person are effective measures	70	20	10
Condom is an effective barrier	52	33	15

collected data in three ways—through personal interviews, telephone interviews, and responses to newspaper questionnaires. Six hundred and eighty-one subway users (352 men and 329 women, 35% of the total) were interviewed directly. Six hundred forty-four (206 men and 438 women, 33% of the total) were selected at random from the telephone directory and interviewed by phone. Finally, 636 people (463 men and 173 women, 32% of the total) were chosen from newspaper questionnaire respondents.

Of the 1,961, 976 (50%) said AIDS was a form of cancer, 788 (40%) said it was not, and 197 (10%) said they did not know (Table 2). As indicated in the table, 86% said AIDS was an infectious disease, but a surprising 36% thought it was curable. Nevertheless, a majority of those surveyed were certain that AIDS led to death and believed that homosexual males and prostitutes were more likely to contract the disease than any other group. Two-thirds of the respondents felt that AIDS could infect anyone, and over half feared that they or a member of their family might contract AIDS for one reason or another.

Nearly all those interviewed were aware of the major transmission pathways, over 90% indicating the disease could be transmitted through sex with an infected person, receipt of a contaminated blood transfusion, or use of contaminated syringes or needles. In addition, 89% stated that AIDS could be transmitted perinatally.

Many also believed incorrectly that AIDS could be transmitted to a person donating blood (75%), casually at work (43%), or casually by a neighbor (25%). (The percentage thinking it possible to acquire HIV infection through blood donation has been shrinking recently as a result of national blood bank campaigns.)

Two-thirds of the respondents said there was no vaccine against AIDS. Over two-thirds felt that either celibacy or a monogamous sexual relationship with someone free of the AIDS virus were means of avoiding HIV infection, and 52% felt that condoms were an effective barrier against HIV.

Seventy-one percent of the respondents reported that they had acquired AIDS information through educational messages, while 67% said they had acquired it by reading newspapers.

The Dominican Republic

A survey of reported changes in public knowledge, attitudes, and practices related to AIDS was carried out by de Moya and Brea de Cabral (4) under the sponsorship of the National Program for the Control of Sexually Transmitted Diseases and AIDS (PROCETS) in November 1987 in 24 districts of Santo Domingo. A questionnaire containing 94 queries was administered to 469 people (182 men and 287 women) at least 18 years of age. The results were compared to those of a 1985 survey of 945 adults (446 men and 499 women) conducted under similar conditions using the 1966 Kasl and Cobb model of preventive health behavior applied to AIDS.

In both surveys, respondents were stratified by sex and age (into groups 18–24 years old and ≥ 25 years old). For the purpose of this overview, however, the answers received from all groups have been combined and averaged.

Nearly 90% of those interviewed said they read newspaper and magazine materials on AIDS carefully—an 8% increase over 1985. Also, 35% believed one of their friends could contract AIDS, as compared to 26% in 1985. Though few of the respondents (12%) knew anyone with AIDS, this was nevertheless a dramatic increase over the situation in 1985, when nearly 98% of those interviewed said they knew no one at all with the disease. Also, a quarter of the respondents thought they could contract AIDS, as compared to 17% in 1985.

Table 3. Data from the Dominican Republic obtained through 1985 and 1987 surveys conducted in Santo Domingo (4).

	Respondents (%)	
	1985 (n = 945)	1987 (n = 469)
Signs and symptoms believed commonly found in AIDS patients:		
Weight loss	68	90
Diarrhea	55	84
Fever	64	79
Hepatitis-jaundice	43	60
Cough	32	51
Skin lesions	33	48
Swollen glands	39	45
Nocturnal sweats	29	29
AIDS transmission pathways believed important:		
Sex with prostitutes	93	97
Sex with homosexuals	96	97
Blood transfusions	94	97
Intravenous injections	88	95
Sex with foreign tourists	80	89
Mother-to-child (perinatal) transmission	60	84
Groups believed especially vulnerable to AIDS:		
Prostitutes	94	98
Men who have sex with other men	96	97
Blood transfusion recipients	89	95
Intravenous drug abusers	76	93
Children of infected parents	62	83
Alcoholics	25	19
Misconceptions—AIDS can be transmitted by:		
Public toilets	51	35
Working near someone with the disease	53	29
Poorly washed drinking glasses	47	22
Restaurants	25	11
Shaking hands	13	4
Measures recommended to avoid acquiring AIDS:		
Monogamous relationship	88	93
Community organization	90	90
Seeking blood transfusions from known persons	80	87
Use of condoms	56	71
Safer sex practices	45	38

In addition, the interview subjects were asked to select from a list the signs and symptoms they felt to be most frequently found in AIDS patients. Their answers, in decreasing order of prominence, are presented in Table 3.

A considerable share of the respondents (42% in 1987, 32% in 1985) said they thought AIDS killed in less than a year. However, fewer thought a lot of people would die from AIDS in the Dominican Republic (21% in 1987, compared to 56% in 1985). Since knowledge of AIDS became public, only 4% of the study subjects said they were more worried than before, while 8% said so in 1985.

As Table 3 shows, high percentages of the respondents knew HIV was being transmitted through intravenous injections, sexual intercourse, blood transfusions, and the perinatal route. In this connection, the percentages noted in the table cited the various categories of people listed as being most vulnerable to AIDS.

There were some slight changes in respondents' misconceptions about casual contagion. In 1987 only 4% believed AIDS could be transmitted by shaking hands, compared to 13% in 1985. Surprising proportions still believed AIDS could be transmitted by public toilets (35%), working near someone with the disease (29%), poorly washed drinking glasses (22%), and restaurants (11%). However, as Table 3 indicates, these percentages were all down considerably from 1985.

Asked about what they would do to keep from acquiring AIDS, 93% of the respondents opted for being in a monogamous relationship with someone free of the disease, 90% indicated they would organize themselves into health protection groups, 87% said they would seek blood from known persons if they had to have a transfusion, 71% said they would use condoms, and 38% (as compared to 45% in 1985) said they would engage in safer sex practices such as masturbation and would refrain from oral-genital contact.

Haiti

A small-scale survey of 250 factory workers and 50 professionals employed in the private sector was conducted in Port-au-Prince, Haiti, in September-October 1987 (5). The survey was sponsored by the Groupement de Lutte Anti SIDA (GLAS), an anti-AIDS organization. The questionnaire employed, which had been designed by Price Waterhouse, was translated into Creole, pretested on several categories of workers, and found to be more effective in eliciting candid responses when administered over the telephone than when it was administered face to face. The questionnaire was therefore administered by telephone—in Creole to the 250 factory workers and in French to the 50 professionals, because the professionals felt more comfortable with the latter language.

This survey, the first of its kind in Haiti, did not select a study population that was particularly representative of the national

Table 4. Data from Haiti derived from a 1987
and professionals in Port-au-Prince (5).

138

Sources of information about AIDS:	
Radio	
Television	
Friends or family members	
Respondents affirming that:	
They cannot tell who has AIDS	
AIDS is a common disease	
They know someone who has AIDS	11
Respondents affirming that the following are AIDS signs and symptoms:	
Diarrhea	73
Weight loss	62
Cutaneous lesions	60
Fever	29
Thinning hair	26
Respondent statements regarding treatment of AIDS patients:	
Medical care is effective	76
Prayers and voodoo are effective	27
Medical treatment is useless	23
Respondents affirming that the following preventive measures are effective:	
Monogamous relationships	82
No sex with prostitutes	44
No sex with homosexual men	29
Use of condoms	25
Avoidance of medication administered by syringe	12
Avoidance of blood transfusions	8

population. (A large-scale national survey was conducted in early 1988, and the findings of that survey will be forthcoming soon.)

The questions asked sought to test the study subjects' knowledge of AIDS, knowledge of HIV transmission via sexual intercourse and injections, fear of the disease, and desire for self-protection against HIV infection.

As Table 4 indicates, the largest percentage of respondents said they had heard about AIDS over the radio, while lesser percentages said they had learned about it from television or from friends or family members. Most (70%) said they thought AIDS was a common disease, though only 11% said they knew one or more people with it. Even more (79%) felt they could not tell if someone had AIDS, even in the advanced stages, though most knew at least three AIDS symptoms (see the signs and symptoms referred to by the study subjects in Table 4).

those interviewed said AIDS was invariably fatal. Regard-
at could be done for those with AIDS, 76% recommended
cal care, 27% looked to prayer or voodoo practices, and 3%
ored going abroad for care. Half felt medical treatment only
elieved the patients' symptoms without curing them, and 23%
believed medical treatment was completely useless.

Regarding transmission, various percentages of the respondents
believed AIDS could be transmitted by sex only (27%), by germs or
microbes only (19%), by sex and germs (27%), or by a combination of
factors, one of them being the supernatural nature of the disease
(17%). It is also true, however, that the study subjects felt those most
likely to acquire the disease were people going to houses of prostitution (68%), gay and bisexual men (65%), promiscuous people (53%),
individuals having sex with people with AIDS (28%), and drug
addicts (24%).

Two-thirds of the respondents said they were extremely afraid of
contracting AIDS. In all, 84% expressed the belief that it was a fatal
disease, while only 2% said it was a shameful disease and 2% said it
was a scary disease. Nearly all those interviewed said that people
with AIDS should be extremely careful not to transmit the disease to
someone else.

The methods of prevention affirmed by the respondents are shown
at the bottom of Table 4. Almost all respondents knew what a condom
was. Eighty-five percent of the men said they knew how to use one,
while 67% of the women said they did not. In most cases, it was the
men who took responsibility for purchasing prophylactics. The men
who did not favor using condoms said that they were in a monogamous relationship.

Discussion and Conclusions

Public awareness and knowledge of AIDS seem to be increasing in all
four countries, especially in regard to the general characteristics of the
disease and its modes of transmission and prevention. The four surveys reviewed here indicated that, on the whole, the study populations had received a high degree of exposure to AIDS information.
The knowledge imparted included basic information about AIDS
(such as who can get it, primary transmission routes, and non-

transmission routes) and was reflected both in the survey subjects' attitudes toward those with clinical disease and in their specific and personal behavior patterns.

Changes observed in behavior patterns included the following:

- Changes were seen in the effective knowledge of the sampled populations, especially among homosexual and bisexual males and young people 15–25 years old. In some countries (notably Brazil and Haiti), the survey data indicated that prostitutes were relatively ill-informed, perhaps because their exposure to AIDS information and education was less marked. This indicates that effective strategies are needed to reach this closed group.
- Slight attitude changes were perceived in the countries that had collected data in 1985 and 1987, but not enough information was at hand to assess the extent of the changes. On the whole, people with AIDS were still regarded negatively and stigmatized in all four countries—especially in the Dominican Republic and Haiti, where practices based on a supernatural understanding of phenomena are common.
- No real evidence was found that indicated improved practices by the general population. Nevertheless, some changes were observed in the homosexual/bisexual groups in Brazil and (to some extent) in the Dominican Republic. These changes included greater condom use, reduced numbers of sexual partners, and a lower frequency of high-risk sex acts. An apparent decline was also observed in the practice of prostitution in Brazil. However, there is no concrete evidence suggesting that these changes were sustained or that they were solely due to AIDS-related information-education campaigns.

This lack of dramatic short-term changes in behavior should not be taken as indicating failure of AIDS-related health education. Changes in sexual behavior take time to come about, and it may be hard to determine when and how they will occur. National information campaigns can teach protective practices, debunk myths, and affect the behavior of individuals who see themselves at risk. Even if such individuals can only be reached by improving general awareness and knowledge, such improved awareness and knowledge is a definite and necessary step toward the ultimate goal of obtaining lasting behavioral change.

References

1. Brandt, A. The syphilis epidemic and its relation to AIDS. *Science* 239:375–380, 1987.
2. *Folha de São Paulo.* Tudo sobre AIDS. São Paulo, 22 February 1987.
3. Mexico, Secretaría de Salud, Subsecretaría de Servicios de Salud, Dirección General de Epidemiología. Encuesta para medir el grado de conocimento sobre el SIDA. Mexico City, May 1987.
4. De Moya, A., and M. Brea de Cabral. Psicología social del SIDA en jóvenes y adultos en Santo Domingo. Programa de Control de Enfermedades de Transmisión Sexual y SIDA, Santo Domingo, 1985 and 1987.
5. Groupement de Lutte Anti SIDA (GLAS). Sondage d'opinion auprès des employés du secteur privé. Port-au-Prince, October 1987.

Bibliography

Dawson, D. A., M. Cynamon, and J. E. Fitti. AIDS knowledge and attitudes for September 1987: provisional data from the National Health Interview Survey. *Vital and Health Statistics of the National Center for Health Statistics: Advancedata*, no. 148, 1988.

Doll, L. S., and L. L. Bye. AIDS: where reason prevails. *World Health Forum* 8:484–488, 1988.

Eisenman, D. We need safer blood—and the way to get it is to screen out the risky donors. *Washington Post*, 10 April 1988.

Fineberg, H. V. Education to prevent AIDS: prospects and obstacles. *Science* 239:592–596, 1988.

Parris, F. Names project quilt is powerful symbol of AIDS crisis. *Nan Monitor* vol. 2, no. 2, Winter 1988.

Job Soames, R. F. Effective and ineffective use of fear in health promotion campaigns. *Am J Public Health* 78(2):163–167, 1988.

AIDS: SOCIAL, LEGAL, AND ETHICAL ISSUES OF THE "THIRD EPIDEMIC"

SUSAN SCHOLLE CONNOR

A nurse in the United States was told she had tested seropositive for the human immunodeficiency virus (HIV) after working on the ward with AIDS patients. She has told her story throughout the country: how she changed her life, and how her life changed. She stopped having any physical contact with her husband or children—she wouldn't even kiss them. She became excessively concerned with personal hygiene and used a separate set of dishes. She found her co-workers, all very sympathetic to her, were wary of working with her in the hospital. Her neighbors treated her with special caution and exaggerated courtesy. She was depressed and angry and very fearful. Her story has a happy ending. She was a false positive. She was not infected. The numerous tests had been wrong. But she has used her experience to educate—the public, health workers, anyone she can reach—about what it might feel like to be infected with HIV. (In addition, living in the litigious United States, at last report she was considering suing the laboratories that had identified her as seropositive.)

This nurse's experience is not unique. AIDS is now found throughout the world. It is a justifiably frightening disease, appearing invariably fatal. We are all afraid of AIDS, just as we are all afraid of cancer. But, unlike cancer, we can get AIDS from other people. It is a contagious disease in a generation that, at least in the developed world, has become accustomed to living without fear of death from contagion. It is merely human nature, then, to fear contact with a person who might be a "carrier" of this disease.

This fear leads to what Dr. Jonathan Mann, Director of the World Health Organization (WHO) Global Program on AIDS, has termed the "third epidemic":

The third epidemic closely follows the first two, of HIV infection and AIDS. It is the epidemic of economic, social, political, and cultural reaction. In the words of Javier Pérez de Cuéllar, Secretary-General of the United Nations, "AIDS raises crucial social, humanitarian, and legal issues, threatening to undermine the fabric of tolerance and understanding upon which our societies function." (1)

This article discusses a few of the more critical social, legal, and ethical issues raised by AIDS. Clearly, however, it is impossible to cover all such issues in a brief article, or to truly analyze the substantial moral questions, about which much has been written by sensitive experts. With this apology for cursory treatment, we will cover essentially the following questions:

1. What is the best public health approach to people with HIV infection and AIDS? What rights should they have?
2. Who should be tested for AIDS on a mandatory basis?
3. Who has the right to know if someone has HIV infection or AIDS? Is there a duty to warn?
4. How can society be protected against people who irresponsibly, perhaps even deliberately, set out to infect others?

All of these questions involve essentially the same analysis. First, where do we draw the line between the rights of the individual and the rights of society? Second, how do we balance those interests? Third, what is the best way to protect individuals at risk and society as a whole against the spread of AIDS? And fourth, what relevant scientific evidence exists regarding transmission, prognosis, treatment, testing, behavior modification, counseling, education, and information transfer?—for ultimately it is science that must determine policy and therefore law.

All these considerations are extremely critical in the case of HIV infection and AIDS, where the scientific evidence points to spread from intimate behavior censured by most societies (homosexual contact, intravenous drug abuse, extensive heterosexual contact). The level of social tolerance or disapproval varies widely from country to country, and every nation also has different traditions governing the strength of individual rights versus those of society at large. There are some absolutes accepted throughout the world, enshrined in human rights conventions and declarations. But those texts leave a lot of room for interpretation. The job of WHO is to define those absolutes from the public health perspective, to elucidate the best way of protecting public health from a scientific standpoint. That is the subject of this paper.

Question 1

What is the best public health approach to people with HIV infection and AIDS? What rights should they have? The best way to protect the health of all the people is to allow people with HIV infection and AIDS to live normal lives to the extent their health permits. Discrimination and stigmatization will hurt, not help, the general public as well as those infected.

The third epidemic has led to some truly horrifying abuses. Adults and children only suspected of being HIV-positive have been denied housing, schooling, employment, and even burial. Health care workers have refused to treat them. Even in the most theoretically enlightened societies, fear has led to hysteria. The home of two hemophiliac boys was burned when they tried to enroll in the local school. Employees have been summarily dismissed. Insurance companies have refused to issue insurance policies to men living in areas known for homosexual activity. Landlords have evicted tenants who have tested seropositive.

Sometimes these abuses have occurred even though local law made them illegal. In many countries, laws and court precedents prohibit discrimination on the basis of handicap or illness (although few or none of those laws specifically bar discrimination for HIV infection or AIDS). Freedom from discrimination on the basis of handicap is deemed a fundamental human right. Worldwide, this has become the modern view.

International human rights conventions and declarations, which set the standards for human rights around the world, were adopted before it became clear that discrimination based on handicap or illness should be made clearly and specifically illegal. Yet the underlying theory of human rights is that no one should be treated unfairly or unequally because of race, religion, national origin, or *other status* unrelated to qualifications or actions. This sentiment, so strongly held in the modern world, applies to HIV infection and AIDS.

The World Health Organization has taken a very strong stand on this, even though human rights (while implicit in the very raison d'être of the international public health agency) do not usually command explicit WHO attention. This strong WHO concern for the right to be free of discrimination is based on more than a general preference for human rights. Experience around the world has shown that the only way to combat an escalated spread of HIV infection depends on public cooperation. Risky behavior must change—particularly risky behavior by people already infected. The changes in behavior involve intimate moments, and there is no way that society can *force* "safe sex" practices without applying unthinkably draconian measures. (Even the draconian measure of quarantine cannot ensure risk-free behavior.) Moreover, AIDS is an illness, not a punishment or a crime.

WHO experts in public health, epidemiology, infectious diseases, health education, and disease prevention—as well as in law, psychology, and sociology—have exhaustively reviewed the potential policies for preventing and controlling AIDS. These experts have been assembled from every type of culture and from countries in all stages of development. Their reports have been debated in worldwide meetings. The essentially universal conclusion has been that respect for human rights is more than a humane approach, it is the only approach capable of effectively combating AIDS.

The reason is plain enough. If people at risk fear losing their jobs, housing, schooling, and participation in normal activities, besides eventually losing their lives, they will not come forward for testing and counseling. Nor will they be reachable by the public health authorities, who will be unable to warn others of potential exposure through blood transfusions or intimate activity. This is the main public health reason for avoiding discrimination and stigmatization. Fortunately, this conclusion coincides with promises made by virtually all the world's countries to respect individual human rights and to treat all people equally, regardless of status.

WHO's initial position against discrimination was affirmed by the World Summit of Ministers of Health on Programs for AIDS Prevention that was held in London early in 1988 (see pp. 361–365 in this volume). There, delegates from 148 countries representing the vast majority of the world's people declared that "We emphasize the need in AIDS prevention programs to protect human rights and human dignity. Discrimination against, and stigmatization of, HIV-infected people and people with AIDS and population groups undermine public health and must be avoided" (2).

The World Health Assembly, the prime WHO governing body comprised of representatives of all the WHO Member States, issued a resolution at its 1988 session that was similarly strong and explicit:

The Forty-first World Health Assembly . . . strongly convinced that respect for human rights and dignity of HIV-infected people and people with AIDS, and of members of population groups, is vital to the success of national AIDS prevention and control programs and of the global strategy:

Urges Member States, particularly in devising and carrying out national programs for the prevention and control of HIV infection and AIDS:

1. To foster a spirit of understanding and compassion for HIV-infected people and people with AIDS through information, education, and social support programs;
2. To protect the human rights and dignity of HIV-infected people and people with AIDS and of members of population groups, and to avoid discriminatory action against and stigmatization of them in the provision of services, employment, and travel;
3. To ensure the confidentiality of HIV testing and to promote the availability of confidential counseling and other support services to HIV-infected people and people with AIDS; . . .

The resolution asks the WHO Director-General to take all measures necessary to advocate the need for this respect for human rights, to cooperate with other relevant organizations in fostering this respect, and to stress to Member States and others "the dangers to the health of everyone of discriminatory action against and stigmatization of HIV-infected people and people with AIDS and members of population groups." The Director-General is also asked to report annually to the World Health Assembly, starting in May 1989, regarding implementation of the resolution, which means that all countries of the world will be asked to report their social responses regarding AIDS to WHO (3). This resolution represents the most comprehensive and official policy statement possible within the constitutional framework of the World Health Organization.

In July 1988, WHO and the International Labor Organization convened a three-day expert Consultation on AIDS in the Workplace. At this meeting, 36 medical, public health, labor, government, union, and business representatives from 18 countries concluded that "workers with HIV infection who are healthy should be treated the same as any other workers," and that "a worker with HIV-related illness, including AIDS, should be treated like any other worker with an illness." They also stressed the need to avoid discrimination, to educate workers and their families about HIV and AIDS, to provide social security and occupation-related benefits for HIV-infected employees, to provide reasonable alternative working arrangements if a worker's fitness is impaired by HIV-related illness, and to avoid holding HIV infection as a reason for termination of employment (4).

The reason for the importance of this benign policy is that most people with HIV are between the ages of 18 and 45. They are in their economically productive years. They, their families, and society expect them to be financially independent if they are not in school. Losing the ability to hold a job is devastating in almost every society, akin to losing one's life. And speaking realistically, few alternative means of support exist. Few nations have a social security system strong enough to cover people who, although they have latent disease, may be perfectly able to work for as long as eight to 10 years before they become ill. Moreover, in some countries the prevalence of AIDS is disproportionately high among the most educated young people, whose services the nation can ill afford to lose. Finally, and most crucially, if people know that revelation of HIV infection means job loss, not even those at risk will seek testing, counseling, or information about how to avoid infecting others. Nor will they identify others who should be warned and who may also be infected and spreading the disease.

Regarding pediatric cases, PAHO's 1988 AIDS guidelines state that "children who are infected with HIV should not, in general, be removed from the school system. In special circumstances (poor personal hygiene, behavioral disorders, etc.) an individual decision for attendance should be made by the parents and school medical authorities" (5).

The basic point that bears repeating is as follows: To discriminate against or punish those with HIV or AIDS is bad policy. Besides contravening basic human rights, it seems likely to promote the spread of AIDS.

Question 2

Who should be tested for AIDS on a mandatory basis?   The spread of AIDS will not be prevented by mandatory testing of any group, except for blood/tissue/organ donors, but extensive voluntary testing of certain high-risk groups may be justified as a public health measure.

WHO has defined the term "HIV antibody testing or screening" as follows:

Testing is defined as a serologic procedure for detecting HIV antibody (or antigen) from an individual person, whether recommended by a health care provider or requested by an individual.

Screening is defined operationally as the systematic application of HIV testing, whether voluntary or mandatory, to any or all of the following: entire populations; selected target populations; donors of blood/blood products and cells/tissues/organs (6).

Testing may be entirely voluntary, mandatory (necessary for a benefit or service that the individual has voluntarily requested, though the person can theoretically refuse testing by refusing the benefit or service), or compulsory (required by law regardless of the individual's desire). The line between mandatory and compulsory testing may be illusory in some circumstances (for example, in the case of required premarital testing). Generally, the term "mandatory" as used here will refer to both mandatory and compulsory testing.

The tests generally available as of this writing do not actually detect the HIV virus itself. Rather, they assess the immunologic response by detecting the presence of certain antibodies in the blood. Therefore, there is a "window" of uncertain duration (probably about six months) when the person tested may already be infected, may be able to spread the infection, but will not test positive for the infection. This fact is critical. A seronegative result does not necessarily mean seronegativity.

Besides leaving this window open, the test itself is not always accurate. (Lack of total accuracy is inherent in any laboratory test of this nature.) For that reason, if an initial ELISA test is positive for the presence of HIV antibody, it is recommended in nearly all circumstances that a second ELISA test, followed by a Western blot test, be performed to confirm the subject's seropositivity. While the ELISA tests are generally not costly, the Western blot test is labor-intensive and quite a lot more expensive; but the multiple tests will only be performed if the first test is positive.

Clearly, some truly infected people will be missed because of the window, while others will be missed because they yield false negative results on the first test. The degree of test specificity—100% specificity means all negatives are true negatives—is over 99%; but if a large population is tested, even one false negative in every 200 can add up to a substantial number.

By the same token, the degree of test sensitivity—100% sensitivity means all positives are true positives—while approaching 99%, will still result in a number of false positives (which could lead to the needless sort of devastation suffered by the nurse). False positives become more likely in a low-risk population. Thus, the test cannot guarantee total accuracy, even if correctly done, although it is extremely reliable. (Obviously, if laboratory standards are deficient, the test becomes far less reliable.)

Although other more reliable tests that do test for presence of the virus have been developed, they are quite expensive and are not yet readily available on the international market. Thus, the basic assumption of the WHO recommendations to date on testing and screening is that the HIV antibody test will be performed, leaving the window open to false negative results and recognizing the uncertainties inherent in tests that cannot guarantee 100% sensitivity or specificity. Here the dependence of law and policy on science is clear. If a more accurate test were developed, and if treatment were available, the recommendations might be different.

Are there any circumstances requiring mandatory testing? One answer is obvious. If the state's duty to protect the public health has any meaning at all, government must seek to insure that the supply of *blood and blood products*, so necessary to modern medicine in every country, is free of disease. Hence, purification of the blood supply is a cornerstone of any AIDS prevention program.

In 1987 the World Health Assembly, in endorsing the Global Program on AIDS, reiterated that "information and education on the modes of transmission, as well as the availability and use of safe blood and blood products, and sterile practices in invasive procedures, are still the only measures available that can limit the further spread of AIDS" (7).

Purification of the blood supply is customarily accomplished in two ways: by questioning the donor about high-risk behavior, and by testing the blood units after donation. Many countries have already enacted legislation to require HIV testing (for HIV-1 and/or HIV-2, depending on the nature of the local infection) of all donated blood. At least one country has closed its private blood banks, which had paid donors, because of higher HIV infection rates. Some jurisdictions have closed certain collecting centers for lack of conformity to required testing procedures. Such measures are clearly the most effective. But other countries have not had the means to test all blood units; their laws may only require questioning of donors, or may make it a criminal act to donate blood that is HIV-infected or that comes from a person who has engaged in high-risk behavior. These latter approaches are obviously less effective.

Similar danger to public health is posed by donation of other potentially infected body fluids, tissues, or organs. Where such material is collected, HIV antibody screening is essential, and some countries have already enacted legislation to require it. Fear of infection from such products can be widespread: The director of one respected center for artificial insemination in the United States noted that the first question posed by 90% of the potential recipients was "Have you tested for AIDS?" (8)

Any blood or tissue screening program (as well as any other testing program) must deal with two ethical issues relating to the very basic human right to privacy, issues intrinsically tied to the traditional ethics of the Hippocratic oath. These issues involve *informed consent* and *confidentiality*.

Informed consent means that the patient's right to bodily integrity and personal dignity are recognized: Every person has the basic right to make the decisions about his or her body; and so every person ordinarily has the right to refuse to take a medical test. As with all personal rights, however, this right can only be exercised while respecting the rights of others. In the case of blood donation, the respect for others' rights clearly outweighs the individual's normal right to refuse testing. But the principle of informed consent should nevertheless be followed. That is, the potential donor has the right to know (1) that an HIV antibody test will be performed on the donated blood, (2) whether he or she will be told of the results, (3) who else will be informed of the results, and (4) what the results mean.

The second ethical principle is the need to ensure confidentiality. The trust between physician and patient has been sanctified for thousands of years. It is a basic tenet of the doctor-patient relationship. The need for confidentiality is particularly acute in the case of HIV infection and AIDS, because of the unfortunate fear, discrimination, and stigmatization that may ensue. If the results may not be kept confidential, how likely are people to volunteer for testing, and how likely are they to voluntarily donate the blood needed to save lives?

Confidentiality can be ensured in either of two ways. One way is to keep the testing "unlinked," so that the donor is not identified in any way. A blood unit that tests positive for infection is simply discarded, without knowledge of the donor's identity. Alternatively, the testing can be anonymous, as is customary with most laboratory samples. That is, a number is attached to the donated unit, but only a master list can match the number to the donor. The master list is carefully controlled, and the laboratory technicians and other personnel involved in the collection are unaware of the donor's identity.

The advantages and disadvantages of each procedure are fairly obvious. Unlinked testing is simple and ensures absolute confidentiality. Only an initial ELISA test need be performed, since a mere suggestion of positivity will be enough to justify discarding the donated unit. Unlinked testing thus serves the basic purpose of purifying the blood or tissue supply.

Confidential testing poses some risk of exposing the donor's identity. However, this type of confidential handling of blood samples has been practiced for years in most countries. Like unlinked testing, confidential testing purifies the blood supply, and it has one advantage over unlinked testing; that is, the donor who tests positive can be told and counseled, hopefully causing a link in the epidemiologic chain to be broken. There is also a growing belief that people have the right to know the test results, and that respect for people as individual human beings requires that they be told. In practical terms, the main disadvantages of such testing are that a second ELISA test, followed by a Western blot test, must be performed, and that manpower and time are needed to follow up on seropositive results.

WHO has not yet taken a position on whether unlinked or confidential testing should be undertaken. At present, confidential testing seems to be the norm in the developed countries.

Are there other situations in which mandatory testing is a justified public health measure? Various societies have considered and even legislated requirements for testing such groups as military recruits, prisoners, prostitutes, homosexuals, airline pilots, international travelers, applicants for marriage licenses, all people admitted to hospitals, and all patients at clinics for sexually transmitted disease.

Besides helping to prevent HIV transmission through donated blood, semen, tissues, or organs, such programs can provide epidemiologic data on HIV incidence and prevalence. Despite these advantages, however, screening programs other than serosurveys to determine HIV prevalence appear advisable only in rare cases. In this vein, a WHO meeting of health experts that reviewed screening in 1987 concluded that:

> HIV screening programs present broad problems beyond the simple recognition to infected individuals. Because of the extremely restricted modes of spread of HIV, the privacy of the behavior usually involved in transmission, and the current lack of any specific intervention, screening programs must be approached with great caution. Such programs may be intrusive and cost-ineffective, and may divert human, material, and

financial resources from education programs that are acknowledged to be the primary and most effective preventive measure available (6).

In short, screening programs are expensive, unlikely to reveal all those infected, and cost-ineffective when applied to low-risk populations. Regarding this latter point, one populous state in the United States decided to require premarital screening. After screening many thousands of marriage applicants for 18 months, fewer than 10 cases of HIV infection were discovered. Where the population group to be screened is at high risk, the argument for screening may be slightly stronger; but screening should still be considered more or less as a last resort.

WHO has convened consultations of experts to weigh the merits of screening certain groups considered for screening by various countries[1]—specifically international travelers, prisoners, high-risk groups, and special occupation groups. The WHO experts' recommendations for each of these were as follows:

International Travelers

The 1969 International Health Regulations of WHO, as amended, are designed to provide all the protections appropriate for containing the international spread of infectious diseases. Signatories to the International Regulations are not supposed to require any health documents not required by the regulations. These regulations have not been amended to include AIDS or HIV infection.

The WHO Consultation on International Travel came to conclusions markedly similar to those of the experts who reviewed screening in general. They said:

The diversion of resources towards HIV screening of international travelers and away from education programs, protection of the blood supply, and other measures to prevent parenteral and perinatal transmission will be difficult to justify in view of the epidemiologic, legal, economic, political, cultural, and ethical factors mitigating against adoption of such a policy. No screening program can *prevent* the introduction and spread of

[1]References in this article to practices and laws adopted by various countries and jurisdictions are based on the excellent summaries prepared on a periodic basis by Mr. Sev Fluss of the WHO Health Legislation Unit entitled "Tabular Information on Legal Instruments Dealing with AIDS and HIV Infection, Part I. Countries and Jurisdictions Other Than the USA," and "Part 2. United States of America (Including States and District of Columbia)." These summaries are available from WHO, Geneva.

HIV infection. Therefore the consultation concludes that HIV screening programs for international travelers would, at best and at *great cost*, retard *only briefly* the dissemination of HIV globally and with respect to any particular country (9).

Nevertheless, a number of countries have adopted some form of HIV screening of international travelers, most commonly of foreigners who are seeking to enter the country as immigrants or for extensive periods of time as students or workers. Such screening has not prevented the spread of HIV into these countries.

One motive behind these screening laws has been a desire to avoid the cost of treating AIDS patients from outside the country. Longstanding precedents exist for refusing to allow long-term entry on medical grounds. One of the most sensible policies dealing with this question of costs has been adopted by the United Kingdom. Unlike other nations, the UK does not require an HIV certificate. Instead, the immigration officer has the discretionary authority to order an HIV test. The National Health System, offering free care to all UK residents, will require payment for certain services supplied to foreigners, including treatment for AIDS under this policy. Free health care to nonresident foreigners with AIDS will only cover testing and counseling. The immigration officer may also require proof of a person's ability to pay for other AIDS medical care before allowing entry into the country. Otherwise, the traveler's status with respect to HIV infection and AIDS symptoms will not influence his or her freedom to enter the country.

Prisoners

In some countries, prisoners are considered to be a high-risk group because of homosexual practices within prisons and the high rate of prior intravenous drug abuse found in the prison population. Despite this, the World Health Organization Consultation on AIDS in Prisons concluded that mass involuntary screening of prisoners for HIV infection should not be recommended for the following reasons:

- Prison administrators have the duty to minimize AIDS transmission in prison.
- Prisoners should be treated with the same principles that apply to other HIV-infected persons—including education, testing, confidentiality, health services, and treatment.

- Discriminatory practices, including segregation or isolation, should be avoided, except when necessary to protect the prisoner's own well-being.
- Compassionate early release should be considered for prisoners with AIDS (10).

WHO has not collected any systematic information on the implementation of this recommendation, but it is evident that involuntary screening and segregation of HIV-infected prisoners has occurred in some countries.

High-Risk Behavior Groups

Who is at high risk in any country depends on the epidemiologic pattern prevailing there. Male homosexuals and bisexuals, intravenous drug abusers, their sex partners, and male and female prostitutes generally constitute high-risk behavior groups. Evidence is increasing that people with other sexually transmitted diseases may also be at higher risk, either due to underlying sexual behavior or to increased susceptibility to HIV infection conferred by the sexually transmitted disease itself. Whether perinatal transmission places newborns at high risk depends almost entirely on the epidemiologic pattern found in the specific locality involved.

WHO has not taken a firm position on the screening of high-risk behavior groups, other than to point out the tests' lack of definitiveness; the ethical issues relating to confidentiality and informed consent; and the critical need to avoid diverting resources from the matters of primary concern: education and provision of a clean blood supply (11). Some countries, according to informal information, have adopted policies of screening certain high-risk behavior groups—especially prostitutes, pregnant partners of male bisexuals or intravenous drug abusers, and patients at clinics for sexually transmitted diseases.

Special Occupation Groups

Certain occupation groups have been singled out for HIV testing, either because of potential exposure to needlestick-type injuries or because they are directly responsible for the lives of many others.

Higher-risk occupational categories are customarily considered to include health care workers, emergency workers (policemen and fire-men), morticians, and people caring for infected infants, who may be extensively exposed to infected bodily fluids. Scientific evidence has shown clearly that the risk of needlestick-type injuries is extremely low. WHO has not taken a formal position on this issue, but is expected to hold a consultation jointly with the International Labor Organization on policies toward health care workers. Currently, extensive voluntary testing seems to have become the approach of choice.

The rationale behind proposals to screen the second occupational group—primarily airline pilots and railroad engineers—is based on fear of the AIDS dementia complex, whose effects are still not clearly known. (These effects seem to be both cognitive and affective, poten-tially altering judgment and perception of spatial relations.)

The concern is that a pilot or engineer might be physically asympto-matic while suffering from neurologic damage that could result in harm to others. If this were remotely likely, it would justify testing. However, a WHO interdisciplinary consultative group has concluded that there is no evidence of judgment being affected in physically asymptomatic individuals (12). Hence, the usual periodic medical ex-aminations required for licensing of pilots and engineers should suf-fice to discover early signs of HIV infection, and the public health judgment is that screening of these low-risk groups is unnecessary.

One other special low-risk group, military recruits and personnel, has been considered for mandatory screening. Two reasons are com-monly given for such screening: military personnel must be free from any potential disability, and all military personnel are "walking blood banks." A number of countries have adopted this type of mandatory screening. WHO has not made any recommendation on screening military personnel.

The ethical issues involved in any screening program are essentially the same. Is there protection of confidentiality? Is the test as reliable as possible? Is the person notified of the results in a humane way and provided with education and counseling? Are the human and eco-nomic costs of the testing program far outweighed by the potential benefits to the tested person and to society? What are the conse-quences of false positive and negative results? Are those conse-quences also justified by the potential benefits? What health care or socially useful activities will be deprived of resources by the testing program? And do the potential benefits justify this allocation of scarce resources?

Question 3

Who has the right to know if someone has HIV or AIDS? Is there a duty to warn? The infected person may have a right to know. Health personnel treating the patient have the right to know, as do public health authorities. Also, identifiable people at significant risk have the right to be warned.

WHO has strongly urged its member countries to make AIDS a reportable disease. Most countries have complied, adopting either the WHO or the CDC definition of clinical AIDS. However, few countries have made HIV positivity reportable for epidemiologic surveillance. Reporting is either anonymous (citing the number of cases detected) or confidential (citing the infected person's name but providing restricted access). WHO has not taken a position as to which practice is preferable, and most nations have followed their customary practice for dealing with sexually transmitted diseases. It seems clear, however, that confidentiality must be maintained under any circumstances.

Similarly, WHO does not appear to have a clear position on who, if anyone, has the right to be warned of potential exposure. Few countries have addressed in legislation the issue of contact tracing. The most commonly notified third party is a known sex partner of the HIV seropositive person. If the HIV seropositive person cooperates by naming partners, providing their addresses, and consenting to their being contacted, no ethical problems are posed (assuming confidentiality is maintained). In that case the only remaining question is who has the duty to make the contact: the person tested, the physician, or the public health authorities.

Where the seropositive individual will not consent, however, the conflict between ethical and public health concerns is sharp, and it becomes necessary to ask when the individual's right to privacy (as well as the clear practical need to encourage people to come in for testing) gets overpowered by the need to protect others.

The infected person has a clear moral duty to cooperate with public health authorities and to inform people who may be infected as a result of his or her behavior. While the author is unaware of any WHO guidance on the subject, the position of PAHO's staff on contact tracing is as follows:

> Individuals who are infected should be encouraged to refer their sexual partners and/or drug-sharing partners for evaluation and testing. It is not

possible to trace the contacts of large numbers of individuals. However, under certain circumstances, such as clients of infected prostitutes and interstate contacts, contact tracing may be desirable. Confidentiality must be preserved in all cases. (5)

In cases where the infected person will not consent, some countries are moving toward the position that the physician is obliged to inform a known sex partner. (The American Medical Association has adopted this viewpoint, for instance. Its position is based on ethical and public health principles. But a physician in the United States may also be held legally liable for failure to warn a third party of substantial and direct potential for harm to health under the Tarasoff principle.)

Other countries have a strong tradition of contact tracing by public health officials, whereby the infected person is asked to name sexual partners. In the case of HIV exposure, a public health official contacts those partners, tells them they may have been exposed to HIV (without naming the seropositive person), suggests that they be tested, and gives them AIDS education and counseling. This procedure is very labor-intensive and is not to be recommended solely for HIV, as skilled personnel experienced with sexually transmitted disease prevention and control must be used in order for the program to succeed.

Question 4

How can society be protected against people who irresponsibly, perhaps even deliberately, set out to infect others? Isolation and quarantine of HIV patients is not recommended, but criminal sanctions may be applied against a person who intentionally transmits or clearly intends to transmit HIV to others.

Isolation of AIDS patients in a hospital or other health care facility is a common practice. In this situation AIDS is treated as an infectious disease, and a contamination-free environment is sought to prevent secondary infection of the immune-damaged patient. Isolation and quarantine of individuals infected with sexually transmitted diseases have never been effective in preventing the transmission of infection. Therefore, isolation of an asymptomatic individual, solely on the basis of HIV seropositivity, has been strongly discouraged by WHO. For example, the official statement on Social Aspects of AIDS Prevention and Control by the WHO Global Program on AIDS asserts that

There is no public health rationale to justify isolation, quarantine, or any discriminatory measures based solely on the fact that a person is suspected or known to be HIV-infected . . . Persons suspected or known to be HIV-infected should remain integrated within society to the maximum possible extent and be helped to assume responsibility for preventing HIV transmission to others. Exclusion of persons suspected or known to be HIV-infected would be unjustified in public health terms and would seriously jeopardize educational and other efforts to prevent the spread of HIV (13).

Very few reports of quarantine or isolation based on asymptomatic HIV status alone have been received. Such a practice is not a means of preventing HIV spread because of the inaccuracies of the tests for HIV conversion and the difficulty of policing behavior even in institutional settings. Mandatory screening of virtually the entire population, or at least those identified as being at high risk, would be necessary; and some would inevitably be missed. Also, it is clear that if HIV seropositivity produced total deprivation of liberty, no sane person would voluntarily come forth to be tested. Moreover, unlike the "old" infectious diseases for which quarantine was customary, AIDS has a very long incubation period. So the quarantined person might have to be held eight to 10 years, during which time he or she might be entirely asymptomatic, i.e., apparently healthy.

Quarantine of people with AIDS is no more effective. By the time someone is diagnosed as having AIDS, he or she will be very ill. It is unlikely that further spread of the infection will result from his or her behavior. Therefore, quarantine makes little sense from any public health standpoint. It is a draconian measure, an inappropriate use of the state's police power, and an unwarranted restriction of liberty since it is not needed to protect society from harm.

This situation changes if there is clear evidence that an infected person is one of those rare individuals inclined to recklessly or intentionally infect others. In this case, the presumption that every human being cares for others does not apply, and society is justified in punishing such irresponsible and dangerous behavior, as well as in protecting itself from predictable harm. In this connection, in a few countries prosecutions have been brought for intentional transmission of AIDS, but in most cases the results are not yet known.

In general, however, it is important to note that such cases will be extremely rare. Few human beings set out intentionally, in essence, to kill another human being. Hence, to assume that HIV-infected individuals will act irresponsibly is not only morally wrong, it is factually incorrect. Moreover, the most important point, that has been emphasized repeatedly in this article and by WHO, is that voluntary compliance, voluntary control, voluntary behavior change, and voluntary testing must be the policy to control the spread of AIDS. This approach has been effective. It must be continued.

References

1. World Health Organization. Statement by Dr. Jonathan Mann, Director, Global Program on AIDS, World Health Organization, at an Informal Briefing on AIDS to the 42nd Session of the United Nations General Assembly, 20 October 1987. Mimeographed document. Geneva, 1987.

2. World Health Organization. *London Declaration on AIDS Prevention, 28 January 1988, World Summit of Ministers of Health on Programmes for AIDS Prevention, Jointly Organized by the World Health Organization and the United Kingdom Government, 26–28 January 1988*. Geneva, 1988.

3. World Health Organization. Resolution WHA41.24, Avoidance of Discrimination in Relation to HIV-infected People and People with AIDS, Adopted 13 May 1988. WHO Document A/41/VR/15. Geneva, 1988.

4. World Health Organization. Consultation on AIDS and the Workplace, World Health Organization in Association with the International Labor Organization, 27–29 June 1988, Geneva.

5. Pan American Health Organization. Guidelines for Acquired Immunodeficiency Syndrome (AIDS), 22 October 1987 (corrected version 4 April 1988). Mimeographed document. Washington, D.C., 1987 and 1988.

6. World Health Organization. Report of the WHO Meeting on Criteria for HIV Screening Programmes, 20–21 May 1987, Geneva. Document WHO/SPA/GLO/87.2. Geneva, 1987.

7. World Health Organization. Resolution WHA40.26, Global Strategy for the Prevention and Control of AIDS. WHO Document A/40/VR/12. Geneva, 1987.

8. Schlatt, William, Johns Hopkins University Hospital, Baltimore, Maryland, as reported in the *Washington Post*, Health Section, Washington, D.C., 5 January 1988, p. 16.

9. World Health Organization. Report of the Consultation on International Travel and HIV Infection, 2–3 March 1987, Geneva. Document WHO/SPA/GLO/87.1. Geneva, 1987.

10. World Health Organization. Statement from the Consultation on Prevention and Control of AIDS in Prisons, 16–18 November 1987, Geneva. Document WHO/SPA/GLO/87.14. Geneva, 1987.

11. World Health Organization. *Guidelines for the Development of a National AIDS Prevention and Control Programme*. WHO AIDS Series, No. 1. Geneva, 1988. (*See also* references 6 and 7.)

12. World Health Organization. Report of the Consultation on Neuropsychiatric Aspects of HIV Infection, 14–17 March 1988, Geneva. Document WHO/GPA/DIR/88.1. Geneva, 1988.

13. World Health Organization. Statement on Social Aspects of AIDS Control, 1 December 1987. Geneva, 1987.

PREVENTION OF HIV TRANSMISSION THROUGH BLOOD AND BLOOD PRODUCTS: EXPERIENCES IN MEXICO

JAIME SEPULVEDA AMOR, MARIA DE LOURDES GARCIA GARCIA, JOSE LUIS DOMINGUEZ TORIX, & JOSE LUIS VALDESPINO GOMEZ

This paper explores efforts undertaken in Mexico to prevent and control HIV transmission through blood. Our country faced special challenges regarding both the scope of the problem and the urgency of implementing measures to correct it. Our legislative and technological experiences may benefit other countries.

Supply of Blood Products

To determine the potential magnitude of the problem of HIV transmission through blood, Mexico's blood requirements and how units of blood are supplied must be studied. The yearly demand for blood units per 100 inhabitants in a given country depends on several factors, including the population's age structure and the country's regional medical and surgical care characteristics. In developing countries, where requirements are lower than in developed countries, it is estimated that between one and three units are needed for each 100 inhabitants. In the United States this figure climbs to six units per 100 inhabitants, and in Europe it reaches eight to ten units per 100 inhabitants (World Health Organization figures).

An estimated 700,000 units of blood are transfused in Mexico annually; this figure is lower than the one which would be arrived at by applying the indicators cited above. Before legislative reforms were enacted in Mexico, the country's blood was provided by volunteer donors, by family members, or by paid donors. This last group provided roughly one-third of the total blood supply (approximately 231,000 units).

As a rule, the use of blood products in Mexico, as in many other countries, is not as efficient as it could be, since whole blood is transfused more often than blood components. The small hospitals that perform most of the transfusions lack adequate equipment, leading to waste of the existing supply. Approximately 95% of blood transfusions are carried out this way.

Percentage of AIDS Cases Associated with Transmission Through Blood

The extent of HIV transmission through blood varies according to several factors. For example, the extent of the spread may depend on how advanced control programs are, especially in terms of the capability to detect HIV in blood products, or on the prevalence of infection among the general population.

Two transmission patterns can be detected by analyzing the situation in the Americas, one characteristic of the Caribbean and the other of the rest of the Region (1). Heterosexual transmission predominates in the Caribbean, which means that the prevalence of HIV infection in the general population may be greater. Elsewhere in the Americas, transmission mainly occurs through sexual contact among homosexual or bisexual men, and HIV infection is consequently concentrated in selected groups.

The extent of transmission through blood products that has occurred in recent years is reflected in the number of AIDS cases associated with this type of transmission. In the United States, for example, 3% of all cases (2) are attributed to blood or blood-product transfusions and 1% have occurred in hemophiliacs or those with blood clotting disorders. In Brazil, 5.2% of AIDS cases have occurred in those receiving transfusions and 2.4% in hemophiliacs (3). In Mexico, these percentages are higher; 10% of all cases have resulted from transfusions and 2% have occurred among hemophiliacs.

Epidemiology of HIV Transmission Through Blood in Mexico

As of 1 August 1988, 1,628 AIDS cases had been reported to the General Directorate of Epidemiology. Since the beginning of the AIDS epidemic, the number of cases has risen exponentially, increasing by 10% each month and doubling every 6.8 months. It has been projected that the cumulative number of cases will reach 60,000 by 1991. As in other regions, and as with other sexually transmitted diseases, those most affected are young adults. In Mexico, AIDS has affected men far more than women, at a ratio of 11 to 1. Approximately 76% of adult cases have occurred among homosexual or bisexual men; 11% have occurred in persons who acquired the infection heterosexually; and the remainder, almost 12% of the cases, have occurred among those receiving blood or blood products. Very few AIDS cases have been associated with intravenous drug use, since this type of addiction is rare in Mexico. Among children, transmission through blood predominates. Of 60 pediatric cases notified as of August 1988, 67% were associated with this mode of transmission: 21 cases among hemophiliacs and 19 among children who had received transfusions (4). The high percentage of cases associated with transmission through blood or blood products indicates the extent of the problem.

Studies on hemophiliacs regarding blood transmission of HIV are available (5). In Mexico, the situation among this group is similar to that reported in the United States. The frequency of infection varies from city to city, ranging from 28% in Monterrey to 66% in the Federal District and 67% in Guadalajara.

Prevalence of HIV Infection Among Blood Donors in Mexico

Until very recently, one-third of Mexico's blood supply came from persons who made their living by selling their blood. These persons came from low socioeconomic levels and were habitually unemployed and disenfranchised. Not until May 1986, when screening for HIV infection was first made compulsory for all blood units, did the high prevalence of HIV infection among paid donors surface (6).

This problem is better understood when seen in a worldwide context. The prevalence of HIV infection among donors in the United Kingdom is 0.002%, and in Canada it is 0.008%. In the United States, the situation varies: in Minnesota prevalence has been found to be 0.003%, whereas in New York City, which has one of the highest rates of AIDS cases per million inhabitants in the country, studies indicate a prevalence ranging from 0.1% to 1.6%. Prevalence among donors in Hungary has been reported as 2.8%. The highest figures are from Zaire, with an HIV infection prevalence among donors of 5%. All these studies were conducted between 1986 and 1987.

In Mexico results vary according to the type of donor studied. In one study carried out between 1986 and 1987 among 9,100 paid donors, a prevalence of 7.2% was found.

When these data were analyzed retrospectively, the results became even more alarming—the observed frequency of infection among donors increased from 6% in June 1986 to 54% in November of the same year. Seroconversion was documented in 21% of these subjects during this period.

This frequency of infection was much lower in studies of another type of donor. A study, conducted in the same period, on 319,153 subjects who donated blood in a social security institution revealed a prevalence of infection of 0.67%. The true figure is probably lower, since these results were not confirmed. The majority of these donors were relatives of patients or volunteer donors. Another study that investigated the frequency of infection in 9,772 family-member donors revealed a prevalence of 0.12%. Lastly, an investigation of 3,314 volunteer donors showed a frequency of 0.09%.

In order to investigate the reasons for the high prevalence of HIV infection in paid donors a study was performed on 50 seropositive donors and on 50 seronegative donors who were used as controls (7). Similar risk factors for HIV infection were found in seven seropositive and in seven seronegative donors. However, a correlation was found between the presence of HIV infection and a history of four or more monthly donations (50% of the seropositives versus 14% of the seronegatives, odds ratio = 5.4, 95% CI = 1.9–16.3). It is feasible, therefore, that once the infection was introduced into the blood or plasma bank, the donors were being infected at the blood bank.

The sale of blood was organized by private companies that processed the plasma and prepared various blood products, including clotting factors. These products were distributed throughout the country and exported to other countries.

Table 1. Mexico's experience in preventing HIV transmission through blood and blood products: a short history.

1985:	Beginning of screening of donors in Mexican laboratories.
February 1986:	Establishment of the National AIDS Prevention Committee (CONASIDA).
May 1986:	Compulsory screening for HIV infection among donors.
Second half of 1986:	High prevalence detected in paid donors (7%).
November 1986:	HIV infection and AIDS subject to epidemiologic surveillance.
May 1987:	Sale of blood prohibited.
Second half of 1987:	National Network of Detection Laboratories established.
1987:	Promotion of volunteer donation strengthened.
January 1988:	Prevalence of HIV infection in donors is 0.4%.

It is known that not all paid donors were infected and that the problem centered among those who lived in certain metropolitan areas. The average prevalence of around 7% made it evident that paid donors constituted a high-risk group.

Control Measures

Given the magnitude of the problem it was decided that measures to halt it should be undertaken without waiting to discover its cause. Once this political decision was taken, legislative amendments were carried out (Table 1). In May 1987, the executive and legislative branches of government approved a law prohibiting the sale of blood in Mexico. This measure, coupled with compulsory screening for HIV infection in all donated blood units, was designed to ensure a safe blood supply (8). Other measures included establishing the National AIDS Prevention Committee (CONASIDA), instituting compulsory reporting of all AIDS cases (8), and promoting volunteer blood donation campaigns.

CONASIDA includes representatives from public and private health sector institutions as well as experts in the field. A central corps within the health sector was established to oversee health institutions throughout the country and to provide them with support and assistance. CONASIDA's functions include epidemiologic surveillance of the epidemic; supervision and evaluation of all related activities; epidemiologic research; social and educational issues; standards and recommendations to prevent transmission; and collection and administration of funds.

Compulsory screening of blood units is supported by a laboratory infrastructure that was nonexistent in Mexico before this time. Within four months, 70 laboratories capable of screening donors were set up in the country's 32 states. To conduct confirmatory tests and to supervise the screening laboratories, two central reference laboratories also were established. An external proficiency evaluation of outlying laboratories is being planned through the use of serum panels of known HIV antibody status.

Production of blood components is carried out in two blood-processing plants, one public and the other private; both adhere to established international standards. Since the quantity of plasma produced is insufficient, construction of an additional blood-processing plant has been started.

It was feared that the adopted legislative measures might give rise to various problems such as opposition from those who profited from the sale of blood and its products, the emergence of a black market, and a temporary shortage in the blood supply. Fortunately, no serious problems emerged, and blood-bank owners supported the new law. Paid donors, however, offered to illegally sell blood to persons in need of it. This situation has been dealt with through an educational campaign designed to inform the public of the dangers associated with blood acquired in this way. An adequate blood supply has been ensured through volunteer donation campaigns that encourage donations from relatives of those in need of blood, and blood collection centers have been set up in conjunction with the Mexican Red Cross. To save blood, guidelines for appropriate indications for blood transfusions have been distributed to physicians and hospitals. In addition, persons from high-risk groups have been encouraged not to donate blood.

The Current Situation

Implementation of the above-mentioned measures has reduced the prevalence of HIV infection among blood donors to 0.04%.

The percentage of cases associated with transmission through blood or blood products is 12% of all current cases. Previous estimates of the number of these cases that would occur in Mexico by 1991 put that figure at 25%, provided that no control program was established

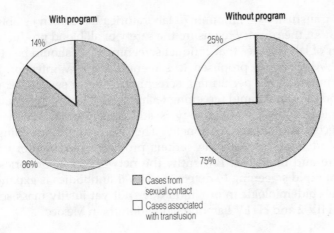

Figure 1. Percentage of cases of AIDS by mode of transmission, projections for 1991.

(9). Current projections indicate that the proportion of cases associated with transfusions will be 14% (Figure 1).

The new law has been in effect since October 1987. Implemented measures have been widely accepted by both the general public and health workers. Screening is performed to detect the presence of specific antibodies in virtually all the blood used for therapeutic purposes; however, in a few small hospitals this testing is still not being carried out. Even though blood-supply shortages were briefly experienced, effective campaigns to promote volunteer donations have solved this problem for now.

Acceptance of reforms by health professionals has resulted in a more rational use of blood and blood products. It has been necessary to make the most efficient use of blood; that is, to ensure that blood components, instead of whole blood, are used for transfusion and that appropriate recommendations for transfusion are being followed. To this end, educational campaigns that foster rational use of blood products have been provided to health personnel through courses and the distribution of handbooks.

Problems and Alternatives

All blood used for transfusion should be screened for HIV infection. The problem rests in those small hospitals, located far away from screening laboratories, that must deal with emergencies requiring urgent transfusions. Although 70 laboratories have been established throughout the country to ensure the safety of all blood products, the number of laboratories that conduct screening tests should be at least tripled. Alternatives proposed to screening for HIV infection in all blood units include performing screening tests on several sera at a time and the use of rapid screening techniques. The first alternative is a technique whose methodology is still controversial and has not been recommended internationally. The use of rapid screening has several advantages given the serious problems of laboratory infrastructure and financing. Presently, the network of laboratories that perform rapid screening to detect the HIV-1 antibodies is expanding. Current epidemiologic information does not yet justify mass screening for HIV-2 and HTLV-I among blood donors in Mexico.

The Need to Evaluate the Control Program

It is important to assess the impact that the above-mentioned measures have had on several indicators. In order to evaluate the short-term effects, the percentage of units that are effectively screened must be determined. This makes it possible to determine the effectiveness of the law requiring HIV-infection screening among blood donors. For the medium term it is useful to determine the prevalence of HIV infection in blood donors. Long-term information will be provided by changes in the number of cases. Over the coming years, the number of cases associated with transmission through blood may even increase; nevertheless, this percentage should eventually diminish over time.

Conclusions and Recommendations

Governments all over the world are responsible for ensuring a blood supply free from HIV infection. Some simple measures require only political will for implementation. Promoting self-exclusion of persons with risk behaviors is efficient and should be recommended. Inactivating the virus in blood products is easy to carry out and also very effective. Prohibiting the sale of blood wherever it occurs is also highly recommended. The most efficient means of ensuring a safe blood supply is by screening all blood intended for transfusions

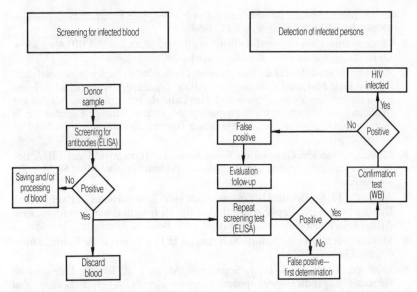

Figure 2. Model for a blood screening strategy.

(Figure 2). Although this measure may place burdens on programs in developing countries, it will, in all cases, be less expensive than the eventual hospitalization of patients.

In the absence of vaccines or drugs, prevention of the spread of AIDS must rely on education and sanitary precautions. The first can be achieved by changing individual behavior, whereas the second involves society as a whole. In developing countries, AIDS competes with other diseases for scanty health resources.

We are convinced that in Mexico it is possible, both technically and politically, to prevent HIV transmission through blood, and that this effort must be undertaken by those in charge of national health institutions and must be supported by international organizations.

References

1. Mann, J. M. The Global Picture of AIDS. Paper presented at the IV International Conference on AIDS, held in Stockholm, 12–16 June 1988. Book of Abstracts 1, p. 105.
2. Centers for Disease Control. *AIDS Weekly Surveillance Report*. United States AIDS Program, 6 June 1988.

3. Brazil, Ministério de Saúde. Secretaria Nacional de Programas Especiales de Saúde. *SIDA Bol Epidemiol* 1:12, 1988.

4. Mexico, Dirección General de Epidemiología. Situación del SIDA en México hasta agosto de 1988. *Bol Mens SIDA* 2:387–399, 1988.

5. Ambriz, R. Prevalencia de Infección en Hemofílicos. Paper presented during the First National Congress on AIDS, organized by Asociación Mexicana de Epidemiólogos, Sociedad Mexicana de Inmunología, Asociación Mexicana de Infectología, Agrupación Mexicana para el Estudio de la Hematología, Asociación de Medicina Interna de México, and held in Cocoyoc, Mexico, 1987.

6. Mexico, Dirección General de Epidemiología. Transmisión del SIDA por sangre y hemoderivados. Actividades de Prevención. *Bol Mens SIDA* 1:41–48, 1987.

7. Avila, C., H. Stetler, E. Dickinson, et al. HIV Transmission in Paid Plasma Donors in Mexico. Paper presented at the IV International Conference on AIDS, held in Stockholm, 12–16 June 1988. Book of Abstracts 2, p. 345.

8. Mexico, Secretaría de Salud. Reformas a la Ley General de Salud. *Diario Oficial*, 27 May 1987.

9. Valdespino Gómez, J. L., J. Sepúlveda Amor, J. A. Isazola Licea, et al. Patrones y predicciones epidemiológicos del SIDA en México. *Salud Publica Mex* 30(4): 567–592, 1988.

THE CANADIAN NATIONAL AIDS PROGRAM

A. J. CLAYTON & A. S. MELTZER

AIDS has been designated a top priority in Canada and, over the last six years, policy has been directed toward containing the spread of the disease, both nationally and internationally. The responsibility of addressing the problems of this emerging illness at the federal government level fell to the Laboratory Center for Disease Control (LCDC), Health and Welfare Canada, which established a reporting system in 1982. For the next four years, the national program was coordinated through the office of the Director General, LCDC. In 1986, in response to the greatly increased requirement for federal activity, a National AIDS Center was created within LCDC. At the same time, the laboratory aspects of AIDS and human immunodeficiency virus (HIV) infection were managed at LCDC through the Bureau of Microbiology. In mid-1987, however, it was evident that the problem of AIDS was sufficiently large and complex to require that the federal government response in the areas of coordination, education, and scientific activities be orchestrated by one center.

In July 1987, the Deputy Minister of the Department of National Health and Welfare announced the creation of the Federal Center for AIDS (FCA), within the Health Protection Branch.

Structure and Functions of the Center

The Center currently employs 40 people and has six bureaus, as outlined in Figure 1. The role of the FCA is to coordinate all federal

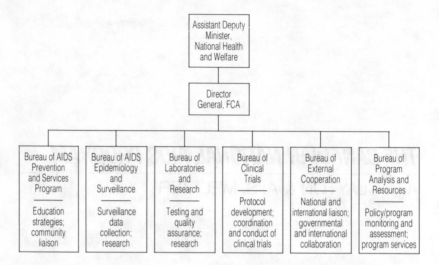

Figure 1. Administrative structure of the Federal Center for AIDS (FCA).

governmental activities with respect to the promotion of public education programs and the coordination of preventive and social health activities. The FCA also promotes clinical trials of drugs and vaccines, stimulates and encourages epidemiologic studies, and works to maintain and improve national surveillance. Other important activities of the Center include coordinating research funding and community-based support groups, providing information services, and establishing and maintaining liaison with ten provincial and two territorial governments, as well as with nongovernmental organizations. Financial support given to the World Health Organization's Global Program on AIDS (WHO-GPA), together with liaison with national organizations, completes the spectrum of the Center's activities.

Bureau of Program Analysis and Resources. As the HIV epidemic spreads, there is an increasing need to develop highly innovative, proactive, and comprehensive policies and programs. Such an approach demands a high level of coordination, and the Bureau of Program Analysis and Resources was established to initiate and enhance policies and programs. The Bureau continues to provide a focus for policy-related issues, and its increasing profile testifies to the need to develop sound policies for all HIV-related activities and programs. The primary functions of the Bureau are policy and program development, monitoring and assessment, and the provision of appropriate program services. Such an approach acknowledges the importance of providing an integrated framework for HIV-related policy development. The monitoring component includes the capacity to conduct in-depth reviews of the human resource and financial implications of proposed national program initiatives. In addition, the Bureau plays an important coordinating role, particularly with reference to human resources and financial planning connected with new initiatives and programs of other bureaus. Through a newly introduced Contribution Program, the Federal Center for AIDS will be better able to strengthen a wide range of programs and projects.

Bureau of AIDS Prevention and Services Program. The national AIDS program places a high priority on preventing AIDS and HIV infection. The Bureau of AIDS Prevention and Services Program focuses on education and awareness strategies, liaison with health care workers and community groups, and the psychosocial aspects of the problem. One priority is delivery of a national education and awareness program. In this regard, the FCA has initiated a national consultation with the education community, which will provide an opportunity for national education organizations, provincial and territorial ministries of education, and the federal government to formulate and implement a comprehensive strategy for AIDS education of schoolchildren and adolescents. Funds have also been provided to carry out the Canada Youth AIDS Survey. In this study, which is being conducted by Queen's University, Kingston, Ontario, 40,000 subjects—including students in grades 7, 9, 11, and first year of university, 1,000 "dropouts," and 700 street youths—have been interviewed. A similar survey of adults commenced in the fall of 1988. In parallel with the above activities, educational brochures covering a wide range of AIDS-related issues are being prepared. These publications will complement the guidelines that have already been developed for health care workers and other professional groups. The Bureau has close ties with nongovernmental organizations, including community groups and specific national agencies such as the Canadian Hemophilia Society, Canadian Medical Association, and Canadian Dental Association, and has conducted a wide range of activities in association with such bodies.

The educational activities of the FCA are complemented by the Canadian Public Health Association (CPHA) AIDS Education and Awareness Program, which is being supported by a Health and Welfare grant over a five-year period. The program includes a clearinghouse for AIDS information, a series of scientific symposia for health professionals, a number of public forums, and a newsletter.

In an effort to permit health care workers and other professional groups to play a greater role in preventing HIV infection, the Bureau has developed a comprehensive set of definitive guidelines. Support has also been provided for workshops and seminars for specific groups such as hospital staff, educational authorities, and police. The need to enhance programs in the psychosocial area is fully recognized. For example, an Expert Working Group in Palliative Care has produced an important report entitled "Caring Together," which is expected to lead to a series of demonstration projects in selected cities.

Bureau of Epidemiology and Surveillance. This Bureau conducts an AIDS surveillance program designed to monitor temporal trends in reported AIDS cases and assess the extent of the disease. Numerous studies have been undertaken in this regard. A study of the risk of HIV infection in health care workers who have been exposed to HIV-infected blood or body fluids is being conducted, using a standardized data collection mechanism. A collaborative study of women attending sexually transmitted disease clinics has been completed. The Bureau is also involved in epidemiologic research with independent investigators. Priority has been placed on determining the prevalence of HIV infection in Canada. This research will include population-based estimates as well as special studies of specific groups such as injection drug users.

Dissemination of information from the Bureau is achieved via an electronic bulletin board, which provides immediate access to Canadian, U.S., and international AIDS statistics, news releases, announcements of forthcoming AIDS conferences, the *Canada Diseases Weekly Report,* and the U.S. Centers for Disease Control *Morbidity and Mortality Weekly Report.* As of 19 September 1988, there were 2,003 confirmed cases of AIDS in Canada.

Bureau of Laboratories and Research. Two divisions comprise this Bureau: retrovirology and immunology. By virtue of being the focal point for the Center's role as a World Health Organization Collaborating Center for AIDS, the primary activity is provision of reference services to provincially designated laboratories conducting HIV antibody screening tests. An extensive array of services is available, including immunoblotting using whole viral lysates and recombinant antigens, antigen capture neutralization assays, peptide mapping of viral isolates, virus isolation, T-cell subset analyses, quality assurance programs, and the serodiagnosis of human retroviruses, including HIV-1, HIV-2, and HTLV-I. In addition, diagnostic kits and commercially produced reagents are evaluated, and proficiency testing and quality control are offered at the national level.

The Bureau collaborates closely with national and international researchers. Current activities include AZT dose-toxicity studies, research to determine the immunogenicity and safety of a candidate HIV vaccine, evaluation of the polymerase chain reaction (PCR) test, research on the prevalence of HIV infection in selected populations, and a study to assess the validity of recombinant protein-based tests. Also, scientific support is provided for the National Immune Study of Hemophiliacs and the Vancouver Lymphadenopathy AIDS project. Many researchers have completed extended stays in the faculty to learn protocols and methods for virus isolation and to acquire techniques for the serodiagnosis of HIV infection and use of recombinant antigens as diagnostic tools. The Bureau has a strong interest in strengthening international scientific collaboration, as exemplified by its extensive input to the FCA/PAHO Workshop on HIV Screening, which took place in Canada in August 1988. The event enabled directors of national HIV screening programs in 25 countries of the Americas to exchange information and develop strategies for HIV surveillance and quality control testing.

Bureau of External Cooperation. The main objective of the Bureau is to enhance and support governmental liaison and national and international collaboration, particularly with reference to policy and programs. It provides the supporting substructure for the Federal/Provincial/Territorial Advisory Committee on AIDS, and coordinates special projects associated with the Committee, such as the formulation of guidelines for organ donation and tissue transplantation in light of the HIV infection crisis, and the development of a policy statement on the confidentiality of HIV antibody test results. Liaison responsibility between the FCA and the National Advisory Committee on AIDS (NAC-AIDS) rests with the Bureau. This Committee was established in 1983 to advise the Minister of National Health and Welfare regarding the implementation of medical and other strategies for the diagnosis, treatment, control, and prevention of AIDS in Canada.

A close working relationship exists with major international agencies, particularly with the WHO-GPA and PAHO, exemplified by the above-mentioned workshop on HIV screening sponsored jointly with PAHO. The Bureau also participates in and coordinates Canadian input for WHO-GPA consultations and workshops to ensure that Canada's contribution to the global effort is adequately represented and utilized. For example, a counseling manual on hemophilia and

HIV infection was developed for the WHO-GPA Hemophilia/HIV Workshop, which was held in Tokyo, Japan, in August 1988; and a workshop for short-term consultants was held in Ottawa, Canada, in October 1988, also in collaboration with the WHO-GPA. Such activities are complemented by close working relationships regarding AIDS with agencies like the Canadian International Development Agency (CIDA) and the International Development Research Center (IDRC), and with embassies.

At the international level, the Bureau participates in the exchange of scientific, medical, and epidemiologic data with international and national organizations. The Bureau is also responsible for the development of policy positions on issues like HIV antibody testing and confidentiality that require collaboration and monitoring with other governments and with organizations such as WHO. Close links with Canadian universities and nongovernmental organizations (NGOs) are also maintained. For example, in September 1988, the Bureau participated in a workshop on the role of NGOs in AIDS programs in developing countries, held at McMaster University, Hamilton, Ontario. Briefings on issues surrounding HIV infection are provided for government personnel posted abroad, and the Bureau also coordinates Canadian training programs for overseas health professionals.

Bureau of Clinical Studies. Its function is to promote studies on drugs and vaccines, which includes improving access to new therapies, providing input for research protocols, advising the pharmaceutical industry and researchers regarding clinical trial procedures and regulatory requirements, and facilitating access to research funding. The Bureau also establishes committees to determine priorities and develop appropriate drug protocols for use at the national level. As a central information agency, it provides authoritative information to physicians, patients, the media, and the general public. Also, the Bureau initiates and coordinates multi-center collaborative studies and plays a strong role in the development of government policy on AIDS drugs.

Other Components of Canada's AIDS Program

Research continues to be a keystone of the national program. The National Health Research and Development Program (NHRDP), Health and Welfare, has conducted special competitions to stimulate and support HIV-related research in Canada. Such funding initiatives are closely coordinated with the Federal Center for AIDS and cover public health, epidemiological, clinical, biomedical, and laboratory AIDS investigations. Special training and career awards for AIDS researchers complement the program.

The national AIDS program received Can$39 million for the period 1986–1991 for research, education, community groups support, laboratories, and operational costs. On 8 June 1988, the Minister of National Health and Welfare, the Honourable Jake Epp, announced that the government's AIDS program funding had been increased by an additional Can$129 million over a five-year period. Research is a high priority in the program, and Can$35 million of this additional funding is targeted for a wide range of research activities, including trials of new AIDS drugs, research on potential vaccines, improved diagnosis, and epidemiologic research. Innovative projects at the community level will be supported by Can$20 million in contributions aimed at enhancing programs to prevent the spread of HIV infection and to provide care in the community for persons with AIDS. Regarding health and social sector support, Can$10 million will be allocated for the training of health care and social service workers, the development of innovative service models, educational materials and guidelines for service support to volunteer organizations, and workplace initiatives. Can$6 million will be used to strengthen Canada's participation in international scientific efforts, such as the WHO-GPA.

Canada's provincial and territorial governments have played important roles in the development of AIDS control programs. Close collaboration has been a key to these activities, particularly the education and awareness components, and has encouraged a sharing of information and enhanced the impact of national and regional programs. The Federal/Provincial/Territorial Advisory Committee on AIDS acts as an important focus for the discussion of national and provincial HIV-related issues. In addition, the Committee has put together expert working groups to prepare position papers on selected topics, such as confidentiality in HIV testing and the implications of HIV infection for organ donation and tissue transplantation. The provinces and territories have also implemented a wide range of innovative educational programs and other activities, including AIDS hotlines, videos, support to community groups, AZT clinical trials, epidemiologic surveillance, and the establishment of multidisciplinary advisory committees. AIDS is a notifiable disease in all provinces and territories.

From the time AIDS was first reported in Canada, community-based AIDS groups across the country have played a crucial role in the development of AIDS programs. In addition to their advocacy role, such groups have extended their activities to include education, counseling, and support programs. Linkages with other community-based organizations have proved extremely useful and have enhanced the impact of preventive and support projects. The Canadian AIDS Society serves as the umbrella organization for 32 community-based AIDS groups.

It is generally acknowledged that AIDS control and research programs cannot be conducted in isolation if the HIV pandemic is to be overcome. Canada, as an active member of WHO and PAHO, is firmly committed to the philosophy of international cooperation. Through CIDA, Canada donated Can$5 million to the WHO-GPA in 1987 and a similar amount in 1988. Also, Canada will host the Fifth International Conference on AIDS in Montreal in June 1989. Such commitments demonstrate Canada's determination to play a significant role in the global struggle to control HIV infection.

Part II

ROUND TABLE

Round Table

AIDS PROJECTIONS ARE TOO HIGH

Among the many projections that epidemiologists have made for the future incidence of AIDS in the United States, those of one senior epidemiologist stand out as consistently more moderate. He is Alexander D. Langmuir, chief epidemiologist from 1949 to 1970 for the Centers for Disease Control (CDC) in Atlanta, Georgia, USA. He is now engaged in what he terms an "active retirement," during which he has been following, among other things, the AIDS surveillance reports from the CDC and the AIDS literature. From time to time he has expressed his views when requested, for example to B. D. Colen, science editor of Newsday, *in an interview published 13 October 1987, and in testimony given to the U.S. Presidential Commission on the Immunodeficiency Virus Epidemic in Washington, D.C., on 10 December 1987. The following article has been condensed from these two sources. It is published here with Dr. Langmuir's permission.*

My long-held view, which is now becoming widely known, is that most of the projections of the incidence of AIDS in the United States are too high.

The active practice of epidemiology has been my professional career for 50 years. During this time I have become increasingly intrigued with epidemic theory, namely, the effort to divine the laws governing the occurrence and course of epidemics and to express them in mathematical terms. Progress in this field over a century and a half has been disappointingly slow. The factors involved are too complex, varied, and intangible, and the measurements are too imprecise to be amenable to mathematical expression, even with the aid of computers.

Back in 1840, however, a great epidemiologist in London named William Farr made an observation that in a very special way has stood the test of time. He noted that epidemic smallpox seemed to follow an orderly path. He fitted a curve to his data which we now recognize to be a normal curve, the simple Gaussian "cocked hat" curve that provides the basis for classical statistics. His later admirers promulgated Farr's Law, which simply states that the rise and fall of an epidemic follows the lines of a normal curve.

During an epizootic of cattle plague in London in 1865–1866, when the incidence seemed to be increasing disastrously, Farr predicted that the epizootic would soon crest and rapidly decline. He was right. Thus began the hazardous game of predicting the course of epidemics.

I am known among my friends as temerarious Alex, foolishly courageous in making predictions. I have been right some of the time, and wrong on many occasions. I persist in this trait for several reasons. First of all, it is exciting to be at the cutting edge of an unresolved epidemic problem and sometimes even over the edge. More seriously, to make reasonably responsible predictions about a disease demands at least the beginning of an understanding of the underlying theory of the disease. When predictions are fulfilled, one gains confidence in going forward toward a more complete theory. When predictions fail, one picks up the pieces, reevaluates the basic premises, and starts over.

Regarding AIDS, my feeling is that the epidemic is not about to break out of the recognized high-risk groups and overwhelm the rest of the population. At present, the weekly AIDS surveillance reports issued by the U.S. Centers for Disease Control (CDC) have a category called "heterosexuals." It is a small group, about 4% of the total. The report's footnotes show that about 50% of this group is made up of spouses and sexual partners of homosexuals/bisexuals, intravenous drug abusers, hemophiliacs, and transfusion recipients—the four high-risk categories. The other half are individuals with extensive overseas contacts of some kind; they have been born in or lived for years in certain Third World countries. They may not know how they got their infection, but the CDC classifies them as heterosexuals. The important point is that this "heterosexual" group is small and is not increasing significantly faster than the other, more frequent categories of cases. The long-predicted breakout of the epidemic to the general population has not materialized. In my opinion, this would have occurred by now if it were going to happen at all.

More specifically, studies of homosexuals have shown that those at greatest risk are those who engage in receptive anal intercourse. This and the inoculation of contaminated blood by intravenous drug abusers appear to be the dominant ways that the AIDS virus spreads. Thus, spread to the general population seems most unlikely.

The epidemic theorist must be concerned primarily with the rate at which a disease spreads. To have an epidemic, one case must give rise to more than one case, not necessarily a lot more, but at least a little bit more. If, on the average, one case gives rise to less than one case, the epidemic dies out. Everything I have seen says that, outside of the known high-risk groups, the rate of AIDS' spread is insufficient for epidemic survival.

I first indulged my obsession concerning AIDS in October 1985. I was "drafted" by Dr. Fred Robbins, then President of the Institute of Medicine of the National Academy of Sciences in Washington. He was organizing a panel discussion at the annual meeting on the epidemiology of AIDS. He asked me to open the discussion and to "be provocative." I quoted William Farr as the basis for questioning the commonly held view that the incidence of AIDS would continue its geometric increase to the point of Black Death.

Considering the four transmission categories separately, none could continue increasing geometrically for long. Most of the multi-partnered homosexuals are already infected. We are still seeing new cases in this group because the incubation period is longer than anticipated. We will not know how many cases will occur until we have measured the incubation period more accurately. But, essentially, new infections among homosexuals will only be arising among new homosexuals, to be measured roughly by the birth rate. This situation does not spell continued geometric increase.

Identical reasoning applies to the other transmission categories: I.V. drug abusers, hemophiliacs, and transfusion recipients. I stated categorically, on the basis of my epidemiologic judgment, that no biological system, surely not an epidemic, can increase geometrically for long. In fact, the then already well-known "increase in the doubling time" precluded such a conclusion. I even hazarded a forecast—prediction is too strong a word—that the epidemic would crest in "mid-summer of 1986." This caused no ripple of interest in the panel. They went on discussing other matters. No mention was made of it in the book summarizing the whole meeting.

Table 1. Semiannual incidence of AIDS in the United States from 1982 through 1986, by year of diagnosis and transmission category.[a]

Year	Half-year	Male homosexuals/bisexuals	I.V. drug abusers	Male homosexual/bisexual drug abusers	Transfusion recipients	Hemophiliacs	Heterosexuals[b]	Unknown	Total
1982	Jan–June	223	56	23	1	2	34	14	353
	July–Dec	399	109	71	7	4	33	20	643
1983	Jan–June	754	216	117	13	8	66	33	1,207
	July–Dec	982	296	160	27	4	65	46	1,580
1984	Jan–June	1,618	410	214	40	24	96	72	2,474
	July–Dec	2,118	553	300	49	25	120	75	3,240
1985	Jan–June	2,982	755	343	103	34	153	91	4,461
	July–Dec	3,735	951	378	106	68	193	154	5,585
1986	Jan–June	4,570	1,142	528	183	60	278	190	6,951
	July–Dec	5,496	1,263	610	202	82	315	259	8,227
Total		22,877	5,751	2,744	731	311	1,353	954	34,721
Percentage		65.9	16.6	7.9	2.1	0.9	3.9	2.7	100.0

[a]Figures corrected for delayed reporting due to the lag from the date of diagnosis to the date the report was received by the CDC. The corrections were made specific for each transmission category and month of diagnosis.
[b]The heterosexual category consists of contacts of AIDS-infected persons plus individuals exposed overseas.

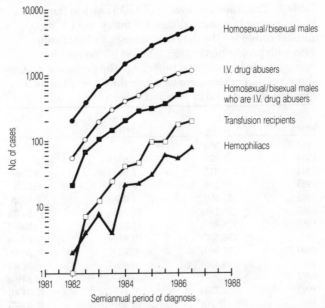

Figure 1. Trends in the semiannual incidence of AIDS in the United States from 1982 through 1986, by year of diagnosis and transmission category. The data charted have been corrected for delayed reporting.

It is just as well. The forecast missed. The incidence continued to increase, to some alarmingly, although the rate of increase steadily dampened and the doubling time lengthened. I was wrong.

My colleague Dennis Bregman and I have persisted. Reassessment of our failure led to what we think are clear explanations. In 1985 I had grossly underestimated the length of the incubation period. I had assumed it was two to three years. In this error I had ample company. We now believe it is 8 to 10 years and highly variable.

The second error was an underestimate of the lag in reporting due to the long interval between the date of first diagnosis and the date the report is received by CDC. This gave a false sense of an impending turnover in the curve.

Bregman and I now present what we believe to be adequately adjusted data in Table 1. The data, graphed in Figure 1 on a standard semilogarithmic scale which shows relative change and reflects comparative trends, reveal the steep upward trends in 1982, 1983, and 1984—the logarithmic phase of the epidemic. Then all of the curves veer off to the right with increasing speed.

Table 2. The annual incidence of AIDS cases in the United States among homosexual/bisexual males and I.V. drug abusers combined, by date of diagnosis, in 1982 through 1986 with projections to 1995. The 1982–1986 data have been corrected for delayed reporting. The projected data, shown in parentheses, are based on the assumption of a constant second ratio in 1985 and 1986.

Year	No. of cases	First ratio[a]	Second ratio[b]
1982	881		
1983	2,525	2.8661	
1984	5,213	2.0646	0.7203
1985	9,144	1.7541	0.8496
1986	13,609	1.4883	0.8485
1987	(17,197)	(1.2636)	(0.8490)
1988	(18,450)	(1.0729)	(0.8490)
1989	(16,807)	(0.9109)	(0.8490)
1990	(12,999)	(0.7734)	(0.8490)
1991	(8,536)	(0.6567)	(0.8490)
1992	(4,759)	(0.5575)	(0.8490)
1993	(2,253)	(0.4734)	(0.8490)
1994	(979)	(0.4019)	(0.8490)
1995	(340)	(0.3413)	(0.8490)

[a]The first ratio is measured by dividing the number of cases in a specified year by the number in the preceding year. It expresses one plus the rate of change, e.g., 2.8661 equals 186.61% increase.
[b]The second ratio is measured by dividing the first ratio for any specified year by that for the preceding year. It expresses the acceleration (deceleration) of the rate of change. For all normal curves the second ratio is a constant less than 1.0.

The curves are astonishingly parallel, a phenomenon we did not expect to find but which we believe to be of great significance. The essential congruity of the curves must mean that some overriding force, or rather a composite of many forces (in mathematical terms a vector or resultant), is exerting an approximately equal effect on all four transmission categories in spite of the wide divergence among these groups.

Any epidemiologist who accepts William Farr as a role model cannot resist the temptation to apply his law to these data. To obtain the most stable data for curve fitting, we have combined the number of cases in homosexuals/bisexuals and I.V. drug abusers into annual totals, shown in Table 2. Using the simplest of arithmetic procedures, we have fitted a normal curve. The fit is excellent, as shown in Figure 2. The projected crest occurs in 1988 and the ensuing decline is symmetric, reaching a low point by 1995. The total projection for

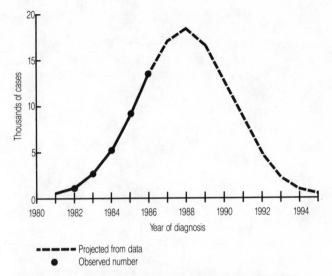

Figure 2. A projection of the annual incidence of AIDS cases in the United States among homosexual/bisexual males and I.V. drug abusers combined, by date of diagnosis, in 1982 through 1986 with projections to 1995. The 1982–1986 data have been corrected for delayed reporting. The projected curve is based on the assumption that the average of the second ratios for 1985 and 1986, namely 0.8490, will remain constant through 1995.

homosexual/bisexual and I.V. drug abuser cases is 130,000. Since this estimate applies to 90% of the total cases, the estimate must be increased by at least 10%.

We make no claim of great precision for this projection. In fact we assume a wide range. We rather expect from general considerations that the decline will not be wholly symmetrical. Rather, it will probably be slower. We have not included any allowance for a continuing endemic incidence although from considerations already mentioned we expect it to be low. The important point is that if Farr's Law has any reasonable validity, the epidemic should crest at an early date and then progressively decline. The total number of projected cases will be about 150,000, approximately half the figure of most projections that have been made so far. Time will tell.

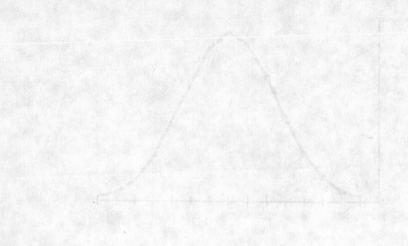

Commentaries

PROJECTION OF AIDS CASES, USA

JAMES CHIN

Since the initial recognition of AIDS in 1981, this worldwide epidemic (pandemic) has been beset by some extreme misconceptions. Among the first of these misconceptions was the belief that AIDS would only be a disease of homosexual/bisexual men and intravenous drug users. When this was shown not to be true, some "scientists" began to spread the alarming misconception that within a couple of decades AIDS would kill almost every man, woman, and child on this planet. That extreme view, based more on social-political motivation than fact, has been dismissed as science fiction by the medical and scientific communities.

Although the ultimate dimensions of the AIDS pandemic are not yet known, our current solid knowledge of HIV transmission and our understanding of the first five to ten years of the natural history of HIV infections enables us to begin to forecast the general scope of the AIDS problem with increasing confidence for up to the next five years.

Virtually all AIDS researchers and public health epidemiologists are predicting that in most areas of the world there will be a five- to tenfold AIDS case increase within the next five years. However, one solitary yet highly respected voice has been raised to challenge this mainstream scientific thinking regarding the future increase. Dr. Alexander Langmuir, former chief epidemiologist for the United States Centers for Disease Control (CDC), has predicted that the AIDS epidemic in the United States will peak in mid-1988 and virtually disappear as a public health problem by 1995. This paper will critique Dr. Langmuir's prediction and provide a simple model that projects an AIDS case increase in the United States similar to that estimated by the current AIDS staff at CDC.

Problems Associated with the Use of Reported AIDS Case Data

In countries where clinical diagnosis and reporting of AIDS cases are relatively accurate and complete, the observed pattern and prevalence of the reported cases can be used as a reasonable approximation of the actual number of cases that have occurred. However, even with the best of surveillance systems the pattern and number of reported cases must be interpreted with extreme caution. In the United States, which probably has the most accurate and complete reporting system for AIDS cases, there are strong indications that during the last year or two there have been changes in diagnostic procedures and in reporting delays that could greatly distort the true temporal pattern of the actual occurrence of AIDS. It must be fully understood that although reported AIDS cases may to some extent represent the pattern of AIDS occurrence, this pattern is overlaid to varying degrees by vagaries of diagnosis and reporting. Thus, when the curve of *reported* AIDS cases is used to project future *occurrence* of AIDS cases, the accuracy of such projections must be seriously questioned.

Even if some "adjustments" are made for reporting delays, based on calculations of average *past* reporting delays, there is no assurance that such adjustments will adequately correct for *current* or *future* reporting delays or changes in diagnostic procedures. Any statistical projection or "curve-fitting" must also be consistent with what is known about the epidemiology and natural history of HIV infections.

Langmuir and Bregman's AIDS Prediction and Their Prediction Model

Doctors Langmuir and Bregman used a Gaussian curve fitted to the log of *reported* AIDS cases for projecting the future incidence of AIDS in the United States. They did not comment on whether such a projected normal, bell-shaped curve was consistent with what is now known about HIV infections and AIDS. They admitted that their first attempt at fitting such a curve grossly underestimated the average

AIDS incubation period. Their first prediction, that the AIDS epidemic in the USA would crest in "mid-summer of 1986," was wrong. Now they are confident that they have adequately adjusted for reporting lags, and they believe the incubation period for most AIDS cases is about eight to ten years. Based on experience from their prior attempts, they predict the crest will occur in 1988. In addition, they project that the total number of AIDS cases in the United States by 1995 (when they also predict the disease will virtually disappear) will be approximately 150,000.

If Doctors Langmuir and Bregman are correct, it will not be because of their use of Farr's Law, which is inconsistent with current epidemiologic thinking on HIV infections and AIDS. Farr's Law may have been applicable to smallpox and cattle plague epidemics that, when introduced into a population, spread rapidly, peaked, and then dissipated with no new incident infections because all the susceptibles were "consumed." Farr's Law does not apply to those diseases that are most similar to AIDS, such as hepatitis B, gonorrhea, and other sexually transmitted diseases that have reached high endemic levels in many human populations throughout the world.

HIV infections are presumably life-long, and the infected person is potentially infectious until death—a death that may not occur for a decade or two. Since most AIDS modelers now believe that the average incubation period from infection to the development of AIDS is some eight to nine years, Dr. Langmuir and Dr. Bregman, if they persist in applying Farr's Law to AIDS, should reset their predicted cresting to the early 1990s, and should readjust the right side of their projected curve to increase the number of total AIDS cases well beyond 200,000.

Short-term Forecasting of AIDS

What are reasonable estimates and projections for AIDS cases in the United States? A simple model is proposed here to forecast the number of AIDS cases expected in any given population for up to five years. Four basic assumptions and estimates, based on our current understanding of the epidemiology and natural history of HIV infections, are needed to operate this model. These are as follows:

1. *The number of HIV infections in the population must be estimated.* Using a variety of methods and assumptions, the CDC has estimated that as of 1987 there were at least one million HIV-infected

Table 1. An estimate of the annual numbers of new and cumulative HIV infections in the United States in 1980–1987, accepting the estimate of 1,000,000 infected persons as of 1987 and distributing those cumulative cases on an appropriate asymptotic curve.[a]

	HIV infections	
Year	New infections	Cumulative infections
1980	5,000	5,000
1981	25,000	30,000
1982	70,000	100,000
1983	175,000	275,000
1984	250,000	525,000
1985	225,000	750,000
1986	150,000	900,000
1987	100,000	1,000,000

[a]Data are insufficient to allow choice of a specific asymptotic curve, but for a short-term forecast the number of cases projected would be about the same regardless of the asymptotic curve selected.

persons in the United States. This conservative estimate is used in the proposed model.

2. *The year when HIV infection probably began to spread extensively in the population has to be estimated.* This model takes the year 1980 as the likely period when HIV infection began to spread extensively in the United States.

3. *The number of people infected each year (in the case of the United States, from 1980 through 1987) needs to be estimated.* The available epidemiologic cohort data indicate a majority of the HIV infections in the United States were transmitted before 1985. Thus, the cumulative HIV infection curve from 1980 to 1987 was not exponential or linear but asymptotic in shape. Using this latter assumption, the one million HIV infections estimated to have occurred in the United States as of 1987 can be distributed into annual infected cohorts back to 1980, as has been done in Table 1.

4. *The annual rate of progression after HIV infection to the development of AIDS needs to be estimated.* This progression has been estimated at about 15–20% after five years and up to 50% within 10 years. The specific annual progression to AIDS has been documented for a relatively large San Francisco cohort of homosexual men, and has reached about 40% after almost eight years. The annual rate of progression to AIDS after HIV infection for this model (Table 2) has been adapted and extrapolated from these data (San Francisco City Clinic cohort study, G. W. Rutherford, personal communication).

Table 2. Estimated annual rates of progression to AIDS following HIV infection. The figures shown have been adapted and extrapolated from progression curves reported for HIV-infected homosexual men.

Years after infection	% annual rate of progression to AIDS
0	0.0
1	0.5
2	2.0
3	3.0
4	4.0
5	6.0
6	7.0
7	8.5
8	9.0
9	9.5
10	10.0
11	11.0

By applying these annual progression rates to the development of AIDS for each of the HIV-infected cohorts starting in 1980, the number of AIDS cases can be estimated by year up to 1991 (Table 3). These calculations indicate that, at a minimum, close to 250,000 AIDS cases can be expected in the United States by the end of 1991. It needs to be noted that this simple model does not take account of new HIV infections occurring after 1987, nor does it consider the probability that

Table 3. A projection of AIDS cases in the United States in 1980–1991 based on the assumptions and figures shown in Tables 1 and 2.

Year	Projected AIDS cases	
	New cases	Cumulative cases
1980	0	0
1981	25	25
1982	224	249
1983	993	1,242
1984	3,186	4,430
1985	7,996	12,426
1986	15,527	27,953
1987	24,803	52,756
1988	35,252	88,006
1989	45,634	133,642
1990	54,044	187,686
1991	59,890	247,576

progression to AIDS could increase markedly above 50% of those infected after 15 to 20 years.

Obviously, the assumptions and estimates in this model will need to be changed when and if additional data warrant any change. Also, the model should be of greatest utility in those countries where the reporting system is not considered sufficiently reliable to attempt statistical extrapolation from the local pattern of reported cases.

Conclusions

To sum up, Dr. Langmuir and Dr. Bregman will be proven wrong again in their prediction. The incidence of HIV infection in the United States has probably decreased in recent years; but, because of the very long incubation period for the development of AIDS, the peak or cresting of AIDS cases will, at the earliest, occur in the early 1990s. Thereafter, AIDS cases will continue to occur at a relatively high endemic level well beyond the year 2000. HIV infection and AIDS in the United States will probably continue to be primarily concentrated among homosexual/bisexual men and I.V. drug users. However, heterosexuals with multiple sexual partners are at a low but measurable risk now; if they persist in their behavior, they will be placing themselves at increasing risk of HIV infection in the future.

AIDS PROJECTIONS, A JAMAICAN PERSPECTIVE

J. PETER FIGUEROA

I have read Alexander Langmuir's views on the AIDS epidemic with care and respect. However, I do not agree with him that the AIDS epidemic in the United States will crest soon (in 1988) or that the projected number of cases will be as low as one-half the presently accepted figure.

Dr. Langmuir bases his views upon Farr's Law that epidemics rise and fall in a normal curve, as well as upon analysis of AIDS incidence data for the United States from 1982 through 1986. His previous forecast, that the epidemic would crest in "mid-summer of 1986," was wrong. His explanation for the miscalculation is a "grossly underestimated" incubation period and a "lag in reporting."

My own view is that AIDS projections, whether for the U.S. or any other country, must be made with caution because our information regarding several critical variables is limited. We do not know the extent of human immunodeficiency virus (HIV) infection in most population groups, or the duration and intensity of the infectivity of HIV-positive persons, or whether all HIV-infected people will develop AIDS (and if so over what time period). Nor are we sufficiently familiar with patterns of sexual activity to accurately predict the number of AIDS cases in any given country.

Nevertheless, we do have enough information to consider Dr. Langmuir's forecasts erroneous. In the first place, the AIDS epidemic is the terminal clinical manifestation of a significantly more widespread but silent epidemic of HIV infection. As there are many HIV-infected people for every person with AIDS (WHO estimates that there are 50 to 100 HIV-positive people per AIDS case), it is logical to assume that the number of AIDS cases will continue to increase over the next few years.

Although the extent of HIV infection in most populations is simply not known, the prevalence studies that have been done have found the level of HIV infection, particularly among high-risk groups, to be almost invariably increasing. Thus, people newly infected with HIV are continually being added to the pool of people out of which the AIDS epidemic grows.

Furthermore, even though the relative proportions of people belonging to the various transmission categories in the United States may not have changed, it would be wrong to conclude that they will not. For instance, the data from the English-speaking Caribbean are showing "a shift from predominantly homosexual spread, seen earlier in the AIDS epidemic, towards a pattern of predominantly heterosexual transmission" (1). The absolute number of heterosexuals with AIDS in the United States is increasing, and there are clear potential routes of HIV infection into the heterosexual community. These include sex with infected bisexuals, prostitutes, injecting drug abusers, and people from countries where HIV infection is prevalent. In my view, it is only a question of time before AIDS due to heterosexual transmission accounts for a larger proportion of cases in the United States.

Within this context it is useful to briefly describe the AIDS epidemic in Jamaica in order to discuss projections in that country.

Sixty-three AIDS cases had been reported in Jamaica (population 2.36 million) as of 31 July 1988, yielding a cumulative AIDS rate of 2.7 cases per 100,000 inhabitants (Table 1). Forty-six of those with AIDS (including children under five years old) were males and 17 were

Table 1. AIDS cases in Jamaica, by year of reporting and sex of patients, 1982–July 1988.

Year	Sex of patient		Annual total	Cumulative total
	Male	Female		
1982	1	0	1	1
1983	0	0	0	1
1984	1	0	1	2
1985	4	0	4	6
1986	5	0	5	11
1987	20	13	33	44
1988	15	4	19	63
Total	46	17	63	63

Table 2. Sexual preferences of AIDS patients in Jamaica, 1982–July 1988.

Classification of patient	Cases	
	No.	(%)
Heterosexual	32	(50.8)
Male	*18*	*(28.6)*
Female	*14*	*(22.2)*
Homosexual	12	(19.0)
Bisexual	5	(7.9)
Child (pediatric case)	8	(12.7)
Unknown	6	(9.5)
Total	63	(100)

females, so that the male/female ratio was 2.7 to 1. As of 31 July 1988, 44 of these 63 people had died, yielding a case fatality rate of 70%.

Nearly all the initial AIDS patients in Jamaica acquired their infections abroad, mainly in the United States. These people included roughly equal numbers of homosexuals and heterosexuals—mainly migrant farm workers employed in Belle Glade, Florida, for four to six months each year. It was not until early 1987, when the number of AIDS cases increased sharply, that the first female (the common-law wife of a migrant farm worker) and the first child with AIDS were diagnosed. In all, 22 of the 63 people with AIDS acquired the infection abroad, while in 24 cases the infection was acquired locally and in 17 cases the area of acquisition is unknown.

As Tables 2 and 3 indicate, the epidemiologic pattern of AIDS in Jamaica is quite different from that found in the United States and Europe. Of the 63 cases, 18 (28.6%) occurred in adult male heterosexuals and 14 (22.2%) in adult female heterosexuals, as compared to 12 (19.0%) in exclusively homosexual males and five (7.9%) in bisexual males. In six cases (9.5%), the patient's sexual preferences are unknown. Thus, heterosexual transmission appears to have been nearly twice as common as homosexual transmission, accounting for 65.3% versus 34.7% of the AIDS cases in adults with known sexual preferences.

Three Jamaican risk groups have emerged in cases where heterosexual transmission is responsible for AIDS—these being migrant farm workers, prostitutes, and sailors. The well-recognized association between HIV infection and promiscuity is the most likely explanation for AIDS developing in these risk groups. However, a number of the migrant farm workers denied promiscuity while admitting to

Table 3. AIDS cases in Jamaica by risk group, 1982–July 1988.

Risk group	Cases	
	No.	(%)
Homosexual males	12	(19.0)
Bisexual males	4	(6.3)
Bisexuals/I.V. drug abusers	1	(1.6)
Heterosexuals	20	(31.7)
Migrant farm workers	*9*	*(14.4)*
Prostitutes (female)	*7*	*(11.1)*
Sailors	*4*	*(6.3)*
Children of HIV-positive mothers	8	(12.7)
Blood transfusion recipients	2	(3.2)
Unknown	16	(25.4)
Total	63	(100)

occasional heterosexual relations in Belle Glade, Florida, where there is a relatively high level of HIV infection among prostitutes.

The eight children with AIDS all acquired the infection through maternal-infant transmission. The high proportion of cases in this category (12.7%) is consistent with a pattern of predominantly heterosexual HIV transmission. The only case involving intravenous drug abuse occurred in a bisexual who acquired AIDS abroad. (I.V. drug abuse is not a problem in Jamaica.) The two infections transmitted by blood transfusion were passed before December 1985, when screening of all blood donations was introduced.

HIV testing in Jamaica has revealed a mixed picture (Table 4). In 1985 none of 4,000 food service workers island-wide and in 1986 none of 239 prisoners were found to be infected, while the level of HIV infection among 2,400 sexually transmitted disease (STD) clinic attendees was relatively low (0.375%). However, 0.265% of all blood donations tested from December 1985 through April 1988 were ELISA-positive (the estimated percentage of true positives based on this figure is 0.125%), a rate higher than that found in the United States; and during 1985 HIV infection was clearly well-established within the homosexual community. During 1985–1987, 12,000 to 15,000 migrant farm workers were tested annually before departing for the United States. Of the 31,552 tests performed in that period, 0.18% were positive by ELISA, for an estimated prevalence in those workers ranging from 0.38% to 0.475%. It is expected that approximately 94% of the positive results will be confirmed.

Table 4. Results of HIV testing in Jamaica.

Test period	Group tested	No. of tests	No. positive (by ELISA)	% positive
12/85–4/88	Blood donors	47,978	127	0.265
1985–1987	Farm workers	31,552[a]	57	0.18
1985	Food service workers	4,000	0	0
1985	Homosexuals	123	18[b]	14.6
1985–1986	Sexually transmitted disease clinic attendees	2,400	9[b]	0.375
1986	Prisoners	239	0	0

[a] 12,000 to 15,000 workers tested annually.
[b] Confirmed by Western blot.

In assessing the spread of HIV infection in Jamaica, it is important to consider prevailing patterns of sexual activity. Sexual intercourse begins young, with some 46.3% of the boys and 15.3% of the girls having sexual intercourse by age 14 (2). A random nationwide survey of the knowledge, attitudes, and practices of 1,200 subjects concerning AIDS/STD in Jamaica in 1988 indicated that 23% of the males and 2% of the females surveyed had had sex with more than one partner within the four weeks preceding the interview (3). Although 95% of all the respondents had heard about AIDS and 85% knew it to be incurable, 44% still thought it was not possible for them to contract AIDS, and 52% thought what they knew about AIDS would not change their behavior. The study indicated that 37% of the respondents were currently using condoms and 17% were using condoms most of the time. It is also important to note that there is a high incidence of STD in Jamaica, estimated at three times the combined reported rates of 474.8 cases per 100,000 for gonorrhea and 120.8 cases per 100,000 for syphilis in 1987 (4).

Given the pattern of AIDS in Jamaica, there are absolutely no grounds for complacency concerning the likely course of the epidemic. We are convinced that we will continue to see an increasing number of cases over the next several years, despite concerted control program and educational efforts. It is no comfort that the cumulative AIDS rate per 100,000 population was only two cases in Jamaica as of December 1987, as compared with 19 in Trinidad and Tobago, 20 in Barbados, and 25 in the United States. For reasons not fully understood, the AIDS epidemic in Jamaica is lagging about two years behind those in Trinidad and Tobago and Barbados. However, we have no doubt that an increasing number of AIDS cases will arise out of the hidden but exploding HIV epidemic.

Making specific projections of the number of AIDS cases expected in Jamaica is quite different than anticipating the general course of the epidemic. Three approaches have been used to make such projections. The first simply doubles the number of cases each year over a five-year period beginning with 30 cases in the year ending in September 1987. This approach forecasts 60 cases in September 1988, 120 cases in September 1989, and 960 cases in September 1992.

The second approach estimates the number of HIV-positive individuals by risk group and the number of AIDS cases that can be expected among these individuals by the end of 1992. Using this approach, it has been estimated that there were 3,681 HIV-positive persons in Jamaica as of September 1987 and that some 1,105 AIDS cases would arise within this group by 1992, assuming 30% progression to AIDS within five years (5).

The third approach uses a simplified projection model that assumes an initial number of HIV-positive people in the population, an annual rate of increase in the number of HIV positives, and an annual rate of conversion of HIV infections to AIDS. These three variables can be adjusted as more information becomes available (5).

The real problem is that for accurate projections to be made, one requires data on the prevalence and incidence of HIV infection that are not readily available. For instance, we have no idea of current levels of HIV infection among prostitutes or their customers, two key groups in the spread of HIV infection in Jamaica. We also have no current information on HIV infection among homosexuals, sailors, informal commercial importers (who travel frequently), workers in the tourist industry, etc. Plans are in place for doing a number of baseline KAP (knowledge-attitude-practice) studies and serosurveys among these high-risk groups, so as to provide a basis for developing better-targeted interventions. Nevertheless, important gaps will remain in the data base upon which projections must depend.

In the final analysis, public health practitioners around the world must decide about the likely course of the AIDS epidemic in their countries and take appropriate measures to control the spread of HIV. Given the nature of the HIV and AIDS epidemic, Dr. Langmuir is indeed bold in predicting an early cresting of the epidemic in the United States.

■ ■ ■

Acknowledgments: I wish to acknowledge the work of my colleagues, in particular Dr. M. Bullock-DuCasse and Dr. A. Braithwaite.

References

1. Caribbean Epidemiology Center. AIDS in the Caribbean: An update. *CAREC Surveillance Report* 14(5), 1988.
2. National Family Planning Board in collaboration with D. Powell, J. Jackson, V. James, C. Watson, L. Morris, and A. Whatley. Young Adult Reproductive Health Survey, Jamaica, 1987, Preliminary Report, September 1987. Mimeographed document. National Family Planning Board, Kingston, 1987.
3. Ministry of Health of Jamaica, Market Research Services Ltd., and The Futures Group (SOMARC). Jamaica AIDS/STD KAP Study 1988. Kingston, 1988.
4. Braithwaite, A. STD Control Programme Annual Report 1987. Ministry of Health of Jamaica, Kingston, 1988.
5. Jillson-Boostrom, I., E. Boostrom, and J. P. Figueroa. Simplified Approaches to Estimating Trends in Cases of AIDS. Paper presented at the IV International Conference on AIDS held in Stockholm, 12–16 June 1988. Book of Abstracts 2, Abstract 4691, p. 234.

CHANGING PATTERN OF HIV TRANSMISSION IN THE CARIBBEAN

DAVID C. BASSETT & JAI P. NARAIN

Dr. Langmuir succeeds admirably in showing that any prediction regarding AIDS, unless stated very cautiously and for the shortest term, must be subject to serious doubt. His own detailed predictions are for the United States, with Pattern I transmission, and not for Africa and the Caribbean with Pattern II.

His paper contains some rather obvious truths, such as that a geometric progression cannot continue indefinitely in a finite population, and at least one "feeling" which many would agree with—that AIDS is not about to overwhelm the general population of the United States. Sexually transmitted diseases (STDs) have never overwhelmed whole populations, but neither have they gone away even when readily treatable.

It would be splendid if the right-hand side of Langmuir's Gaussian curve really represented the future of the epidemic, but there are reasons to doubt this. If the epidemic were to peak in 1988, the curve for HIV infection should have peaked some years ago—perhaps before the disease was recognized—and the incidence of seroconversion should have been declining since. Is there evidence of this?

Further, the left-hand side of his curve may not truly represent events to date, and may have led to the false expectation that the epidemic would peak in the immediate future.

Dr. Langmuir's feeling that AIDS will remain within recognized risk groups seems to dismiss the half of heterosexual cases that would particularly interest us in the Third World—those with no known contact with the recognized risk groups.

Obviously, risk groups are not homogeneous. For example, within the category of homosexual males, promiscuity varies from person to person. Ignoring, for the moment, differences in sexual practices, it can be anticipated that the most promiscuous will, in general, become infected first. Imagining a "promiscuity distribution curve" of some shape or other (it hardly will be a normal distribution), the first cases and the highest rates of transmission will be at the high, right-hand end of the curve. While there are no useful data from which to plot this curve, it is reasonable to postulate a declining rate of transmission, but among larger and larger numbers of susceptibles, as we move from right to left along the curve until that point at which the doubling time exceeds the mean incubation period (or the sexually active survival time of the HIV-infected, assuming some never develop AIDS itself). Presumably, the epidemic will not spread into the less promiscuous part of the homosexual risk group beyond that critical point.

The effect of new homosexuals entering the population is dismissed by Dr. Langmuir as insufficient to maintain geometric increase, but that is hardly the same as being unable to sustain an incidence of new infections.

If we apply the "promiscuity distribution" concept to the group of heterosexuals without known contact with other risk groups, we once again have no data to plot a real curve, but we know that heterosexual transmission occurs and that the most promiscuous at the right-hand tail of the curve will be at greatest risk. How far to the left along this imagined curve can transmission be sustained?

Recruits to heterosexual behavior—the great majority of young persons of either sex—will in some societies appear further to the right in their youth than they will in maturity. Thus, if there were data, "promiscuity distributions" could be plotted for each sex, for each sexually active age group, each culture, religion, socioeconomic group, occupation, et cetera.

For each imagined curve, the question again would be: How far to the left is HIV transmission sustainable, and what part of the population lies under the residual part of the curve and can be regarded as not at risk?

One can accept Dr. Langmuir's point that a peak must be reached at some time, but his date for the event and his guess as to what the rest of the curve will look like do not seem well founded.

The left-hand side of his curve may begin too vertically and may end too horizontally. If we accept the fact that early in the epidemic diagnostic capability increased with time, the 1982 notifications may be well below the actual number of cases, even after including retro-spective diagnoses. In subsequent years, this discrepancy would diminish. The proportion of diagnosed cases that were notified may have peaked once diagnostic proficiency was generally established in the United States, but may have declined since then. Substantial underreporting is accepted as a fact: With little to gain and much to lose, some patients can be expected to try avoiding diagnosis (and thus notification also).

Has the proportion of cases being notified fallen as the absolute numbers have continued to rise? If this has occurred, it is not only late notification but non-notification that may have artificially flattened the upper part of Dr. Langmuir's curve, exaggerating whatever real lengthening of the doubling time may have occurred. The true curve may still be closer to the linear than Langmuir has calculated; the gradient may be less and the peak may not yet be in evidence.

Any attempt to predict the impact of AIDS on the general popula-tion of the United States must be based on available information on heterosexual transmission of AIDS cases, which has tended to occur with disproportionate frequency in two minority groups—blacks and Hispanics. These two groups account for 26% and 13% of the AIDS cases, respectively, compared with the overall proportion of blacks (12%) and Hispanics (6%) in the U.S. population (1), and account for 70% of the cases in heterosexual men, 70% of those in women, and 75% of those in children. The number of U.S.-born women with heterosexually acquired AIDS has been increasing (2), and women and children are the fastest growing groups of persons with AIDS. Most importantly, studies suggest that in some areas of New York, HIV seroprevalence in women of child-bearing age ranges from 2% to 5.9% (3), indicating that the level of infection in some heterosexual populations is high and will result in an increasing number of AIDS cases among heterosexual men and women and their children in the future.

The changing epidemiology of AIDS in the Caribbean may have important lessons for us. Analysis of data on reported AIDS cases suggests that transition from homosexual/bisexual to heterosexual transmission can occur, and once that happens, transmission in the latter population may take place quite rapidly and efficiently (see the article on pages 61–71 in this volume). In countries with smaller and more homogeneous populations, such as those in the Caribbean, this transition and its aftermath can be noticed more easily than in large countries, especially since, in our opinion, the AIDS epidemic is still at the initial stages.

AIDS in the 18 English-speaking Caribbean countries and Suriname (populations ranging from 8,000 to 2.3 million) was first reported in 1983. Until 1985, reported cases were among homosexual or bisexual males only. Thereafter, the heterosexually acquired cases started to increase. In Trinidad and Tobago they constituted 13% of the total in 1985; this proportion increased to 25% and 47% in 1986 and 1987, respectively. As a result, greater numbers of women with AIDS were reported, and the male to female ratio declined from 5.9:1 in or before 1985, to 3.3:1 in 1986, and 2.4:1 in 1988. By September 1988, 52% of cases reported from Trinidad and Tobago and a majority of the cases reported from the Bahamas were among heterosexual men and women. Similarly, an initial transition from predominantly intravenous drug-related AIDS to heterosexually acquired cases has been seen in Bermuda. In 1985, 80% of reported cases from Bermuda were among intravenous drug users. This has now declined, with a concurrent increase in the proportion of heterosexual contact cases from 6% in 1985 to 24% in 1987.

In Guyana, on the other hand, which only started reporting cases in 1987, most cases (all but 2%) are in males, predominantly among homosexuals or bisexuals. Given our experience in the Caribbean, this is likely to change in the future.

The underlying reason for this initial transition has been transmission from bisexual males to women, since most bisexual men in the Caribbean tend to be married. Further spread was probably facilitated by the sociocultural and sexual behavior of the population (4, 5). Important factors affecting transmission include fragile male–female relationships, men having multiple partners, teenagers engaging in unprotected sex, and the increasing incidence of other sexually transmitted diseases, particularly syphilis. Given the size of the heterosexual population, it is inevitable that transmission will continue to increase and the number of AIDS cases among heterosexual men, heterosexual women, and children will continue to grow.

Whether patterns in the United States will follow those seen in the Caribbean will be determined largely by the sociocultural and sexual behavior of various population groups in that country.

We agree that, based on current data, the number of cases among homosexuals in the United States will slow gradually as a result of the "exhausting of susceptibles" and perhaps also due to the impact of health education campaigns directed toward the homosexual population. However, heterosexual transmission may continue to increase in the foreseeable future. This is likely to be an area of great concern, especially because of the number of susceptibles and because of the relatively low emphasis that public education has placed on hetero-sexual transmission so far. Therefore, the importance of heterosexual transmission must be stressed worldwide, and this problem should be emphasized when charting the future course of action in our fight against AIDS.

References

1. Selic, R. M., K. B. Castro, and M. Pappaioanou. Distribution of AIDS cases, by racial ethnic group and exposure category, United States, June 1, 1981–July 4, 1988. *MMWR* 37(SS-3):1–10, 1988.

2. Chamberland, M., L. Conley, and T. Dondero. Epidemiology and Evolution of Heterosexually Acquired AIDS—United States. Paper presented at the IV International Conference on AIDS, Stockholm, 12–16 June 1988. Book of Abstracts 1, Abstract No. 4107, p. 264.

3. Centers for Disease Control. Human immunodeficiency virus infection in the United States: A review of current knowledge. *MMWR* 38(56, Suppl.):30–31, Dec. 1987.

4. Jagdeo, T. P. Myths, misconceptions and mistakes: A study of Trinidad adolescents. The Family Planning Association of Trinidad and Tobago, 1986.

5. Kerr, M. *Personality and Conflict in Jamaica*. Collins, London, 1963.

WHO IS REALLY RIGHT?

JAIR FERREIRA

Dr. Langmuir's presentation addresses the highly controversial subject of AIDS projections in the United States. It is Dr. Langmuir's personal view that no communicable disease has an incidence that progresses geometrically over the long run. This is quite true, and I fully agree with him; no communicable disease until now has ever behaved this way.

Dr. Langmuir further argues, with much reason, that the modes of AIDS transmission are unlikely to affect with any great intensity groups other than those already involved. So far the figures bear him out, for in heterosexuals, for example, the frequency of the disease, though somewhat higher, has not risen as much as it was expected to rise a few years ago. In general, the heterosexual case of AIDS is still the exception, male homosexuals/bisexuals and intravenous drug abusers remaining the two major groups at risk in the United States.

We have lately seen the rate of increase of AIDS cases among homosexuals decline, but this is counterbalanced by progressively greater increases among intravenous drug abusers, so the rate of increase for these two groups combined has held more or less steady as a proportion of all new cases.

Proceeding from this point, Dr. Langmuir makes a projection utilizing a normal curve, the type of curve followed by most infectious disease epidemics—notably those of acute diseases with incubation periods shorter than that of AIDS. In this respect it appears that Dr. Langmuir may be somewhat optimistic in predicting that the incidence of AIDS cases among homosexuals and intravenous drug abusers will peak in 1988, turn downward in 1989, and descend to almost zero by 1995.

In my view, AIDS more closely resembles a chronic disease, and so the incidence curve should level out to a plateau—a plateau that will probably persist for many years at a high and stable rate. The downturn in this curve, coming sooner or later, could well occur very late, in which case the incidence of AIDS in the United States could stay high for many years without any further marked increase.

Regarding the first part of Dr. Langmuir's presentation, I fully agree that predictions based on geometric progressions are probably in error, but I differ on the use of a normal curve as he has suggested for making a short-term projection. Perhaps a closer approximation to reality could be obtained by using a logistic curve, at least for the middle term during which the disease reaches a plateau. That plateau would be the limit of the logistic curve, a limit that should be possible to estimate when the rate of increase in the disease incidence has been decelerating for three years in succession.

As Dr. Langmuir says, only the future will tell who is really right.

Part III

ABSTRACTS AND REPORTS

STATUS OF THE AIDS EPIDEMIC

Seven years have passed since the United States Centers for Disease Control reported the occurrence of an unusual disease in five homosexual men in San Francisco. This was the first awareness of an epidemic that is now known to have begun before 1981 with the silent spread of the human immunodeficiency virus (HIV) throughout the world during the mid- to late 1970s. The magnitude of HIV's spread can still only be estimated. According to the World Health Organization, 5 to 10 million people are currently infected worldwide, and, using the best available data, the Pan American Health Organization estimates that 2.0 to 2.5 million of those infected people reside in the Region of the Americas.

Current Knowledge About AIDS

A vast amount of information has been gathered about HIV and many significant advances have been made in understanding the virus's genetic composition and how it interacts with human cells.

Sources: Pan American Health Organization, Acquired Immunodeficiency Syndrome (AIDS) in the Americas (Document CD33/21 and Annex), Washington, D.C., 11 August 1988; *and* AIDS in the Americas, Presentation to the XXXIII Meeting of the Directing Council by Dr. Ronald St. John, Program Coordinator, Health Situation and Trend Assessment, Pan American Health Organization, Washington, D.C., 28 September 1988.

However, the knowledge that has emerged leads to the sobering conclusion that public health interventions will be more complex and
difficult than had been thought. For example, the virus has an
impressive ability to change its outer envelope, the part of the virus
which is essential for its attachment to cells and which is very active
immunologically. One single amino acid change in the envelope glycoprotein may result in a total loss of reaction with antibodies produced by the host. These changes take place with amazing frequency
as the virus makes mistakes—in its favor—during replication. Various
new mechanisms have been described by which the virus can incorporate itself into a number of cells other than lymphocytes, its primary targets. Moreover, laboratory studies suggest that under certain
conditions, the human immune response itself may contribute to
enhancement of viral replication in human monocytes. Finally, many
areas of the viral structure which contribute to its infectiveness are
not readily accessible to the immune system.

There is considerable optimism regarding the possibility of developing chemotherapeutic approaches to contain, retard, or stop the
currently inevitable deterioration of the human immune system.
However, much more pessimism exists regarding the possible development of a vaccine. Even if a vaccine were available which adequately stimulated the production of antibodies, it might not protect
against infection by this virus.

It is now clear that the asymptomatic infected person is not disease-
free; the slow, steady, progressive deterioration of the immune system and the inevitable progression from an asymptomatic infected
state to AIDS may take much longer than was originally supposed.
Roughly 3% of infected people develop AIDS per year; only about
18% to 20% of those infected will develop the disease within five
years and 48% within 10 years. It is estimated that the median time
from infection to disease may be as long as 14 years. The implication
is that asymptomatic infected persons who may have no reason to be
tested for AIDS may remain undetected and infectious for a very long
period of time. Also, infected people must be persuaded to change
their lifestyles and sexual behaviors and sustain those changes for a
very long time.

Evidence has also come to light that a small number of infected
people may lose their antibody production when the virus goes into a
dormant phase, a phenomenon that has been found in both adults
and children. In these people, the virus enters quietly and may
undergo rapid proliferation with a readily detectable antibody
response. Then follows a gradual slowdown in replication and finally

a truly dormant period of unknown duration with a concomitant shutdown of the antibody response. Thus, an infected, antibody-positive person may no longer be detectable by currently available tests, but nevertheless remains infectious.

In summary, the more that is learned, the more apparent it is how difficult and complex the fight against AIDS will be. ⚐

Current Situation in the Americas

The Pan American Health Organization initiated AIDS surveillance throughout the Region of the Americas in 1983. Only officially reported cases of full-blown AIDS have been tabulated, and, as elsewhere in the world, the number of reported AIDS cases grossly underestimates the magnitude of the problem. As of 30 September 1988, 89,834 cases of AIDS had been reported in the Americas, and of those cases, 48,374 had died.

Table 1 reveals the large differences that exist between different subregions in totals of cases reported. The Andean group of countries had reported 746 cases as of 30 September 1988, and the Southern Cone countries had reached a total of 339, while Brazil had reported 4,153 cases. In the Central American countries and Panama, there had been 428 reported cases, while the total in Mexico was 1,642. The Latin Caribbean, which includes Cuba, the Dominican Republic, and Haiti, had reported a total of 2,261 cases, and the non-Latin Caribbean countries 1,124 cases. North America had reported a total of 79,141 cases, the great majority of those from the United States of America. Five countries—the United States, Brazil, Canada, Haiti, and Mexico—had contributed approximately 96% of the total number of cases in the Region (Figure 1).

The percentage increase between 1986 and 1987 in the number of reported cases in the subregions is shown in Table 2. Although reported cases from North America increased by 13%, several other subregions experienced much more dramatic increases, for example, 213% in the Southern Cone countries, 155% in the Latin Caribbean, and 117% in the Central American Isthmus.

This epidemic has been tracked by monitoring the total number of accumulated cases since 1981, but comparisons based on the total number of cases are not particularly useful because they do not take into account the size of the populations out of which the cases arise. A better method of comparison is provided by calculating the ratio of

Table 1. Cumulative reported AIDS cases and deaths for subregions and countries of the Americas, as of 30 September 1988.

Country/subregion	Cases	Deaths
Latin America[a]	9,569	3,309
Andean Area	746	332
Bolivia	8	6
Colombia	308	70
Ecuador	45	26
Peru	122	65
Venezuela	263	165
Southern Cone	339	187
Argentina	197	112
Chile	100	44
Paraguay	8	8
Uruguay	34	23
Brazil	4,153	1,902
Central American Isthmus	428	225
Belize	9	8
Costa Rica	79	39
El Salvador	43	16
Guatemala	46	36
Honduras	186	87
Nicaragua	1	0
Panama	64	39
Mexico	1,642	319
Latin Caribbean[b]	2,261	344
Cuba	34	8
Dominican Republic	566	59
Haiti	1,661	277
Caribbean	1,124	636
Anguilla	1	0
Antigua and Barbuda	3	2
Bahamas	236	116
Barbados	67	45
Cayman Islands	4	2
Dominica	6	6
French Guiana	113	78
Grenada	16	5
Guadeloupe	74	36
Guyana	40	19
Jamaica	72	44
Martinique	38	22
Montserrat	—	—
Netherlands Antilles	26	16
Saint Lucia	10	7
St. Kitts and Nevis	14	5
St. Vincent and the Grenadines	13	5
Suriname	11	11

Table 1. (*Continued*)

Country/subregion	Cases	Deaths
Trinidad and Tobago	336	206
Turks and Caicos Islands	5	3
Virgin Islands (UK)	—	—
Virgin Islands (US)	39	8
North America	79,141	44,429
Bermuda	92	71
Canada	2,156	1,189
United States of America[b]	76,893	43,169
Regional total	89,834	48,374

Source: Pan American Health Organization. AIDS Surveillance in the Americas. Health Situation and Trend Assessment Program, PAHO/WHO Global Program on AIDS in the Americas. Data through 30 September 1988, as received by 31 October 1988.
[a]French Guiana, Guyana, and Suriname included under Caribbean.
[b]Puerto Rico included under USA.

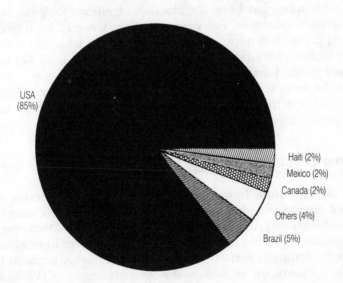

Figure 1. Distribution of reported AIDS cases, by country in the Americas, based on information as of 30 September 1988.

Table 2. Number of AIDS cases and ratios per million population in 1986 and 1987, with percentage increase.

	1986		1987		
Subregion/country	Cases	Cases per million pop.	Cases	Cases per million pop.	% increase
Latin America	1,807	4.5	3,337	8.1	80
Andean Area	111	1.3	246	2.9	123
Southern Cone	42	0.8	129	2.5	213
Brazil	844	6.1	1,574	11.1	82
Central American Isthmus	62	2.3	139	5.0	117
Mexico	440	5.4	451	5.4	0
Latin Caribbean	308	13.2	798	33.7	155
Caribbean	252	35.1	393	53.9	54
North America	15,886	59.5	18,111	67.2	13
Regional total	17,945	26.5	21,841	31.7	20

reported cases in a given calendar year to the median population estimates for that year. This ratio, shown in Table 2, reveals that prevalence is highest in North America, with 67.2 AIDS cases per million population, and that the non-Latin Caribbean area, with 53.9 cases per million in 1987, is second.

Even this subregional average obscures significant differences that exist between countries. For example, there were 11.1 AIDS cases reported per million population in 1987 in Brazil, while the ratios in French Guiana, Bermuda, and the Bahamas ranged from 240 to 400 cases per million inhabitants.

With the exception of Montserrat and the British Virgin Islands, AIDS cases, and thus evidence of the spread of HIV, have been found in all the countries and territories of the Americas.

Patterns of Transmission

Sexual transmission. Initially, AIDS cases in Latin America were reported among male homosexuals and bisexuals with a history of travel outside Latin America and the Caribbean. Sexual transmission among males continues to be the predominant pattern in most countries in the southern part of South America (Chile, Argentina, Uruguay, and Paraguay), as well as the Andean countries (Venezuela, Colombia, Ecuador, Peru, and Bolivia).

Seroprevalence studies of HIV in some groups of homosexual and bisexual men, most of them volunteers, have disclosed rates of infection of 8.3% in the Dominican Republic in 1986, 20% in Costa Rica in 1985–1986, 37.5% in Brazil in 1987, and 30.9% in Mexico in 1987. Although these rates are far below the very high rates (above 70%) of HIV infection found among some homosexual groups in some areas of the United States, the difference may only indicate the later introduction and spread of HIV infection among homosexual men in Latin American and Caribbean countries. Indeed, HIV prevalence rates found in prospective studies have risen from below 5% to 10–20% in some countries, such as Argentina and Uruguay.

The proportion of cases in which heterosexual transmission of HIV is implicated is still below 10% of all cases in most countries of Latin America. However, in the Caribbean and parts of Central America, significant numbers of AIDS cases and HIV infections in women are being detected. As an example, 24 cases of AIDS were diagnosed in Jamaica in 1987, of which 10 occurred in women.

Studies of HIV infection rates in female prostitutes have found rates ranging from zero in some studies in Mexico and Argentina to 49% in one limited study in Haiti.

Transmission associated with blood and blood products. In some countries, notably Costa Rica, Mexico, Brazil, and Jamaica, between 5% and 10% of all cases of AIDS are presumed to be secondary to blood transfusions. HIV antibody prevalence among blood donors is highly variable, ranging from 0.00% among 4,000 donors in Argentina and 0.1% in more than 1,400 blood samples tested in Barbados to as high as 1.6% in the Dominican Republic and 7.3% among some paid blood donors in high-risk areas of Mexico City.

The contribution of contaminated needles and syringes to the transmission of the AIDS virus among I.V. drug abusers appears to be less significant in Latin America than in the United States. Less than 1% of AIDS cases are believed to be associated with I.V. drug abuse in Latin America, as opposed to 17% in the USA.

Transmission in children. Cases of perinatal transmission in Latin America and the Caribbean have been few so far. For example, less than one-fifth of cases in infants and children have been associated with perinatal transmission in Brazil. In Mexico, 16% of cases occur in infants of infected mothers. However, limited studies in Haiti have found prevalences of HIV infection of 3% to 8% in pregnant women. The small number of reported cases in women and children may be related to the recent introduction of the virus into these two groups, as well as inadequate surveillance methods for identifying such cases.

The majority of cases in children outside the United States have thus far been associated with transfusion of blood and blood products, and in rare cases with sexual abuse and child prostitution. In contrast, more than 75% of pediatric cases in the United States can be traced to a parent with proven HIV infection or who engages in a high-risk behavior, principally I.V. drug abuse.

The Global AIDS Situation

As of 30 September 1988, 142 countries had reported 124,959 cases of AIDS to WHO's Global Program on AIDS (Table 3). As a result of underreporting and underdiagnosis, this total probably represents a two- to fourfold underestimate of the actual number of cases. Figure 2 illustrates the evolution of the epidemic, based on case reports, and the distribution of those cases by region.

In Europe, 28 countries have reported over 14,600 AIDS cases. The incidence rates per million population have been highest in France, Switzerland, and Denmark. WHO estimates that about 500,000 persons in Europe are infected with the AIDS virus, and that close to 20,000 cases of AIDS will have occurred there by the end of 1988.

The number of African countries reporting AIDS cases to WHO has increased substantially in the past year. In the most recent tabulation, 45 countries reported over 19,000 cases of AIDS.

So far, the number of cases reported from both Asia and Oceania has remained fairly low, with only two countries in Oceania (Australia and New Zealand) reporting substantial numbers of cases. Many of the Asian AIDS cases have been linked to persons who had visited areas where AIDS is more prevalent.

In Europe, Australia, and New Zealand, as in the Americas, most AIDS cases have occurred among homosexual and bisexual men and intravenous drug users between the ages of 20 and 49. The proportion of cases acquired through heterosexual contact in these areas is estimated at about 5%. In Africa, however, heterosexual transmission is a major factor in the spread of HIV, along with transfusion of unscreened blood and use of unsterilized needles or syringes. Perinatal transmission is also a significant problem in Africa. In some urban areas, HIV infection has been found in up to 20% of pregnant women.

Table 3. Cumulative reported AIDS cases for countries and regions worldwide, as of 30 September 1988.

Country/region	Number of cases
Africa	19,141
Algeria	13
Angola	65
Benin	15
Botswana	34
Burkina Faso	26
Burundi	1,408
Cameroon	53
Cape Verde	4
Central African Republic	432
Chad	7
Comoros	1
Congo	1,250
Côte d'Ivoire	250
Djibouti	—
Egypt	6
Equatorial Guinea	—
Ethiopia	54
Gabon	18
Gambia	52
Ghana	145
Guinea	10
Guinea-Bissau	29
Kenya	2,732
Lesotho	2
Liberia	2
Libyan Arab Jamahiriya	—
Madagascar	—
Malawi	2,586
Mali	29
Mauritania	—
Mauritius	1
Morocco	12
Mozambique	10
Niger	9
Nigeria	11
Reunion	3
Rwanda	987
Sao Tomé and Principe	1
Senegal	131
Seychelles	—
Sierra Leone	5
Somalia	—
South Africa	135

Table 3. (*Continued*)

Country/region	Number of cases
Sudan	68
Swaziland	14
Togo	2
Tunisia	21
Uganda	4,006
United Republic of Tanzania	3,055
Zaire	335
Zambia	993
Zimbabwe	119
Americas[a]	89,834
Asia	278
Afghanistan	—
Bahrain	—
Bangladesh	—
Bhutan	—
Brunei Darussalam	—
Burma	—
China	3
China (Province of Taiwan)	1
Cyprus	5
Democratic People's Republic of Korea	—
Democratic Yemen	—
Hong Kong	13
India	9
Indonesia	3
Iran (Islamic Republic of)	—
Iraq	—
Israel	65
Japan	90
Jordan	3
Kuwait	1
Lebanon	5
Malaysia	3
Maldives	—
Mongolia	—
Nepal	—
Oman	6
Pakistan	6
Philippines	15
Qatar	21
Republic of Korea	3
Singapore	4
Sri Lanka	1

[a]See Table 1 for country totals.

Table 3. (*Continued*)

Country/region	Number of cases
Syrian Arab Republic	4
Thailand	8
Turkey	9
Viet Nam	—
Yemen	—
Europe	14,623
Albania	—
Austria	202
Belgium	368
Bulgaria	3
Czechoslovakia	11
Denmark	301
Finland	32
France	4,211
German Democratic Republic	6
Germany, Federal Republic of	2,307
Greece	127
Hungary	13
Iceland	6
Ireland	49
Italy	2,233
Luxembourg	12
Malta	12
Monaco	1
Netherlands	573
Norway	90
Poland	3
Portugal	152
Romania	8
San Marino	—
Spain	1,471
Sweden	217
Switzerland	502
USSR	4
United Kingdom	1,669
Yugoslavia	40
Oceania	1,083
Australia	988
Cook Islands	—
Fiji	—
French Polynesia	1
Kiribati	—
Mariana Islands	—
New Caledonia and Dependencies	—

Table 3. (*Continued*)

Country/region	Number of cases
New Zealand	89
Papua New Guinea	4
Samoa	—
Solomon Islands	—
Tonga	1
Tuvalu	—
Vanuatu	—
World total	124,959

Source: World Health Organization. Acquired immunodeficiency syndrome (AIDS)—data as of 30 September 1988. *Wkly Epidemiol Rec* 63(41):309-310, 1988.

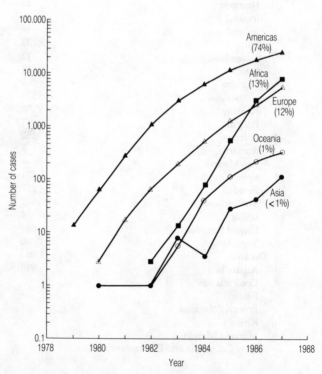

Figure 2. Reported cases of AIDS, by region, 1979-1987.

Outlook for the Future

In the coming years, the situation will get worse. The number of people infected with HIV is increasing, since transmission is still taking place. The vast majority of infected people will progress to disease. Thus, given the long period between infection and disease, the number of cases of AIDS will continue to increase for some time in spite of prevention efforts already underway.

This disease will have repercussions for the basic legal, moral, and religious principles of society. Its impact on health care services and the burden that caring for affected people will place on society will be enormous. In economic terms alone, the cost would be very high even if an effective preventive measure were found tomorrow. AIDS cannot be approached with a traditional vertical disease-control mentality. Community participation, full commitment on the part of the health sector and other sectors such as education and finance, and planning for the future will be essential to minimize the impact of AIDS on all societies.

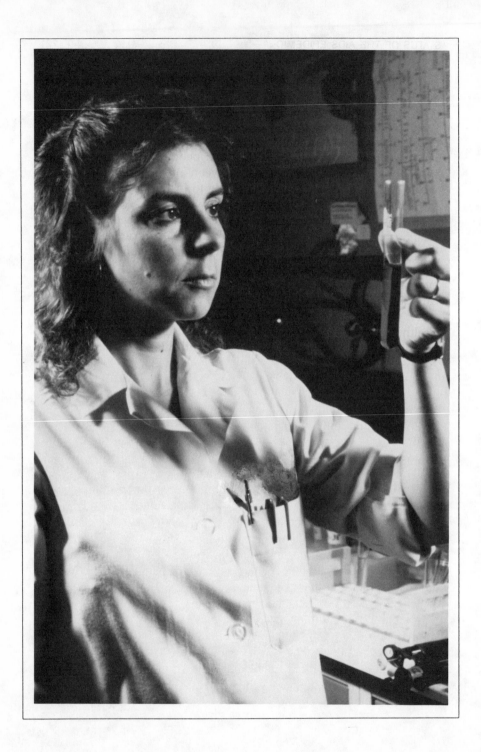

THE WORLD HEALTH ORGANIZATION'S GLOBAL PROGRAM ON AIDS

As many as 100 million persons may be infected with HIV by 1991. As many as three million new AIDS cases may occur between 1987 and 1991 among persons already infected by HIV in 1986. No vaccine will be available for widespread use. For each AIDS case, there may be up to 100 HIV-infected persons.

Even accepting that these projections are tentative and issued with great caution pending the collection and analysis of more worldwide epidemiological data, the numbers are still staggering. Without question, the epidemic of infection by HIV and related retroviruses is an international health problem of extraordinary scope that demands unprecedented and urgent global responses. The World Health Organization (WHO), fulfilling its constitutional mandate to direct and coordinate international health, has responded by establishing its Global Program on AIDS (GPA).

In late 1983, as soon as it became clear that AIDS was a worldwide health problem, WHO began to consider how it could best confront this epidemic. By early 1986, having determined that an AIDS program would be useful, a small unit was set up at the Organization's headquarters in Geneva. In May of that year, the World Health Assembly, in resolution WHA39.29, requested that the Director-General search for ways to increase the scope of the Organization's cooperation with its Member States and mobilize extrabudgetary resources for this purpose. In January 1987, the WHO Executive Board supported the priority granted by WHO to this global health problem by endorsing the strategy adopted for the then Special Program on AIDS. The Program was formally established on 1 February 1987, and during its short existence, it has amassed an impressive list of accomplishments: It has designed a global AIDS strategy, has raised funds to implement it, and has garnered the support of all nations.

The Program's goals, strategy, and activities, as well as its operational organization, reflect current knowledge of the HIV pandemic and are designed to reduce, and ultimately stop, the spread of the disease and to foster, gather, and exchange new information in order to better understand the epidemic, to accurately predict its course in the future, and to help develop new and better ways to fight it.

GPA has three goals—preventing new HIV infection; caring for those already infected, both medically and in terms of support and counseling; and harnessing all national and international efforts toward the struggle against AIDS. These goals are guided by two major thrusts: first, to support national AIDS prevention and control programs, and second, to provide global leadership and foster international cooperation and collaboration.

Since AIDS will not be stopped in any single country unless it is stopped in all countries, the Global Program's direct support to countries for establishing or strengthening national programs is critical to its global AIDS fight. WHO has designed a blueprint for such programs and provides both technical and financial support to countries throughout the world. To date, national AIDS committees have been established in more than 150 countries. Out of 136 countries that have requested collaboration, Global Program staff have visited 115, and the remaining 21 visits were scheduled for the third quarter of 1988. The Program also has completed more than 300 consultant missions which have resulted in 80 short-term (6–12 months) and 22 medium-term (3–5 years) national program plans; 31 additional countries are currently working toward medium-term plans. Throughout the world, national AIDS programs are being rapidly established with the Global Program's technical and financial support.

Support for national programs must be coupled with strong international leadership. So that the best information on AIDS can be shared worldwide, GPA collects and exchanges information on cases, on studies of virus infection, and on issues of social and behavioral practice. In collaboration with world-renowned scientists, the Program has generated guidelines and consensus statements on issues such as HIV and international travel and on screening criteria for HIV infection. A global AIDS data bank has been organized to allow for the vital exchange of information as the disease is tracked. In addition, the Program also has pursued joint efforts with other WHO units and programs, with United Nations agencies, with international finance agencies, and with nongovernmental organizations. Some of these efforts will investigate the economic and demographic impacts of AIDS, as well as modeling the epidemic to help predict its future course.

The Program's conceptual framework is embodied in six strategies: prevention of sexual transmission, prevention of transmission through blood, prevention of perinatal transmission, prevention of transmission from HIV-infected persons through use of therapeutic agents, prevention of HIV transmission through the development and delivery of vaccines, and reduction of the impact of HIV infection on individuals, groups, and societies. Epidemiological studies throughout the world have identified only three ways in which the HIV virus spreads from person to person—by sexual contact, whether heterosexual or homosexual; by parenteral contact with contaminated blood, blood products, or donated semen and organs; and from mother to child before, during, or shortly after birth. This information is invaluable because it shows how new HIV infections can be prevented; the first three strategies address this. Efforts to develop therapeutic agents to reduce or eliminate HIV in infected persons and, ideally, to develop a vaccine capable of protecting persons against HIV infection should be emphasized; the fourth and fifth strategies deal with this. Even though no vaccine seems possible for the near future, the first candidate AIDS vaccines have been prepared with unprecedented speed, and initial human studies are already under way. In addition, remarkable progress has been achieved toward treating AIDS with drugs such as zidovudine (AZT). Finally, the sixth strategy addresses what has been called by some "the third AIDS epidemic," the epidemic of economic, social, political, and cultural reaction to HIV infection and to its subsequent and inevitable progression to AIDS.

The Program is directly attached to the Office of the Director-General, and its operations are organized in seven major components: national program support; surveillance, forecasting, and assessment; health promotion; social and behavioral research; biomedical research; epidemiological support and research; and management, administration, and information.

The national program support component is charged with providing technical and financial support to Member States, in collaboration with Regional Offices, in the planning, design, implementation, strengthening, monitoring, and evaluation of all components of national AIDS prevention and control programs. The surveillance, forecasting, and assessment unit is responsible for collecting, analyzing, and disseminating data that will subsequently be used to assess the future impact of AIDS on health care systems, national economies, and demographic patterns.

The health promotion component develops, promotes, and helps design, implement, and evaluate health promotion efforts that use behavioral change strategies and communication techniques. This component has pursued joint educational efforts with other United Nations agencies as well as other governmental and nongovernmental organizations, has organized an exhibit, and has developed a brochure and poster with the message "AIDS: A worldwide effort will stop it." Other activities include the publication of a quarterly newsletter, *AIDS Health Promotion Exchange*, intended for health education professionals working in national AIDS prevention and control programs. This newsletter emphasizes the exchange of innovative ideas and reports on the results of health promotion programs. The Royal Tropical Institute in the Netherlands is collaborating with the Program to produce this publication.

Three organizational components—social and behavioral research, biomedical research, and epidemiological support and research—are charged with coordinating, promoting, and supporting research and development in their respective fields. Social and behavioral issues have been given special prominence, including questions such as perceptions of AIDS and responses to it, educational strategies to prevent AIDS transmission, and the disease's impact on demography and on social structures, especially families. A consultation convened in May 1987, which gathered 20 participants, including epidemiologists, psychologists, anthropologists, social demographers, and economists from 12 countries, identified four major research areas: high-risk behavior and situations, perception and knowledge in relation to behavior and risk, responses to epidemics—traditional and anticipated, and the effect on family life and social structures. The social and behavioral research unit of GPA has established multidisciplinary technical working groups to further develop a wide spectrum of research or training areas. Several institutions are also being assessed for designation as WHO collaborating centers in this area. The unit also has addressed such issues as sexual behavior and HIV transmission, prostitution and HIV transmission, and intravenous drug use and HIV infection. The Global Program has a unique potential to provide a global forum for the exchange and validation of technical information and expertise, and it can facilitate the development and improvement of diagnostic reagents and antiviral agents and vaccines, as well as their safe and ethical transfer to all countries in the world. Among other efforts, the biomedical research component has worked to coordinate vaccine development, to help assess and exchange reagents needed for biomedical research, to evaluate diagnostic assays for HIV infection, and to help develop new techniques for laboratory diagnosis of HIV infection.

In addition to these operational components, the Program counts on two important additional sources of support. A Global Commission on AIDS has been constituted, bringing together experts in health, social, economic, legal, ethical, and biomedical fields to review and interpret global trends and developments related to HIV and other human retrovirus infections; to conduct scientific, technical, and operational reviews and evaluations on the content and scope of the Program; to provide expert guidance for global activities; to advise WHO's Director-General on priorities in the Program's scientific and technical components; and to provide the Director-General with a continuous evaluation of the scientific and technical aspects of the Program. The other source of support rests on WHO's Collaborating Centers on AIDS. Support activities from these designated centers include assisting Member States in initial studies or surveys on AIDS; assisting countries to develop laboratory capabilities by providing technical expertise, training, and proficiency testing; providing reference materials and reagents; and conducting quality control for national reference laboratories. To date, there are collaborating centers in each of the six WHO Regions.

The following paragraphs highlight some of the Global Program's salient activities during 1987 and 1988.

World Summit of Ministers of Health on Programs for AIDS Prevention. WHO and the Government of the United Kingdom jointly organized the summit in London, in January 1988. The meeting, attended by 114 Ministers of Health, delegates from 148 Member States, and representatives of organizations within the United Nations system and from other intergovernmental and nongovernmental organizations, unanimously endorsed the "London Declaration on AIDS Prevention," which states that with no vaccine or cure for AIDS, "the single most important component of national AIDS programs is information and education. . . ." The summit declared 1988 a year of communication and cooperation about AIDS, and the Director-General announced that 1 December 1988 would be "World AIDS Day." (See pp. 361–365 in this volume for a report on the summit.)

WHO/United Nations Development Program (UNDP) alliance to combat AIDS. To ensure the best possible coordination among all those working to combat AIDS, to address the concerns of many countries about uncoordinated or inappropriate offers of external assistance, and to respond to the insistence of donor agencies for well-coordinated activities in countries as a prerequisite for their support, WHO's Director-General has completed negotiations with the Administrator of UNDP to combine the strengths of that agency and the Global Program on AIDS.

World Bank. The World Bank is collaborating with the Program in studies on the economic impact of AIDS in the developing world and on the demographic impact of AIDS. During the first quarter of 1988, the initial development phase was completed of a model for estimating direct-treatment costs and indirect costs from years of social and economic productivity lost due to HIV infections and AIDS.

Global Blood Safety Initiative. The Global Program on AIDS is coordinating a Global Blood Safety Initiative to safeguard blood from the possibility of serving as a vehicle for transmission of HIV and other viruses such as hepatitis. The initiative will soon be launched by a consortium of participants, including the Program, the WHO Health Laboratory Technology unit, the League of Red Cross and Red Crescent Societies, the International Society for Blood Transfusion, and the UNDP. This effort is based on the conviction that a long-term reduction in the transmission of diseases, including HIV infection, through blood can only be effectively achieved by establishing blood transfusion systems capable of implementing adequate quality-control measures, including screening, on a routine and sustained basis. UNDP has made a pledge of US$700,000 to the Program for the initial costs of this activity.

Criteria for screening programs for HIV infection. A meeting to consider the complexities of screening for HIV infection was convened by the Global Program in Geneva, in May 1987. Twenty-one participants from 17 countries attended the meeting, including epidemiologists, virologists, experts in legal medicine and ethics, social and behavioral scientists, and disease control specialists. The meeting developed a comprehensive list of criteria which should be closely observed in the planning of any HIV screening program. These criteria are designed to serve public health interests while protecting human rights.

WHO Collaborating Centers on AIDS. In June 1987, the third meeting of the collaborating centers was held in Washington, D.C., where three consensus statements were adopted on transmission of HIV, HIV infection and health workers, and present and future developments in laboratory testing for HIV. The collaborating centers have been working with the Program in training laboratory workers, preparing documents, evaluating test kits, and preparing and standardizing reagents and reference material. Several centers have provided technical support for epidemiological assessments in some African countries and the formulation of short-term plans of action.

Prevention of HIV transmission through injections. In July 1987, the Global Program convened a meeting within WHO on preventing HIV transmission through injections and other skin-piercing procedures. In a "note verbale" issued to all ministers of health in Member States, the Director-General recommended, among other things, that injections and other skin-piercing procedures be restricted to situations where there is no other alternative.

HIV and routine childhood immunization. To address concerns regarding immunization of children who are HIV infected, a consultation was jointly sponsored by the Global Program on AIDS and the Expanded Program on Immunization (EPI). The meeting, held in Geneva in August 1987, was attended by 13 participants from eight countries and included immunologists, virologists, disease control specialists, infectious disease specialists, and experts in immunization and epidemiology. Participants endorsed the recommendation of EPI's Global Advisory Group to immunize HIV-infected children with EPI antigens, except for those with clinical manifestations of AIDS, for whom BCG is to be avoided.

Prevention and control of AIDS in prisons. In November 1987, in Geneva, a consultation on prevention and control of AIDS in prisons was convened by the Program. The meeting developed a detailed consensus statement specifying that the general principles adopted by national AIDS programs should apply to prisons.

The struggle against AIDS in the future will, most assuredly, make increasing and more wide-ranging demands on individual countries. WHO's Global Program on AIDS has shown what can be done in a short time when individual countries' efforts are unified.

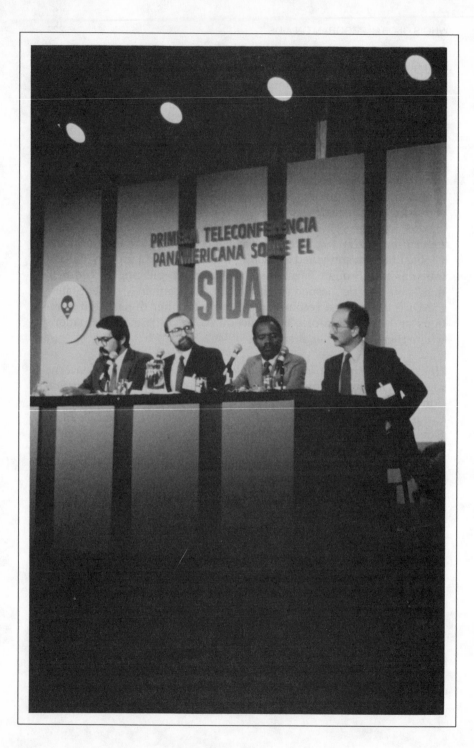

THE RESPONSE TO AIDS IN THE REGION OF THE AMERICAS

Even before the formal organization of the Global Program on AIDS (GPA) by the World Health Organization in early 1987, countries in the Americas were beginning to develop a wide variety of activities for the prevention and control of HIV infection and AIDS. In 1987 and 1988, the Pan American Health Organization (PAHO) collaborated with nearly all the countries in the Region of the Americas to consolidate those activities into national AIDS prevention and control programs. These programs, which can be differentiated into short-term programs (encompassing 6 to 12 months) and medium-term programs (covering 3 to 5 years), follow the general guidelines developed by WHO for AIDS prevention and control strategies. Every country in the Region now has at least a short-term program in operation, and PAHO is providing technical collaboration in the preparation of medium-term programs.

In addition to national plans, PAHO has collaborated with its Caribbean Epidemiology Center (CAREC) and WHO in a subregional AIDS prevention and control initiative for the Caribbean Area. In November 1987, a Caribbean-wide workshop was held to discuss and organize the preparation of a coordinated subregional approach,

Sources: Pan American Health Organization, Acquired Immunodeficiency Syndrome (AIDS) in the Americas (Document CD33/21 and Annex), Washington, D.C., 11 August 1988; *and* AIDS in the Americas, Presentation to the XXXIII Meeting of the Directing Council by Dr. Ronald St. John, Program Coordinator, Health Situation and Trend Assessment, Pan American Health Organization, Washington, D.C., 28 September 1988.

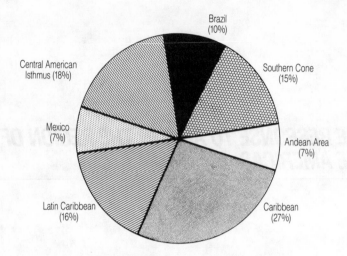

Figure 1. Distribution of funds allocated by PAHO/WHO to the countries for combating AIDS in the Americas, by subregion.

which potential donor agencies were invited to review. At a meeting of donors in October–November 1988 the countries were to present consolidated subregional medium-term plans in order to secure full financing for the period covered by those plans.

Informal evaluation of some of the early national plans revealed some problems. Even though initial funding was provided swiftly by WHO through PAHO, there were delays in fully utilizing the available funds in some countries, caused in some cases by lack of political will and in others by lack of installed capacity to deal with the problem. For example, many countries must set up new laboratory facilities, which requires significant lead time for personnel training and purchasing of supplies.

Funding

Initial funding for the rapid implementation of national activities was obtained from the GPA, and a total of US$6.99 million was distributed to 30 countries and CAREC during 1987–1988. An additional US$1.3 million was obtained for regional activities in support of national programs. Thus, of the total of US$8.3 million received, 84% was spent in support of national programs. The Caribbean Area received the largest proportion (27%), followed by Central America (18%) and the Latin Caribbean (16%) (Figure 1).

PAHO estimates that its requirement for both regional activities and support of country activities will be approximately US$35 to US$40 million over the period 1989–1991. An estimate of the total external and internal funding required for AIDS prevention and control is not possible at this time. So far, projections have concerned start-up costs, not longer-term funding needs. The countries have been asked to develop three-year plans indicating both their funding requirements and their commitments. PAHO recognizes the additional financial burden imposed by HIV infection on already strained budgets, but believes the countries must search for financial support of their national programs from local sources, in addition to depending on funds provided by WHO/PAHO.

Regional Support for National Programs

Like the other WHO Regional Offices, PAHO, as Regional Office for the Americas, executes regional activities for the control of AIDS. The objectives and strategies of the regional attack on AIDS are conceptually identical to WHO's global objectives and strategies. The PAHO Regional Program on AIDS provides technical assistance and financial support for the formulation and execution of national programs through a variety of activities.

Technical cooperation. PAHO is working to mobilize a staff of experts to manage the program and provide direct technical cooperation to Member Countries in support of the planning, execution, evaluation, and financing of national AIDS prevention and control programs. Although the GPA is centralized in Geneva, PAHO is responsible for the recruitment and selection of regional posts related to AIDS prevention and control. The staff will be assisted by a cadre of specially trained short-term consultants who have helped Member Countries in the development and refining of national AIDS programs and will be available to monitor and evaluate national and regional efforts to prevent AIDS.

Dissemination of information. The Regional Program has provided and will continue to provide the latest scientific literature to the staff and scientists of national programs to keep them up-to-date on epidemiological, biological, clinical, laboratory, and educational/behavioral aspects of AIDS and HIV infection. It has forwarded documents, policies, and statements developed by WHO through global consensus. In addition, PAHO produced "Guidelines for AIDS Prevention and Control," which has been reviewed, updated, and distributed to all the countries (see pp. 241–246 for a summary).

Major efforts have been made to distribute AIDS educational materials and information to the countries. Two AIDS information/education exchange centers have been set up, one at CAREC and the other in Mexico, and three other subregional centers, strategically located throughout the Region, are planned. The purpose of the centers is to collect, evaluate, and disseminate AIDS information and educational materials from as many countries as possible to assist other Member Countries in formulating their own AIDS education programs. The AIDS education effort must be innovative, and sharing of materials developed in a variety of settings by different countries will broaden perspectives and stimulate creativity. As countries develop specific educational messages which are acceptable to their cultures and particularly to high-risk population groups, a mechanism must be established for the exchange of these materials between countries, and existing facilities will be utilized as much as possible in this exchange. The Regional Program will provide financial and technical support to the subregional centers.

Another effort to promote AIDS education was the First Pan American Teleconference on AIDS, broadcast in September 1987 from Quito, Ecuador. The teleconference reached over 650 sites throughout the countries and territories of the Western Hemisphere. This initiative allowed approximately 45,000 health workers to participate in a PAHO/WHO technical scientific meeting (see pp. 247–264 in this volume). The Second Pan American Teleconference is scheduled to take place in Rio de Janeiro, Brazil, in December 1988. PAHO will sponsor other AIDS teleconferences as appropriate.

PAHO has participated in numerous national and international congresses, meetings, and workshops. It will continue to keep professionals throughout the Region informed of relevant scientific seminars and other forums. Periodic national and international meetings of persons involved not only in national AIDS programs but also in other health sector activities that feel the impact of AIDS, such as maternal and child health, blood banks, and human resources development, will be organized in order to share knowledge.

Research. Through a contract with the National Institute of Allergy and Infectious Diseases (NIAID), U.S. National Institutes of Health, PAHO is involved in research into the epidemiology of HIV and other retroviruses. This research, which will be done in collaboration with national scientists, will focus on four areas: seroprevalence of the infection in population groups at high, medium, and low risk; the natural history of the disease and its relationship to other endemic diseases; factors contributing to the heterosexual transmission of AIDS; and factors involved in perinatal transmission of AIDS. In the future, PAHO plans to expand its research efforts to include studies on the behavioral and social aspects of AIDS.

Training. Five international laboratory workshops have been held since early 1987 to disseminate AIDS laboratory technology to Member Countries. Although the Organization will continue to provide occasional international courses as the need arises, the Regional Program will direct its future support toward training done at the national level within the context of a country's AIDS prevention and control program. PAHO will provide short-term consultants and generic training materials.

Regional monitoring. PAHO will continue to monitor the AIDS situation through regional surveillance and to provide statistical and analytical support for the strengthening of national surveillance efforts, including standardization of case definition. PAHO is exploring coordination of an electronic AIDS information bulletin board and periodically will provide Member Countries with regional and subregional analyses of the AIDS situation. Monitoring with regard to AIDS also includes collaborating with Member Countries to evaluate national program progress on a periodic basis.

Regional coordination. The Regional Program on AIDS has established working relationships with the United States Agency for International Development, United Nations Children's Fund, World Bank, Inter-American Development Bank, International Planned Parenthood Federation, International Development Research Center, Canadian International Development Agency, and other major international organizations in the Region to coordinate hemisphere-wide activities as well as technical and financial support for national AIDS prevention and control programs. Through the development of an international AIDS commission, under PAHO leadership, the

Regional Program will continue to share information with other international organizations participating in the effort to stop the spread of AIDS. This commission will serve as a mechanism for coordinating international efforts and preventing duplication. In addition, international meetings will be organized to coordinate interprogrammatic activities within the health sector in support of AIDS prevention.

Goals of the Regional Program

Among PAHO targets in the fight against AIDS for the biennium 1988-1989 are the following:

- All countries will have national programs covering a minimum of three years for AIDS prevention and control. Those programs will be compatible with strategies for health for all by the year 2000 and primary health care, and will be fully integrated within national health systems.
- By the end of 1988, the programs of all countries that received initial funding from GPA will have been evaluated, and long-term financial needs and sources of funding will have been identified. Periodic re-evaluation of national programs will continue.
- By mid-1989, up to five subregional AIDS information/education exchange centers will have been established.
- By the end of 1989, AIDS research projects will have begun in at least 12 countries and a regional AIDS reference laboratory network will be fully operational.
- By the end of 1988, all blood products utilized by the public sector in all countries in the Region will be screened for HIV, and by the end of 1989, all blood and blood products utilized by all sectors in the Region will be screened for HIV.

Official Expressions of PAHO's AIDS Policy

The topic of AIDS was on the agenda at the meetings of PAHO's Governing Bodies in 1987 and 1988. The XXXII Meeting of the Directing Council in September 1987 and the XXXIII Meeting of the Directing Council in September 1988 each adopted a resolution expressing support for the policies and activities of the WHO Global Program on AIDS (previously known as the Special Program on AIDS), and urging specific action on the part of the Member Countries and the Organization in fighting the disease. The text of the resolutions is given below.

Resolution XII: Acquired Immunodeficiency Syndrome (AIDS) in the Americas

The XXXII Meeting of the Directing Council,

Having reviewed Document CD32/10 on acquired immunodeficiency syndrome (AIDS) in the Americas and Resolution WHA40.26 of the Fortieth World Health Assembly;

Recognizing that the AIDS epidemic presents an unprecedented immediate and long-term threat to public health in the Region of the Americas, requiring urgent, coordinated action;

Aware that, under these conditions, special efforts must be made to prevent and control the spread of the disease, yet concerned that these efforts reaffirm human dignity; protect human rights while stressing the social responsibilities of individuals; foster political commitment to health; strengthen health systems based on the primary care approach; and protect freedom of travel, interpersonal communication, and international commerce;

Fully supporting the global response to this problem which is being implemented through the WHO Special Program on AIDS, and recognizing its responsibilities as WHO Regional Committee for the Americas to review annually the situation in the Americas, to monitor the use of regional resources, and to report annually to the Director-General of WHO; and

Aware of the impact AIDS has on health services,

Resolves:

1. To urge Member Countries:
    (a) To develop, implement, and sustain strong national AIDS prevention and control programs along the model recommended by the WHO Special Program on AIDS, adapted to individual national contexts;
    (b) To strengthen national epidemiological surveillance activities in order to improve national programs;
    (c) To mobilize and coordinate the use of national and international resources for the prevention and control of AIDS

while assuring that national health systems are maintained and strengthened in order to combat this epidemic;

(d) To provide accurate information to their citizens about AIDS, strengthening health information through all mass media and health promotion activities, and promoting responsible, appropriate public action to reduce the transmission of the virus and to provide compassionate responses to those with the disease;

(e) To continue permitting freedom of international travel, without restrictions based on human immunodeficiency virus (HIV) infection status;

(f) To provide periodic situation and progress reports to PAHO/WHO, as requested;

(g) To make every effort to develop the Special Program on AIDS within the framework of the policy for health system development and strengthening, making use of the AIDS crisis to promote the needed changes in health services.

2. To request the Director, within available resources:

(a) To coordinate regional AIDS prevention and control activities with the global program in the establishment of a PAHO/WHO Special Program on AIDS;

(b) To provide urgently needed technical support to national AIDS prevention and control programs, including support for implementing, strengthening, and maintaining surveillance systems with appropriate laboratory support services; transmission prevention and control programs; health professional training programs; and research activities needed to define the epidemiology of AIDS;

(c) To develop AIDS control activities, especially those related to health care, together with the development and strengthening of health systems;

(d) To promote, coordinate, and conduct epidemiological studies and related research in order to support regional control efforts;

(e) To disseminate information to the Member Countries concerning technological advances in combating AIDS, epidemiological information about the regional situation, and other information vital for the conduct of national AIDS prevention and control programs;

(f) To develop mechanisms to facilitate the interinstitutional exchange of technical and resource information at the operational level;

(g) To provide annual reports on the regional situation and the use of regional resources to the WHO Regional Committee for the Americas;

(h) To take further steps as may be needed, within his authority, to combat this epidemic.

(Adopted at the seventh plenary session,
24 September 1987)

Resolution IX: Acquired Immunodeficiency Syndrome (AIDS) in the Americas

The XXXIII Meeting of the Directing Council,

Having reviewed the report on acquired immunodeficiency syndrome (AIDS) in the Americas (Document CD33/21);

Recalling Resolution CD32.R12, adopted by the XXXII Meeting of the Directing Council (1987), dealing with AIDS in the Americas, and Resolutions WHA40.26 and WHA41.24 dealing, respectively, with the global strategy for the prevention and control of AIDS and the avoidance of discrimination in relation to HIV-infected people and those with AIDS;

Considering that the AIDS pandemic continues to grow throughout the Region of the Americas, requiring a sustained commitment by every country to control the spread of the human immunodeficiency virus (HIV) and to mitigate the magnitude of the future impact of this disease on health services and national economies;

Recognizing the continued need for joint, coordinated international efforts to prevent and control this disease;

Cognizant of the need for WHO's global coordinating and promoting role through the Global Program on AIDS and the joint work carried out in the Region of the Americas by the Pan American Health Organization; and

Considering the profound impact the care of AIDS patients has on the already stretched national health services and health resources and the need for national AIDS programs and activities articulated with national plans for strengthening health and services,

Resolves:

1. To endorse the objectives, strategies, and targets for the Glo-

bal Program on AIDS in the Americas, as presented in Document CD33/21.

2. To urge Member Countries to:

(a) Make special voluntary contributions for the carrying out of catalytic research and cooperative activities in relation to AIDS in this Hemisphere;

(b) Make available to PAHO human and institutional resources to enable the Organization to better fulfill its mandates in this regard.

3. To request the Director of the PASB to:

(a) Continue to search for funds, in addition to those already approved in the PAHO/WHO regular program budget for the biennium 1988–1989, in support of the efforts of the Member Countries to carry out their short- and medium-term programs for AIDS prevention and control;

(b) Study the feasibility of establishing a revolving fund for the procurement of reagents, equipment, and other critical materials in support of the Member Countries for the implementation of their plans of action against AIDS.

(Adopted at the sixth plenary session,
28 September 1988)

• • •

Given the magnitude of the current and future impact of AIDS on health care services, current and future costs associated with the epidemic, and the current economic difficulties experienced by many countries, it is obvious that political and financial commitment by each and every country will be essential in order to deal with AIDS and attract external funds for AIDS prevention and control. Some countries are already beginning to feel the impact of AIDS on their health care delivery systems. Those countries which have yet to feel that impact must prepare for the inevitable consequences of a relatively broad epidemic of HIV infection. PAHO will continue in a united effort with its Member Countries in the fight to stop AIDS.

PAHO GUIDELINES FOR AIDS

These guidelines were originally prepared in 1985 by an ad hoc expert advisory group brought together by PAHO. The group, made up of scientists, epidemiologists, and disease control specialists from several of the Region's countries, met again in December 1986 to review and update the document. The current guidelines are a result of a subsequent review by the WHO Global Program on AIDS, and eventually will be replaced by guidelines prepared by that program.

The guidelines comprise an introduction and six sections, which deal with the development of national AIDS programs, recommendations for health care workers, prevention, psychosocial aspects, legal aspects, and the socioeconomic and health aspects of AIDS; four appendices contain additional information on AIDS. This abstract presents a condensed version of the section on recommendations for health care workers.

A condensed version of the original guidelines appeared in Spanish in the October 1986 *Boletín de la Oficina Sanitaria Panamericana*.

Source: Pan American Health Organization, Guidelines for Acquired Immunodeficiency Syndrome (AIDS), Washington, D.C., October 1987. A copy of the complete document can be obtained from the Pan American Health Organization, Health Situation and Trend Assessment Program, 525 23rd Street, N.W., Washington, D.C., 20037.

Recommendations for Health Care Workers

Since HIV infection and hepatitis B virus infection share a similar epidemiology—the modes of transmission for both viruses are by sexual contact, by parenteral exposure to contaminated blood or blood products, and from infected mother to child by exposure before, during, or shortly after birth—knowledge gathered about the risk of acquiring hepatitis B in the workplace can effectively be used to understand the risk of HIV transmission to health care workers.

Obviously, for health care workers, exposure to blood, blood products, other specimens, or blood-contaminated needles or instruments from persons at high risk for HIV infection presents a particular risk. However, it should be noted that several studies suggest that the actual risk of occupational transmission is very low, that even among thousands of health care workers with documented parenteral exposure to contaminated blood, only very few have had evidence of HIV seroconversion to date. Furthermore, transmission of HIV in the workplace by casual contact, contaminated food or water, insect vectors, or airborne routes has not been documented.

In any case, patient-care and laboratory personnel should take precautions to avoid bringing their skin and mucous membranes in direct contact with blood, blood products, excretions, secretions, and tissues of AIDS patients or persons likely to be infected with HIV. The precautions outlined below should be routinely enforced, as should other standard infection-control precautions—regardless of whether the HIV-infected person is a patient or a health care worker. All health care workers, including students and hospital staff, should be informed of these precautions and should also study the epidemiology, clinical manifestations, modes of transmission, and prevention of HIV infection. Finally, hospitals and laboratories should tailor these recommendations to their particular circumstances, implementing additional precautions if they consider it necessary.

Precautions Advised in Providing Hospital and Outpatient Clinic Care to HIV-Infected Patients

1. Care must be taken to prevent accidental wounds from sharp instruments such as needles, scalpels, and razor blades that have been contaminated with potentially infectious material and to avoid having open skin lesions come into contact with material from infected patients.

2. Disposable syringes and needles, scalpel blades, and other sharp instruments should be discarded in puncture-resistant containers placed within easy reach. To prevent punctures, needles should not be recapped, bent, broken, or removed from disposable syringes, or otherwise manipulated by hand.

3. Precautions should be taken whenever there is potential exposure to blood or other body fluids. When handling blood-soiled items or equipment contaminated with blood or other body fluids, gloves should be used. If the procedure involves more extensive contact with blood or potentially infected body fluids—for example, when performing certain dental or endoscopic procedures or postmortem examinations—gowns, masks, and eye coverings may also be required. If hands accidentally become contaminated with blood, they should be washed thoroughly.

4. Blood and other specimens should display prominent warning labels, such as "Blood Precautions," and if the outside of the container is visibly contaminated with blood, it should be cleaned with a disinfectant such as a 1:10 dilution of 5.25% sodium hypochlorite (household bleach) in cold water. When transporting blood specimens, they should be placed in a second container such as an impervious bag; this second container should be examined carefully for leaks or cracks.

5. Blood and body-fluid spills should be cleaned quickly with a disinfectant solution (see item 4).

6. Before reprocessing or disposing of articles contaminated with blood, they should be placed in impervious bags prominently labeled "Blood Precautions," or placed in plastic bags of a color that the hospital has designated exclusively for the disposal of infectious wastes.

7. Disposable items should be incinerated or autoclaved and discarded according to hospital policies; reusable items should be reprocessed according to hospital policies regarding items contaminated with hepatitis B virus; and instruments with lenses should be sterilized after use on infected patients.

8. Disposable syringes and needles are preferable; if reusable syringes are used, they should be sterilized before reprocessing. Only needle locking syringes or one-piece needle syringe units should be used to aspirate fluids from patients, so that collected fluid can be discharged safely through the needle when desired.

9. In most countries it is common practice to isolate any patient with a severe, undiagnosed infection in a single room. However, this practice, or special admission policies, are not recommended for HIV-

infected persons—including those with AIDS, except: (a) when a particular superinfection such as tuberculosis requires special isolation precautions; (b) when protective isolation is deemed necessary; (c) when maintaining hygiene standards becomes difficult, such as in circumstances when there is profuse diarrhea, fecal incontinence, uncontrolled bleeding, or altered behavior as a result of central nervous system involvement; and (d) when the severity or terminal nature of the illness requires care in a single room.

10. To avoid mouth-to-mouth contact during emergency resuscitation attempts, mouth pieces, resuscitation bags, or other ventilation devices should be strategically located.

Precautions Advised for Persons Performing Laboratory Tests or Studies

These precautions are intended for both clinical and research laboratories. Since clinical laboratories may not always have biological safety cabinets and other safety equipment, assistance should be sought from microbiology laboratories as needed, to assure that available containment facilities permit safe laboratory tests.

Guidelines for studies involving experimental animals inoculated with tissues or other potentially infectious materials from individuals with known or suspected HIV infection were published in 1982 by the Centers for Disease Control in volume 31 of their *Morbidity and Mortality Weekly Report*, pages 577–580.

1. Mechanical pipetting devices should be used to handle all liquids in the laboratory. Mouth pipetting should not be allowed.

2. Needles and syringes should be handled as stipulated above.

3. Laboratory coats, gowns, or uniforms should be worn while working with potentially infectious materials.

4. Gloves should be worn to avoid skin contact with blood, specimens containing blood, blood-contaminated items, body fluids, excretions, and secretions, as well as with surfaces, materials, and objects exposed to them.

5. Potentially infectious material should be processed and manipulated carefully to minimize creation of aerosols.

6. When conducting procedures likely to create aerosols, including centrifuging, blending, sonicating, vigorous mixing, and harvesting

infected tissues from animals or embryonated eggs, biological safety cabinets (Class I or II) and other primary containment devices such as centrifuge safety cups are recommended.

7. Since fluorescent activated cell sorters generate droplets that could result in aerosols, translucent plastic shielding should be used between the droplet collecting area and the equipment operator to reduce this risk. Primary containment devices should also be used in handling materials that might contain greater quantities of concentrated infectious agents or organisms than those expected in clinical specimens.

8. Following any spill of potentially infectious material and upon work completion, laboratory work surfaces should be cleaned with a disinfectant such as sodium hypochlorite (see item 4 in the previous section).

9. All potentially contaminated materials used in laboratory tests should be sterilized, preferably by autoclaving, before they are disposed of or reprocessed.

10. All personnel should wash their hands after removing protective clothing and before leaving the laboratory.

Precautions for Dental Care Personnel

1. Personnel should wear gloves, masks, and protective eyewear when performing dental procedures or oral surgery. Personnel should wash their hands before and after attending each patient.

2. Dental instruments used for a patient should be sterilized before reuse on another patient.

3. *Use and care of ultrasonic scalers, handpieces, and dental units.* Routine sterilization of handpieces is desirable between patients. However, given the configurations of most handpieces, not all lend themselves to high-level disinfection of both internal and external surfaces (see following paragraph). Therefore, when using handpieces that cannot be sterilized, the following cleaning and disinfection procedures should be conducted between each patient: After use, the handpiece should be flushed (see following paragraph) and then thoroughly scrubbed with a detergent and water to remove adherent material. Then it should be thoroughly wiped with an absorbent material saturated with a chemical germicide that is known to inactivate HIV virus and that is mycobactericidal at use-dilution.

This disinfecting solution should remain in contact with the handpiece for the time specified by the solution's manufacturer. Ultrasonic scalers and air/water syringes should also be treated this way between patients. After disinfection, any chemical residue should be rinsed off with sterile water.

Water retraction valves within dental units may aspirate infective materials into the handpiece and water line; therefore, check valves should be installed to reduce this risk. Even though the magnitude of this risk is unknown, it is prudent to run water-cooled handpieces and discharge the water into a sink or container for 20 to 30 seconds after completing care on each patient. This is designed to flush any patient material that may have been aspirated into the handpiece or water line. In addition, there is some evidence that shows that overnight bacterial accumulation can be significantly reduced by allowing water-cooled handpieces to run and to discharge water into a sink or container for several minutes at the beginning of the workday. Sterile saline or sterile water should be used as a coolant/irrigator when performing surgical procedures involving the cutting of bone or soft tissue.

Precautions for Operative and Obstetric Procedures

1. All health care workers who perform or assist in vaginal or cesarean deliveries must use appropriate barrier precautions, such as gloves and gowns, when handling the placenta or the infant until blood and amniotic fluid have been removed from the infant's skin.

2. Guidelines for HIV disinfection are sufficient and should be followed when disinfecting instruments (endoscopes, bronchoscopes, cytoscopes, fiberoptic scopes) used during invasive procedures in HIV-infected patients. When properly disinfected, these instruments can be safely reused in persons without HIV infection.

FIRST PAN AMERICAN TELECONFERENCE ON AIDS

The First Pan American Teleconference on AIDS took place in Quito, Ecuador, on 14–15 September 1987. An innovative approach to the traditional scientific meeting, it allowed an estimated 45,000 health-care workers at over 650 sites in Latin America and the Caribbean and at over 350 hospitals in the United States to hear presentations by some of the world's leading authorities on AIDS and to participate by posing questions to the experts.

The teleconference was organized by the Pan American Health Organization with technical assistance and support from the Miami Children's Hospital (Global Development Network) and Project Share (Satellites for Health and Rural Education) of International Telecommunications Satellites (INTELSAT), which carried 16 hours of the broadcast free to 30 countries. It was cosponsored by the World Health Organization, the Inter-American Development Bank, the U.S. Centers for Disease Control, the National Institute of Allergy and Infectious Diseases of the U.S. National Institutes of Health, the Latin American Union Against Sexually Transmitted Diseases, the Abbott Wellcome Group, and Electronucleonics Laboratories. The U.S. Agency for International Development also provided some financial assistance.

The objective of the two-day teleconference was to make available the latest scientific and technical information on AIDS to health professionals, researchers, and educators, as well as to decision-makers and the media. In recognition of the impact the media can have in supporting disease-prevention programs in general and the fight against AIDS in particular, press conferences were held at the end of each day. In addition, key speakers gave separate interviews with world media representatives. Because of the broad coverage afforded the teleconference by newspapers, radio, and television, it reached not only the thousands of people who viewed it directly but also millions of others who learned about it through the press.

With assistance from the Ecuadorian Institute of Telecommunications, the teleconference was transmitted live in four languages— English, Spanish, French, and Portuguese. Participants used portable earphones or radio receivers to hear the simultaneous translations. The teleconference consisted of four sessions, each of which included formal presentations, a round-table discussion, and a question-and-answer period during which viewers in the countries receiving the transmission could pose questions via satellite to the panel of experts in Quito. Multilingual volunteers manned the specially installed telephones to receive the questions, and a board of editors sorted them, translated them into the language of the speaker to whom they were directed, and gave them to the session's moderator for presentation to the speakers and the audience in Quito.

The teleconference was inaugurated by Dr. José Tohmé, Minister of Health of Ecuador, who welcomed the participants on behalf of President Febres Cordero. PAHO's Director, Dr. Carlyle Guerra de Macedo, emphasized in his opening remarks the commitment of PAHO and WHO to fighting AIDS everywhere by all available means. He announced that PAHO/WHO had received US$5 million to support AIDS research in Latin America and the Caribbean through a contract with the U.S. National Institutes of Health.

Dr. Ronald St. John, Coordinator of PAHO's Health Situation and Trends Assessment Program and Scientific Director of the Teleconference, was the moderator for the first session, which reviewed the epidemiology of AIDS in the Americas and around the world. During this session, Dr. Jonathan Mann, the Director of WHO's Global Program on AIDS, spoke of the precarious balance required between sounding an alarm against the spread of this lethal disease and voicing optimism that the profound changes needed to stop it can be made. He said that since AIDS is a disease spread by specific, identifiable actions, it is controllable and preventable by changes in human behavior. Presentations on AIDS in Africa and in the Americas followed.

The second session, which focused on virology and immunology, was moderated by Dr. Gloria Echeverría de Pérez of the WHO Collaborating Center on Clinical Immunology in Caracas. This session included overviews of HIV and related viruses, the immunology and pathogenesis of HIV infection, and the clinical spectrum of the infection. One speaker, Dr. Thomas Quinn of Johns Hopkins University, reviewed the natural history of HIV infection and transmission and cautioned that changing people's sexual behavior is not easy. Participants in the round table discussed the clinical and laboratory diagnosis of AIDS, testing methodology, surveillance, and case definition.

Dr. King Holmes of Harborview Medical Center in Seattle, Washington, was the moderator for the third session, on day two of the teleconference. This session addressed aspects of the management of AIDS and HIV infection such as the clinical management of AIDS patients and counseling and long-term care of individuals with AIDS and HIV infection. Also considered were prospects for AIDS prevention, treatment, and vaccine development. In the third round-table discussion, moderated by Dr. St. John, topics ranged from screening for HIV infection to the impact of AIDS on the strategy of health for all by the year 2000.

Dr. Kenneth Castro of the Centers for Disease Control moderated the teleconference's last session on prevention and control, during which presentations were heard on the AIDS education program in Brazil, the protection of blood supplies, training for health personnel who work with AIDS patients, and the psychosocial, ethical, and legal issues surrounding AIDS. The round-table discussion focused on global, national, and regional strategies for the prevention and control of AIDS.

Dr. Lydia Bond, Director of PAHO's AIDS Education, Information, and Counseling Program, introduced two PAHO-produced documentary films during the teleconference. The first dealt with innovative methods for teaching persons who engage in high-risk behaviors how to prevent the disease. The second film described mass AIDS-education campaigns in various countries and illustrated the diverse and sometimes unconventional approaches employed to improve communication about the spread of AIDS.

At the press conference following the last session, Dr. St. John closed the teleconference on a note of guarded optimism based on the enormous progress that has been made in understanding the disease in the few years since it became known.

To assist in evaluating the teleconference, participants were asked to fill out questionnaires. Of the 3,639 completed questionnaires received by PAHO, a sample of 1,211 was selected for analysis. Well over half of the respondents (63%) were physicians, and 18% were nurses. Two-thirds of the respondents had professional contact with

AIDS patients in either a health education, clinical, laboratory, research, or counseling setting. The topics in which participants indicated the greatest interest were epidemiology (27%), AIDS diagnosis (20%), virology and immunology (16%), prevention and control (10%), and public health aspects of AIDS (7%). Suggested improvements included providing better translations, improving the acoustics and transmission of the signal, giving daily summaries of the material presented, and examining some topics in greater depth. These recommendations will be taken into account in the organization of future teleconferences.

Since it was possible to answer only a fraction of the questions received during the question-and-answer periods, PAHO made a commitment to the audience to address others in a question-and-answer booklet on AIDS. In addition, PAHO will make available a series of videotapes based on the teleconference that will cover such topics as the virology and immunology of AIDS, prevention and control, and AIDS in children. Also included in the series will be tapes offering a general introduction to educational teleconferencing on AIDS and an overview of the First Pan American Teleconference.

Questions and Answers about AIDS

The following is a sample of the more than 600 questions that were received during the teleconference. Those questions were grouped and summarized in a document containing some 40 questions and answers. Taken together, they constitute a primer on such topics as the epidemiology of AIDS and human immunodeficiency virus (HIV) infection; current issues in the pathogenesis of HIV infection; the clinical picture of AIDS and its related disorders; present and future therapies; and social, ethical, and legal concerns regarding the spread of the AIDS virus. The responses were compiled from PAHO experts and from currently available information in the medical and scientific literature. The positions of the World Health Organization and Pan American Health Organization are presented when those organizations have made statements on the issue being reviewed.

Where did the AIDS virus originate?

The origin of the human immunodeficiency virus must remain a matter of speculation at the present time. The path of the virus through different geographic areas and populations can be retrospectively studied by serologic testing of banked blood. The accuracy of such work depends on the wide availability of well-preserved human sera that are free of potentially complicating cross-reactive agents. Based on these studies, with their inherent limitations, the earliest evidence of an infected human comes from serum collected in Central Africa in 1959. The prevalence of the virus in surrounding areas was very low until it began increasing in the mid- to late 1970s. Serologic evidence of the virus also began to appear in North America and Europe in the 1970s, with subsequent rapid increases in the prevalence of HIV infection in at-risk populations.

Regardless of the exact geographic location of the first identified case of HIV infection, it is likely that the virus had been present in some isolated human population for many generations. There is ample precedent for rare viruses that infect isolated groups of people but that are not found outside of those groups. Increased travel to and from a previously isolated area can serve as the bridge that allows rare pathogens to escape their confined location. This scenario seems probable in the case of HIV.

It is likely that HIV has infected humans for much longer than since the beginning of the present epidemic. In a series of studies, the RNA sequences of HIV-1 were compared with those of another related human retrovirus, HIV-2, and those of the monkey equivalent of HIV, simian immunodeficiency virus (SIV) to determine relatedness. These studies suggest that as the primates diverged evolutionarily, retro-viruses adapted to each respective branch may have also evolved from a common precursor. There is little reason to believe that HIV only recently entered the human population.

What is the relationship of HIV-2 to the AIDS virus?

A human retrovirus related to HIV-1 was first isolated from patients with an AIDS-like syndrome in West Africa. This second virus, now called HIV-2, has been conclusively linked to a clinical syndrome indistinguishable from AIDS caused by HIV-1. The routes of trans-mission of HIV-2 and its spectrum of disease are similar to those of HIV-1. Little is known, however, about the natural history of infection with HIV-2 and the rates of progression from an infected asympto-matic state to AIDS. Genetic studies suggest that HIV-2 occupies a position genetically intermediate between the simian immunodefi-ciency viruses and HIV-1. HIV-2 antigens cross-react inconsistently with HIV-1 antigens in commonly employed screening tests, which further indicates that HIV-1 and HIV-2 are related viruses.

AIDS caused by HIV-2 is a problem principally in West Africa. Occasional cases of infection with HIV-2 have been reported in Europe, and HIV-2 infection has been suspected in the Americas. A surveillance program for HIV-2 infection in the United States found no cases of infection in a study of over 22,000 individual sera, a preponderance of which were samples from individuals at risk for HIV-1 infection. Effective programs for control of HIV-1 transmission are also anticipated to control the spread of HIV-2.

Does the mutability of HIV present problems in developing a vaccine against the virus?

The genetic variability of HIV has been well documented. Virus isolates obtained from different infected individuals display a great degree of diversity, particularly in the composition of the envelope protein. Because the envelope is a principal antigen leading to the production of neutralizing antibodies in infected individuals, envelope diversity may explain the poor neutralizing activity of antisera raised against individual isolates when tested against other isolates. This diversity of HIV may present difficulties in establishing a common immunogen that could form the basis for a vaccine.

Which cells does HIV infect?

HIV has a selective tropism for cells bearing the CD4 phenotypic marker, which includes the principal target cell of HIV, the T4 lymphocyte. It has been shown that the CD4 marker serves as a receptor for the virus, and its presence on the cell surface is an absolute requirement for infection of human cells. Cells of macrophage/monocyte lineage that also bear the CD4 marker have been found to be infected with HIV in clinical specimens obtained from blood, brain, and various other organs. Despite the characteristic profound depletion of T4 lymphocytes in patients with AIDS, only about one in 100,000 peripheral blood lymphocytes show actual evidence of infection with HIV. The disparity between the devastating immune deficiency seen in AIDS and the very low levels of virus detected in patients remains an unexplained aspect of the pathogenesis of AIDS.

How can the virus be detected in *the individual*?

Culturing the virus from an individual is the definitive proof of infection with HIV. Research laboratories routinely culture the purpose of scientific study, but in clinical practice culture is rarely required to demonstrate infection with HIV. A number of serologic tests have been developed to indirectly detect the presence of the virus. The most commonly used tests are the enzyme immunoassay (EIA or ELISA) and the Western blot. Both of these tests employ disrupted virus particles as a substrate to demonstrate the presence of host antibodies directed against the various viral antigens.

The diagnostic tests passing the United States Food and Drug Administration's (FDA) stringent evaluation for licensing are very accurate (>99.0% sensitivity and specificity). The grave implications of a positive test result, however, have prompted the wide use of a tiered approach in testing for HIV to reduce the risk of false positive results. Initially positive EIA tests are repeated to reduce the risk of laboratory error. Two positive EIA tests are confirmed by the Western blot, a test that detects the presence of specific antibodies directed against individual HIV proteins. The criteria for a positive EIA result have been developed by the manufacturers of each test in extensive clinical evaluations before licensing. These criteria have been further evaluated by ongoing efforts to improve the sensitivity and specificity of the tests. It should be noted that not all EIA and Western blot tests on the market have the same diagnostic accuracy. The clinical validation of any unlicensed HIV diagnostic test kit should be evaluated prior to its use.

Western blot tests licensed by the FDA are also interpreted following the manufacturer's guidelines established through clinical testing. Current guidelines advise that a positive Western blot displays virus-specific bands in a pattern described by the test's manufacturer. Blots revealing the presence of bands that are insufficient to diagnose HIV infection are considered indeterminate; a test is usually scored negative only if no bands appear on the blot. Indeterminate tests are typically repeated at a later date if the clinical circumstances and history suggest an increased risk for HIV infection. The use of highly accurate EIA and Western blot tests in a tiered protocol can yield a false positive rate of only about one in 100,000 persons tested. In some countries, sensitive immunofluorescence techniques have been used in place of Western blotting to confirm a positive EIA result.

...inical manifestations shortly following infection ...us?

...onucleosis-like syndrome has been described in many but not ...patients after a presumed exposure to HIV with subsequent sero-...onversion. An estimated incubation period of three to six weeks precedes the development of an acute febrile illness lasting another two to three weeks. Fever is typically accompanied by chills, diarrhea, arthralgias, and myalgias. Patients commonly report headaches, which at times are associated with meningism. A characteristic maculopapular rash often occurs on the trunk for the duration of the acute illness.

Hematological abnormalities frequently include a mild leukopenia, lymphopenia, and a relative monocytosis. HIV has been isolated from both the cerebrospinal fluid (CSF) and blood at the time of the acute illness, which often presents as a lymphocytic meningitis. Serologic evidence of HIV infection is absent at the time of symptoms, but seroconversion reportedly occurs within two to three months after the illness. The few reports of initial seroconversion confirm the presence of antibodies against the core and envelope constituents of the virus; however, newer laboratory techniques have indicated the presence of viral antigen at the time of presentation and preceding the antibody response.

What is the minimum infective dose of HIV?

The minimum number of viral particles leading to a productive HIV infection that culminates in human disease is not known. Blood transfusion-related cases of AIDS provide indirect information about the circumstances surrounding single exposures that result in HIV infection. These cases prove that single exposures are sufficient to infect a host and ultimately produce AIDS. One study showed that once an infected donor gave blood that led to infection in a recipient, all subsequently donated blood was also infectious. Blood that was most likely to be infectious was donated by individuals who developed AIDS in the next 23 months. In contrast, health-care workers exposed to needlesticks from HIV-infected patients rarely develop HIV infection. The risk of infection from the small amounts of blood contained in a typical needle (approximately one microliter) is estimated to be less than 1%. It is likely, therefore, that a single inoculum of blood will result in infection only if it is sufficiently large and delivered parenterally.

The risk of infection through sexual transmission can only be estimated. Studies of long-term monogamous heterosexual partners of persons with AIDS have found that only two-thirds or less of the partners show signs of infection despite months to years of unprotected sexual activity. Studies in homosexual men have demonstrated that the likelihood of seropositivity rises with increasing numbers of different sex partners, but there has been no consistent correlation between seropositivity and the length of a relationship with a single partner or the number of sexual encounters with that partner. Perhaps genetic and environmental factors interact with differences in HIV strains to determine susceptibility in any given individual.

Are some individuals more likely to be infected with HIV than others?

The most important risk factors for infection are behaviors that allow an uninfected person to be exposed to an infected individual. Numerous investigations have attempted to identify genetic predispositions for infection when exposure to HIV takes place. Early reports identified plasma proteins called group components that seemed to confer relative resistance to HIV-1 infection; however, these reports remain unconfirmed in follow-up studies.

The lack of association between either the length of a sexual relationship or the number of exposures to a single individual and the risk for HIV seroconversion implies that other biological determinants may influence transmission during exposure to an infected individual. Some studies have shown a link between infection with other sexually transmitted diseases and risk of HIV infection, independent of the total number of sexual contacts. In addition, a history of genital ulcerative disease prior to HIV infection has been found in some groups studied. It is possible that lesions present in mucous membranes or skin at the time of an exposure to HIV increase the likelihood of infection.

Does the serologic response to the virus determine an individual's prognosis?

Researchers are attempting to identify a serologic pattern that characterizes the course of infection with HIV. Initial indications are that early in infection there is a burst of viral protein production that is followed by the development of antibodies against the different viral proteins. Concurrent with antibody production, viral antigen becomes undetectable in most assays. During this interval, patients are often asymptomatic, but virus can be isolated from their peripheral blood.

Before the appearance of clinical AIDS, core antibody levels fall and viral antigen once again becomes detectable. Envelope antibodies often remain at high levels for the duration of infection. Thus, it appears that a fall in core antibody titers associated with a rise in viral antigen levels is a marker for progression of HIV infection to AIDS. At present it is unclear if the core antibody titer falls because of a debilitated immune system, or if it falls because it binds increasing levels of antigen. While these preliminary studies are provocative, the exact relationship of serology to the natural history of HIV infection remains to be firmly established.

Variations in many other serologic and immunologic determinants during HIV infection have been examined with inconsistent results. One reproducible observation is the fall in T4 cell numbers before the appearance of AIDS. The decrease in T4 cells is associated with many immunologic abnormalities that are readily demonstrable in a clinical laboratory.

Have any factors been identified that hasten the course of HIV-related disease?

The long period of apparent viral inactivity after infection and before the development of AIDS or AIDS-related complex (ARC) has raised questions about the possible influence of cofactors on the progression of HIV-related disease. In an effort to identify agents implicated in promoting disease in infected individuals, several prospective studies have examined seropositive patients who went on to develop AIDS or ARC. One large study failed to identify factors that influenced the progression of disease in male homosexuals. Early hypotheses implicating cytomegalovirus and amyl nitrates as catalysts for the development of AIDS have not been confirmed, but pregnancy has been associated with an accelerated disease progression in women who are seropositive when pregnant.

Researchers have demonstrated that HIV has elaborate genetic controls that regulate reproduction of the virus and perhaps determine some of the clinical syndromes of AIDS. Immunologic activation of infected T-cells is known to induce HIV production in these cells, although the link of repeated antigenic stimuli to disease progression has not yet been conclusively demonstrated. Several different potential mechanisms by which agents might activate the virus are under study, but none has been clearly shown to serve as a cofactor.

Are babies born to HIV-infected mothers at risk for HIV infection?

The vast majority of children with AIDS have been born to a parent known to have AIDS or who is a member of a risk group for HIV infection. The isolation of HIV from umbilical cord blood, the presence of HIV in infants delivered by cesarean section, and the presence of a typical malformation in a series of HIV-infected infants show that infants can be infected with HIV in utero. The likelihood of infection in utero has been estimated in small studies to be from 40% to 50%. The small number of HIV-infected infants in the population relative to the number of child-bearing intravenous drug abusers supports these levels of transmission during pregnancy. Reports of mothers giving birth to uninfected infants following the birth of an infected sibling further confirm that in utero infection is unpredictable. Infection during delivery has yet to be demonstrated, but a few case reports of HIV infection linked to breast-feeding have identified breast milk as a potential route of virus transmission. The inactivation of HIV in breast milk by pasteurization or other means has not been described.

Do prisoners represent a high-risk group for HIV infection?

AIDS cases have been identified with increasing frequency in prisons in many countries. The number of HIV-infected prisoners usually reflects the prevalence of HIV in the community from which the prisoners came. The reasons for HIV infection in prisoners vary, but in many countries prison inmates often have a history of intravenous drug abuse or prostitution. In addition, situational homosexuality can occur in prison due to the unique conditions imposed by prolonged incarceration. Thus, prisoners may already be infected with HIV at the time of incarceration or they may become infected during their internment.

In an attempt to deal with HIV infection in prisons, the World Health Organization has developed general guidelines for prison officials and health authorities. Control and prevention of HIV infection are to be undertaken within the context of the need to improve the overall hygiene and health facilities of prisons. Prison officials should recognize their responsibility to minimize HIV transmission in prisons and thereby protect the general community from infection when prisoners are released. Prisoners should have the same right of access as other members of the community to educational programs designed to minimize the spread of the disease. Likewise, they should have access to confidential serologic testing for HIV infection with appropriate pre- and post-test counseling, access to appropriately trained medical personnel for patient services that are equivalent to those given to AIDS patients in the community at large, and access to information on treatment programs with the right to refuse such treatment.

Prisoners should not be subjected to discriminatory practices related to HIV infection or AIDS, including involuntary testing, segregation, or isolation, unless such action is required for the prisoner's own well-being. It is essential that all prison staff receive current information and education on AIDS as part of an effective HIV transmission prevention program. WHO has also recommended that prisoners with AIDS be considered for compassionate early release so that they may die in dignity and freedom.

WHO projects that HIV infection and cases of both AIDS and ARC will increase markedly in the next few years. In facing this problem, it notes that prison officials have the responsibility to ensure the safety of prisoners and staff and to minimize the transmission of HIV in prison. Because transmission of HIV may occur in prison through homosexual acts and intravenous drug abuse, officials are urged to implement education and drug-user rehabilitation programs. Careful consideration should be given to providing condoms in the interest of disease prevention.

What types of behavior or contact do not transmit the virus?

Casual contact of household members with AIDS patients is not associated with HIV transmission. Family contact of several years' duration, which included sharing beds, bathing facilities, toilets, kitchens, eating utensils, plates, and towels, has not been linked to a single case of HIV infection. Studies examining the contacts of AIDS patients note that transmission did not occur even though many of the patients were bathed, dressed, and fed by family members, the patients' clothes were put in the family wash, and family members routinely kissed the patients on the cheek and lips. Other studies have noted the lack of HIV transmission following bites inflicted by both infected adults and children. There are no data to suggest that HIV-infected patients pose a risk of transmitting the virus other than through sexual contact or through the exchange of blood. Accordingly, it is not recommended that authorities impose restrictive measures on HIV-infected patients or limit their nonsexual contact with others in efforts to control the spread of infection.

Have insects been implicated in the spread of HIV?

There is no evidence that biting insects can transmit HIV. The potential transmission of HIV by this route has been investigated in a variety of studies. Laboratory work shows that HIV cannot replicate or survive for prolonged periods of time in arthropods, and epidemiologic studies show that AIDS cases continue to cluster in young adults of reproductive age, with a relative absence of cases in the very young and the very old—age groups that are potential targets for biting insects. The most compelling evidence for a lack of HIV transmission by insects comes from southern Florida, where a detailed investigation in an area with a very high prevalence of AIDS revealed no association of AIDS cases with exposure to insects. Serologic studies to detect exposure to both arthropod-borne viruses and HIV documented no increased incidence of arthropod-borne viruses in HIV-infected compared to uninfected individuals. Also, careful follow-up of all AIDS cases in that area proved that the vast majority of patients came from well-recognized risk groups and that the age distribution of the infected persons did not include the non-sexually active age groups of children and the elderly.

What treatment has been shown to be effective against HIV in infected patients?

The genome of HIV encodes numerous structural and regulatory proteins that provide potential targets for pharmacologic intervention in the treatment of AIDS and its related disorders. Research and clinical trials have concentrated on identifying inhibitors of the viral enzyme reverse transcriptase. This enzyme catalyzes an essential step in the early stages of the reproduction of the virus. Although many agents are being investigated for their ability to interfere with this enzyme, the compound most thoroughly studied has been azidothymidine (AZT). This compound is an analogue of the thymidine that is normally incorporated into the viral RNA. The chemical modification in AZT (loss of the 3' hydroxyl group) prohibits the normal synthesis of viral DNA from the RNA template, and thereby is thought to inhibit replication of the virus.

In double-blind, placebo-controlled clinical studies performed on patients with advanced ARC or with AIDS manifested by recent *Pneumocystis carinii* infection, AZT decreased mortality and the frequency of opportunistic infections. In many patients receiving AZT there was also a transient improvement in T4 cell number and neurologic function. The drug produced numerous toxicities in the form of marked bone marrow suppression, headaches, myalgia, nausea, and insomnia. Despite the high cost of the drug and its significant toxicities, AZT is currently the most efficacious drug available for use in individuals with AIDS or ARC. Its place in the treatment of other stages of HIV infection remains to be established, and such studies are already underway. Other compounds, including dideoxycytidine (ddC), alpha interferon, ribavirin, and tumor necrosis factor, are being evaluated in clinical trials now in progress.

No curative therapy for individuals infected with HIV has been identified. In addition to current antiretroviral therapy, short-term gains in prolonging the life of AIDS patients will center around the development of drugs that effectively treat the debilitating opportunistic infections and malignancies that afflict these patients. Other therapeutic advances will come with a more complete understanding of the life cycle and gene function of HIV, which are currently under investigation in laboratories around the world.

What are the costs of caring for an AIDS patient?

Most published figures for the costs of caring for AIDS patients come from estimates made in the United States. The economic cost of the first 10,000 AIDS cases in the United States, when expenditures for hospitalization and economic losses from disability and premature death are combined, has been estimated at over US$4.8 billion. Of this total, about US$1.4 billion went for payment of expenses directly related to patient care.

Studies have consistently documented the high cost of caring for AIDS patients in the United States, even if the expense of the recently available antiretroviral drug AZT is not included. The studies have shown the costs per patient to range from over US$27,000 per year for inpatient care to over US$46,000 per year of combined inpatient and outpatient care. Innovative community-based programs that supplement hospital care and provide hospice services can decrease the costs of caring for AIDS patients. The actual price of medical care for AIDS patients will vary from country to country, but in no case will it be low. With increasing numbers of AIDS patients, the burden on health services will also increase and the availability of resources to address other health problems will be jeopardized.

Is there an effective prophylaxis against infection with HIV?

Mechanical and chemical barriers such as the condom and some spermicidal gels can provide protection against sexual transmission of the virus. Once the virus breaches these barriers and encounters infectable cells, no known factors—genetic or environmental—confer resistance to HIV infection in humans. Attempts to develop agents that can prevent infection after exposure to the virus have not been successful.

Drug trials currently center on altering the progression of HIV-related disease once infection has occurred. They have not systematically addressed the possible post-exposure protection against HIV provided by agents known to inhibit the virus. The role of immunoglobulins in development of passive protection after exposure has not been sufficiently studied. It has been noted, however, that neutralizing antibodies do occur in HIV-infected individuals, but they do not prevent the ultimate development of AIDS. Their ability to prevent primary infection has not been demonstrated.

What are the prospects for an effective vaccine against HIV?

An intensive search has been mounted to develop a vaccine against HIV. Initial efforts have centered on developing a vaccine based on the virus envelope, which presents the outer protein coat of the virus to the immune system in the absence of an intact infectious virus particle. In the United States and some countries in Africa, early trials have begun in order to assess the ability of these vaccines to promote an immunologic response without adverse side effects.

Several difficulties must be overcome before a safe and effective vaccine is developed. The inherent variability of the virus, especially of its envelope, will present obstacles to the development of a single vaccine that will give protection against all isolates. Additionally, it is likely that the virus is transmitted at least in part by cell-to-cell spread, which could make an antibody-based vaccine inefficient in preventing infection. Another difficulty will be the design and execution of trials to adequately demonstrate that a candidate vaccine is safe and effective. The long incubation period of HIV-related disease will require protracted studies to prove that a vaccine will protect against disease following exposure to the virus.

Should the activities of HIV-infected individuals be restricted?

The legalized sequestering of HIV-infected individuals may significantly deter these people from presenting themselves to health-care providers. Fear of punishment for HIV infection could cause infected persons not to seek medical help when appropriate, not to reveal their potential HIV infection, and not to participate in epidemiologic studies and preventive programs.

Unlike other communicable diseases that are readily spread from person to person, HIV is transmitted inefficiently and only through intimate contact. HIV is not spread by any form of casual contact, and its transmission can be interrupted by changing the behaviors that lead to its propagation. Uninfected individuals will not be at risk for infection unless they engage in sex with carriers of the virus or are exposed to the blood of these carriers. Adequate educational programs that inform the general public as well as at-risk and infected individuals of the mechanisms of HIV infection and that promote preventive behavior should greatly reduce the likelihood of transmission and spread of the virus.

Some countries provide for the detention of infected individuals who flagrantly ignore the risk that they pose to others and are thought to endanger the public significantly. Large-scale detention programs or quarantines have never been shown to reduce the spread of sexually transmitted diseases and are not likely to halt the spread of HIV. In a similar fashion, routine screening of travelers and the prohibition of HIV-seropositive persons from entry into a country is not thought to significantly reduce the introduction of the virus into new populations and is therefore not encouraged. Children who are infected with HIV need not be removed from the school system unless special circumstances such as poor personal hygiene or behavioral disorders are thought to pose a risk to others.

What evidence exists that an educational campaign can modify the risk of HIV transmission?

Programs that provide the public with basic information on AIDS and that describe behaviors known to transmit the virus are primary elements in controlling the AIDS epidemic. The homosexual communities of San Francisco and New York City, two areas with large and well-organized male homosexual populations severely affected by the epidemic, have carried out extensive educational campaigns to prevent the spread of the virus. These programs typically consisted of widespread community participation, the distribution of educational literature, face-to-face counseling, telephone hotlines, support groups, and broadcast media campaigns. Studies to assess the impact of education in these cities have documented a clear reduction in behaviors known to transmit the virus.

A homosexual cohort studied in San Francisco demonstrated a marked decrease in the number of nonsteady sex partners over a period of years, along with a reduction in the number of individuals practicing receptive anal intercourse. Condom use has also increased in some of the populations receiving the coordinated educational barrage. Studies in other cities also demonstrate a reduction in risk behaviors, although the extent of reduction and duration of effect varies from study to study.

Similar attempts to reach the drug-abusing population are underway in some areas. While European and North American studies show that many intravenous drug abusers are aware of the risk of HIV infection, there is scant evidence to indicate that there has been a significant reduction in needle and syringe sharing despite the high levels of awareness. The utility of needle sterilization programs or providing "clean" needles directly to the user is presently under study.

Research performed in the United States has shown that while the public believes that AIDS is the most serious health threat to that nation and while many people display a basic understanding of the illness, misconceptions about the modes of transmission remain widespread. A study of the impact of an advertising campaign about AIDS on a group of young heterosexuals found no change following the campaign in either the frequency of sexual contacts or the use of a condom. It thus appears that information is not enough, and that the intensity of informational efforts and the risk perceived by the population being addressed may influence the effectiveness of any educational program.

How can the fight against AIDS be funded in the Americas?

The AIDS problem in the Americas challenges national health care systems with already limited budgets to develop affordable approaches that will address a wide range of concerns. Any national or local AIDS program will require funding for public educational programs, patient care expenses, HIV screening, professional and technical training, and research and development initiatives. Other costs that are more difficult to cope with are the lost productivity of AIDS patients and the emotional trauma experienced by their friends and families.

Some of the financial burdens of caring for AIDS patients can be confronted by thoughtful community planning that addresses the long-range goal of reducing the number of infected individuals. Alternatives to expensive hospital-based care, including community support groups and hospices for AIDS patients, have been shown to reduce the cost of caring for terminally ill patients. In the absence of an efficacious vaccine or curative therapy, however, AIDS programs must center around prevention of new infections through targeted educational approaches and the screening of blood and blood products.

Financial and technical support for the establishment of national AIDS programs is being provided in part by funds raised by the World Health Organization. While this support is important to begin the fight against AIDS, additional funding and support from national and international sources in the respective countries will be required for operational and basic research to develop new preventive measures, treat infected patients, and develop educational services.

SEXUAL TRANSMISSION OF AIDS

Of the various ways in which HIV can be transmitted, sexual contact is responsible for the greatest proportion of infections. It was initially believed that homosexual males were the only group at risk, but cases of AIDS were soon described in men and women who had become infected via heterosexual contact.

Sexual transmission of HIV is associated with transfer of bodily products; according to the type of sexual contact, vaginal secretions, saliva, urine, semen, rectal mucus, feces, and blood may be transferred. Although HIV has been isolated from all these substances, the mere presence of the virus—for example, in saliva—does not necessarily imply that a substance is an important vehicle for transmission; up to now only blood and semen are known for certain to play that role. Vaginal secretions have been implicated in sexual transmission of HIV, but confirmation is still lacking (1).

Portals of Entry

Several studies have sought to determine the differences in transmission efficiency of different sexual practices and the portals of entry of

Source: Dirección General de Epidemiología, Secretaría de Salud, Mexico. Transmisión sexual. *Bol Mens SIDA* 2(1–2):231–241, 1988.

the virus. Transmission has been found to occur from male to male, male to female, and female to male, with the frequency of transmission varying for each combination.

Anal intercourse. Sexual contact involving penetration of the penis into the rectum carries the greatest risk of transmission of HIV (2). This fact is explained primarily by the nature of the rectal epithelium, which is a layer of simple columnar cells, is richly vascularized, and contains abundant unencapsulated lymphoid tissue. The epithelium is often damaged during rectal penetration, permitting contact between HIV and the cells that have specific receptors on their membranes (CD4 surface marker).

Vaginal intercourse. HIV transmission appears to be less efficient via vaginal coitus owing to the anatomic and physiologic characteristics of the vaginal mucosa, which consists of a flat, stratified, unkeratinized epithelium that provides more resistance to solutions in contact with it.

Although HIV may be present in the female genital tract throughout the entire menstrual cycle, the risk of infection for both the woman and her male partner probably increases during the menstrual period. Hormonal changes that affect the vaginal mucosa permit easier access of the virus to the bloodstream, increasing the possibility of infection for the woman, and contact with blood would pose a potential threat to the male (3).

There seems to be a higher risk of transmission from an infected male to a female rather than the reverse (1), which could be due to the higher concentration of virus in semen as opposed to vaginal secretions. Also, it is likely that sexual relations in which there is contact with the oral mucosa (oral-penile, oral-vaginal, and oral-anal) favor transmission of HIV, although the importance of this route has not been confirmed.

Contributing Factors

An association has been observed between transmission of HIV and some other microorganisms, among which are cytomegalovirus, herpesvirus, Epstein-Barr virus, hepatitis B virus, and the bacterial agents of other sexually transmitted diseases (STDs) such as gonorrhea, syphilis, and venereal lymphogranuloma. The interaction of these cofactors may be due to the fact that the virus multiplies more actively when the immune system is stimulated, as occurs when there are multiple infections, or to the genital lesions produced by these infections, which facilitate entry of HIV.

In addition, a history of infection with microorganisms that cause other sexually transmitted infections may be a sign of risk-generating behaviors, since it indicates greater exposure to such agents, including HIV. In a study by Handsfield et al. (4), there was a relationship between the presence of anti-HIV antibodies and genital ulcers even after adjustment for the number of sexual partners, which suggests that some STDs are in themselves risk factors for infection with HIV.

Exposure to HIV

The number of exposures necessary for sexual transmission of HIV to occur is still unknown. Cases attributable to just one exposure have been recorded, and it is known that the risk increases in direct proportion to the number of sexual contacts with one or more infected persons (2). The problems that arise in trying to determine precisely the relationship that exists between exposures and risk of infection are due to the multiple variables that must be taken into account, such as type of sexual practice, number of exposures, number of sexual partners, phase of the infection, and other risk factors.

In one study of male to female heterosexual transmission, based on the duration and frequency of sexual relations, the risk of acquiring the virus was estimated to be one in 1,000 (5). It has been more difficult to determine the risk of transmission of HIV from female to male, but one prospective study of spouses of AIDS victims found seroconversion in 42% of the men and 38% of the women within one to three years, which may indicate that the efficiency of transmission is similar in either direction (6).

Preventive Measures

Prevention of the sexual transmission of AIDS presents more problems than prevention of any other type of transmission, since it involves one of the most intimate and sensitive aspects of human behavior. As the means of transmission that is associated with the greatest number of cases, it is the one which must receive the most attention. Since there is not yet any effective vaccine or treatment available for AIDS, education and the modification of certain risky sexual behaviors constitute the only methods for preventing and controlling the disease.

Information and education campaigns and prevention programs must promote safer sexual practices, particularly among those persons who engage in high-risk or potentially risky behaviors. In this regard, it has been demonstrated that the risk of transmitting or acquiring HIV infection is substantially reduced by observation of the following general recommendations: a) limit sexual relations to only one partner or reduce the number of partners; b) avoid casual sexual relations; c) use a condom. The last of these recommendations has been widely publicized in educational campaigns the world over as an effective way to reduce the risk of the sexual transmission of AIDS. In addition, the use of certain spermicides, such as nonoxynol-9, has been suggested, since laboratory studies have shown that these substances inactivate not only HIV but also lymphocytes that contain it.

Finally, because evidence suggests that STDs facilitate transmission of HIV, it may be highly useful to incorporate programs of diagnosis and treatment of these infections into AIDS prevention programs.

References

1. Friedland, G. H., and R. S. Klein. Transmission of the human immunodeficiency virus. *N Eng J Med* 317:1125–1135, 1987.

2. Winkelstein, W., D. M. Lyman, N. Padian et al. Sexual practices and risk of infection by the human immunodeficiency virus: the San Francisco Men's Health Study. *JAMA* 257:321–325, 1987.

3. Vogt, M. W., D. J. Witt, D. E. Craven et al. Isolation patterns of the human immunodeficiency virus from cervical secretions during the menstrual cycle of women at risk for the acquired immunodeficiency syndrome. *Ann Intern Med* 106:380–382, 1987.

4. Handsfield, H. H., R. L. Ashley, A. M. Rompalo et al. Association of anogenital ulcer disease with human immunodeficiency virus infection in homosexual men. Paper presented at the III International Conference on AIDS, Washington, D.C., 1–5 June 1987. Book of Abstracts, Abstract F.1.6.

5. Padian, N., J. Wiley, and W. Winkelstein. Male-to-female transmission of human immunodeficiency virus (HIV): current results, infectivity rates, and San Francisco population seroprevalence estimates. Paper presented at the III International Conference on AIDS, Washington, D.C., 1–5 June 1987. Book of Abstracts, Abstract THP.48.

6. Fisehl, M. A., G. M. Dickinson, G. B. Scott et al. Evaluation of heterosexual partners, children, and household contacts of adults with AIDS. *JAMA* 257:640–644, 1987.

7. Feldblum, P. J., and M. J. Rosenberg. Spermicides and sexually transmitted diseases: new perspectives. *NC Med J* 47:569–572, 1986.

8. Hicks, D. R., L. S. Martin, J. P. Getchell et al. Inactivation of HTLV-III/LAV-infected cultures of normal human lymphocytes by nonoxynol-9 in vitro (letter). *Lancet* 2:1422–1423, 1985.

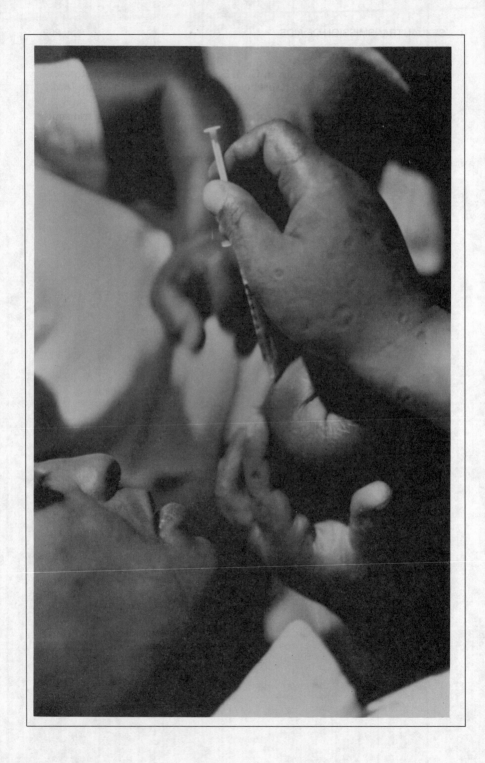

CRITERIA FOR HIV SCREENING PROGRAMS

Screening[1] for infection or disease indicators has undoubtedly bene-fited many public health programs, screened individuals, and the community at large—both when it has been used to detect treatable diseases which are otherwise difficult to recognize and also when it has been used to detect conditions for which there is no therapy. It is not surprising, then, that proposals for screening often arise in the context of the AIDS epidemic and of public health efforts to control its causative agents, human immunodeficiency virus (HIV) and related retroviruses.

Without question, the pandemic spread of HIV infection warrants close monitoring and public health planning. However, any HIV screening program raises delicate and difficult logistical, legal, techni-cal, personal, social, and ethical questions that must be addressed and resolved if the program is to be successful. Because of the restricted modes of HIV transmission, the privacy of the behavior

Source: World Health Organization. Report of the WHO Meeting on Criteria for HIV-Screening Programs, Geneva, 20–21 May 1987. Document WHO/SPA/GLO/87.2. Geneva, 1987.

[1]For the purpose of this report, HIV testing and screening are defined as follows: Testing is a serologic procedure for identifying HIV antibodies or antigens in an indi-vidual, whether recommended by a health care provider or requested by the individ-ual. Screening is the systematic application of HIV testing, whether voluntary or mandatory, to any or all of the following: entire population; selected target popula-tions; donors of blood or blood products and cells, tissues, and organs.

usually involved, and the current absence of any specific therapy, screening programs must be approached extremely carefully. Otherwise, these programs could be intrusive and costly, and could divert human, material, and financial resources from education programs that, to date, have been the most effective weapon against the spread of HIV.

To help ensure that these issues are systematically addressed whenever HIV screening is considered, the WHO Special (now Global) Program on AIDS convened a meeting on "Criteria for HIV Screening Programs" in Geneva, in May 1987. Twenty-one participants from 17 countries attended, including epidemiologists, virologists, experts in legal medicine and ethics, social and behavioral scientists, and disease control specialists. This report outlines criteria which should be considered in planning an HIV screening program, and points out areas that must be addressed before successful and effective public health outcomes can be achieved. Both public health and human rights will best be served by addressing these issues prior to implementing any HIV screening program.

Background

In response to the spread of HIV that the world has experienced during the 1980s, many authorities are considering or implementing programs to halt transmission of the virus. With neither a vaccine nor effective drug therapy in sight for the near future, these programs offer the greatest hope for halting the spread of the disease.

HIV transmission. Epidemiologic studies in Europe, the Americas, and Africa repeatedly have documented only three modes of HIV transmission: heterosexual or homosexual intercourse; contact with blood, blood products, or donated organs and semen (most cases of contact with blood involve transfusion of unscreened blood or the use of unsterilized syringes and needles); and from mother to child before, during, or shortly after birth. HIV is not transmitted by close but nonsexual contact or by food, water, air, or insect vectors. The documented routes of HIV transmission should be considered whenever public policies are developed; for this discussion, it is particularly important to keep in mind that HIV is not transmitted by casual contact with an infected person.

HIV infection. Almost all HIV-infected persons develop antibodies against the virus within a few months. Even though infected persons may appear healthy at the time of testing, laboratory studies have shown that the presence of antibodies indicates current and persistent HIV infection, and these infected persons can potentially transmit the virus to others by sexual contact or through blood by, say, sharing injection equipment. Infants born to HIV-infected mothers have passively acquired antibodies to HIV which may persist for up to one year; about 50% of these infants will themselves be infected, and their antibodies to HIV will persist indefinitely.

HIV serologic testing. Tests to detect antibodies to HIV have been available commercially since 1985, and they have been used for several different purposes. Most countries have first and primarily used them to screen donated blood and plasma and to discard units inadvertently collected from infected persons. Epidemiologists have used the tests to assess the prevalence and incidence of infection in different geographic areas and populations, as well as to better understand the infection's natural history. With this information, areas and groups which need to be targeted with specific educational programs and other prevention efforts can be determined. Health officials and physicians in some countries also have used these tests to help individuals determine whether they have been infected. This sort of testing should be coupled with individual counseling and education, so that persons at risk can reduce their own risk of infection or the risk of transmitting the infection to others.

HIV screening. Several testing and screening programs have been proposed, aimed at reaching as many HIV-infected persons as quickly and as thoroughly as possible. While a well-designed testing program might reduce the incidence of new HIV infections, some screening efforts may be sparked by unfounded concerns about casual transmission of HIV or by the need to appear to be actively fighting the HIV problem. The purposes and objectives of these programs have not always been clearly defined, and the practical, economic, and social costs of implementing them may not have been sufficiently examined.

If testing programs are to be effective, the major problem of disclosing personal information that may result in ostracism or discrimination must be carefully considered and resolved. Alternative approaches should be explored whenever the risks are too many, too great, or when they outweigh the benefits. Failure to do this may lead persons at high risk of infection to avoid testing and would ultimately result in counterproductive programs.

Criteria for Planning and Implementing HIV Screening Programs

What Is the Rationale of the Proposed Program?

The rationale and desired public health outcome of any proposed screening plan should be carefully articulated. Depending on the program's objectives, it should be determined from the outset what counseling and follow-up services will be provided to those who are to be identified and notified of their HIV antibody findings. Addressing social, legal, and ethical ramifications of screening and follow-up programs is a critical part of this assessment. A cost/benefit/risk analysis is also recommended at this initial stage.

Since there is no effective treatment for HIV infections, the public health rationale for HIV screening programs rests on the premise that identifying infected individuals will reduce HIV transmission; HIV screening programs also may help reduce the incidence of new HIV infections by reaching and counseling persons at risk. To do this, however, the type of voluntary or mandatory screening program to be used must both effectively identify persons at high risk of HIV infection and also motivate them to voluntarily change their high-risk behaviors.

Another public health objective is to obtain data on the pattern and prevalence of HIV infection, critical information in drawing up measures to slow the spread of HIV in a given area. Screening of total or selected populations in a newly involved area has been proposed as a way to monitor the silent, early spread of HIV and thus be able to implement specific control measures early on. Some countries have conducted this kind of epidemiologic surveillance by using samples previously collected for other purposes and which have been rendered anonymous.

Even after an HIV screening program is considered justified and necessary for prevention, the following criteria must be resolved before implementing the program. At each stage, the rationale and the possibility of achieving the goals of the program may need to be reconsidered in light of new information on costs, risks, and benefits. Furthermore, it must be borne in mind that screened individuals who are found uninfected but who continue to engage in high-risk behavior remain at risk—the screening program cannot identify persons who become infected after testing unless screening is repeated at intervals.

What Population Is To Be Screened?

Identifying and selecting the target population is a critical aspect of a successful screening program. Each of the following questions must be adequately answered before continuing to design the program.

- What population should be screened?
- What is the relative risk of HIV infection in this population?
- Is the proposed program voluntary or mandatory?
- Does the proposed program allow anonymity or does it require and plan to retain identifying information?
- Can the screening program readily reach the population?
- How will individuals in the target population be identified for screening?
- How will people be notified of the need or obligation to be tested?
- What sanctions would apply to persons failing to comply with obligatory testing?
- Can persons in the target population be reached through traditional medical care sources or is there need for a separate access system?
- Is the site for screening, including pre- and post-test counseling and/or specimen collection, suitable for the target population?
- What is the plan for confirming that a given test result applies to the person being informed?
- How will those already tested be identified?
- What plan has been made for periodic retesting of the screened population?

What Test Method Is To Be Used?

Since no single test, or series of tests, fits all circumstances, the chosen test methods should be tailored to the setting where they will be used. In choosing both primary screening and confirmation test systems, the technical nature of the test system, the availability and disposition of necessary resources, and the characteristics of the target population should be considered. Other, more specific aspects also should be considered in selecting a test or tests:

- Desired characteristics of the test(s), such as whether the test(s) should detect antigens or antibodies, HIV-1, HIV-2, or other related retroviruses; the type and source of test materials required.

- Technical aspects of the test(s), such as design of the test system, type and complexity of required equipment, time and laboratory space required, storage characteristics and stability of reagents, technical skill and training required by technicians.

- Support aspects of the test(s), such as source and reliability of test kits and reagents, stability or electrical source for electronic equipment, calibration requirements, spare parts and availability of service for special equipment.

- Interpretation characteristics of the test(s), such as sensitivity and specificity of the test(s) in the target population (these values and the prevalence of HIV infection in the population determine the predictive value of positive and negative test results).

- Quality control and proficiency evaluation systems to be established in the laboratory.

Whichever system is ultimately selected, there must be access to a regional reference laboratory resource that can evaluate and assess how appropriate assay systems are for the given setting or use, that can provide validation or confirmation testing, that can oversee quality control at screening centers, and that can train staff for local screening centers.

Where Is the Laboratory Testing To Be Done?

Implementing a screening program also will require that an appropriate site be determined for laboratory test facilities. Factors to be considered in making this decision include the scope of the program, its geographic extent, its duration, the percentage of the population to be screened, the existing distribution of technical and human resources, and supply constraints. In addition, the following issues need to be resolved:

- Is the screening test to be conducted where specimens are collected or at a laboratory away from this site?
- Is the test site under national or local government or under private jurisdiction?
- Will the screening tests be processed by a centralized laboratory or by multiple local laboratories?
- What laboratory sites will be used for supplemental tests?
- How will the proposed screening program affect existing laboratory functions?
- Are existing multipurpose serologic facilities suitable or will a separate new facility be needed?
- What safeguards will be taken in labeling and transporting specimens to retain both convenience and confidentiality?
- Are quality control systems for tests and procedures adequate?
- Who is responsible for testing costs?

How Will the Data Obtained from the Testing Be Used?

Since the social and personal consequences of known HIV seropositivity are so profound, exceptional care must be taken in handling laboratory and medical data from HIV testing. If the program has a surveillance function, the suitability of the data for demographic purposes must be assessed at the outset. In addition, the following questions must be resolved:

- What identifying information about screened persons will be collected and maintained with test records?
- How will an individual's data be recorded and how will the cumulative records from the screening program be managed and stored?
- Will the person tested have direct access to the test results and other recorded information?
- How will confidentiality be assured; what legal measures are available or can be introduced to assure it?

- Under what circumstances will persons other than the person tested be allowed to seek and obtain access to the data?

What Plan Will Be Used to Communicate Results to the Person Tested?

On being informed that they are HIV seropositive, persons often experience a profound psychological disturbance, particularly if they were unaware that they were being tested or if they are unprepared for the implications of positive test results. To offset the potential psychological damage, counseling should always be provided before HIV testing is conducted and HIV test results are communicated. Whenever possible, test results should be communicated in person by a trained counselor. In addition to the above-mentioned counseling, other factors to consider and resolve include the following:

- Who will communicate the information?
- At what stage in the screening and laboratory confirmation process will persons be contacted with results?
- If it is impossible to convey results in person, will the information be conveyed by telephone, by mail, or by some other means? Will this differ for positive and negative test results?
- What written record of test results, whether positive and negative, will be provided to the person tested?
- Other than the person tested, who will be informed of test results—physician, spouse, household members, sexual partners? Will program personnel decide this or does control rest with the person tested?

How Will Counseling Be Accomplished?

Counseling is so important that WHO held a separate consultation about it in May 1987. In countries or areas where there are no available counseling services, these need to be developed as soon as possible. It should also be considered that the magnitude of the epidemic has already stressed available counseling services in many countries, and that the demands created by a screening program may compete with those of other programs for scarce counseling personnel. Other considerations include:

- Who will conduct the counseling?
- How will counselors be trained and the adequacy of their performance be assured?
- Where will services be provided?
- How will confidentiality be achieved and maintained in the counseling setting?

What Is the Social Impact of Screening?

Even when test results are negative, the adverse social consequences of participating in a screening program can range from social isolation to economic losses, insurance cancellation, and restrictions in employment, schooling, housing, health care, and social services. These potential outcomes underlie the urgency of dealing with confidentiality and with informed consent prior to beginning testing.

What Legal and Ethical Considerations are Raised by the Proposed Screening Program?

Since HIV screening involves the collection of sensitive medical information, it could result in the infringement of a person's human and legal rights. Someone's right to privacy could be violated if information about HIV test results, or even about the fact that testing was sought or required, is disclosed without the person's authorization or without a clear public health benefit. Human rights are best respected by using the least intrusive measures to accomplish public health objectives. The following legal and ethical questions regarding HIV screening programs must be resolved:

- Is informed consent for the HIV screening test required?
- Are screening test results validated to ensure correct identification of a person with a positive test result?
- Are appropriate supplemental laboratory test procedures used to minimize false positive results that inevitably occur in screening

tests? Individuals falsely assumed to be seropositive may suffer severe and unjust consequences.

- Are there laws and regulations to safeguard against breaches of confidentiality or intentional disclosure of personal information not necessary for public health purposes?
- Will tested individuals be deprived of their legal or social rights?
- Are there laws or regulations to protect against discrimination in employment, housing, insurance, or health care and that provide redress for those who have suffered such discrimination?
- Will all personal identifying information be removed from specimens collected for other purposes before they are tested for HIV?

Conclusions

The meeting participants concluded that ready access to counseling and voluntary HIV antibody testing were more likely to contribute toward reducing the spread of HIV than were universal or targeted mandatory screening approaches. On the one hand, a single screening effort would yield only limited benefits, since screening alone does not result in behavioral changes that ultimately curb HIV transmission to others, and screening of targeted populations might not reach all persons at potential risk of infection, thereby becoming an inadequate public health measure.

The complex issues raised by mandatory screening efforts must be recognized and resolved. If epidemiologic data must be gathered, it should be obtained through methods that do not compromise human rights.

ARMING HEALTH WORKERS FOR THE AIDS CHALLENGE

DANIEL TARANTOLA

Patients with AIDS present health care personnel with a wide range of new problems in biology, therapy, and behavior. But more striking is that AIDS has led to the resurgence of older problems that did not seem to require specific solutions but now threaten to defeat us unless they are addressed. Health personnel—sometimes well-briefed, sometimes forced to interpret the facts for themselves, sometimes completely unequipped—are in the front line of the AIDS battle so far as both action and criticism are concerned, and in every country of the world they are eager for information, education, and support to enable them to meet the challenge posed by a disease that was unknown a few years ago but that today has become a fact of everyday life.

There are several reasons for this thirst for knowledge on the part of health personnel. One is a deep-seated desire to do more and do it better; another is the need to be able to answer questions asked by the public, by their elected representatives, and by the media. For health personnel to be able to perform all aspects of their jobs more effectively, they require easily and quickly obtainable information, appropriate training, and the necessary material and psychological support.

Source: Adapted from "Arming Health Workers for the AIDS Challenge," paper presented at the World Summit of Ministers of Health on Programs for AIDS Prevention, London, 26–28 January 1988.

Rapidly Available, Relevant, High-quality Information

One important characteristic of information about AIDS is its *quality*. The media are frequently criticized for inaccuracy, but they are constantly faced with the problem of confirming the reliability of the information they collect. Where AIDS is concerned, that information usually comes from someone working in the health services or from one of the many research centers, and it is not easy for representatives of the media to assess the source's mastery of his subject. Therefore, health personnel must be able to select good quality information and must act toward the media with competence and a sense of proportion when supplying it to them.

The second important aspect of information sought by health personnel is *relevance*. Recently, a large number and wide variety of AIDS publications intended for health workers have appeared: periodic bulletins, specialist journals, bibliographies, and articles published in professional journals. Information is becoming more and more comprehensive, but it is also becoming more complex and sometimes hard to grasp (AIDS is generating its own jargon). The mode or modes of access to relevant information must therefore be chosen carefully, either by the individual health worker or by someone else. In either case, the purpose of the information selected will be to equip health professionals with knowledge that allows them to carry out their duties more effectively and reliably and to provide the public and policy makers with accurate information.

The third crucial aspect of the information destined for health personnel is the *speed* with which it reaches them, and in this respect workers in the developing countries are at a great disadvantage. Long-distance data processing facilities, direct access to the best sources of information, personal participation in congresses and conferences, and the opportunity for everyday access to a wide range of media all enable the health personnel of industrialized countries to bring themselves rapidly up-to-date. Elsewhere, such opportunities are limited and communications problems can be enormous. Information produced in the country itself does not circulate properly, and several weeks or even months may be required for information from abroad to reach the health team in a rural area. Moreover, prohibitive prices or national restrictions on payments in foreign currencies may prevent staff from subscribing to international journals, so that often the information finally reaches those who desperately need it only when and if local journals publish an update.

Training Geared to Specific Tasks and to Problem-solving

Training, including refresher training, is another essential component of preparing health personnel to deal with AIDS. Since it is likely that in coming years no national health service employee or private practitioner will fail to be involved with AIDS in the course of his or her normal professional activities, the volume of training required is immense. The purpose of this training is not only to prepare staff of every category to perform technical tasks properly, but also to enable them to provide effective and appropriate psychological support for people who undergo a screening test, people found to be carrying HIV, patients with AIDS or related symptoms, and relatives of those patients. The training process must also include instruction on how to counsel people to avoid infection and on how health personnel can protect themselves against infection within their professional environment. Staff must also learn how to provide care to patients and virus carriers and how to motivate and support the infected individual in the battle he or she will have to wage against the disease and against the stigma and rejection that is society's reaction to it.

It is essential to focus the training of each category of health personnel on the specific tasks expected of them and on the particular problems they will have to deal with. In the health sector, the principle of knowing more in order to know better has been broadly accepted, and educators have often lost sight of the fact that knowledge is not an end in itself—it must be applied to performing tasks and solving very specific problems. The advent of AIDS has generated a great deal of knowledge and many new techniques, and it is the health sector's duty to reexamine its approach to staff training so that curricula do not become even more overloaded.

With the problem of AIDS being in the forefront of worldwide concern, health personnel have found themselves under the spotlight before an audience seeking information and guidance. Even though AIDS has dramatic social and behavioral, as well as medical, ramifications, the health services have played the dominant role in making the general public aware of the nature and extent of the AIDS problem, and in every country they are continuing to lay the groundwork for intersectoral mobilization to prevent and control the disease. This is a leadership role to which the health services are unaccustomed and for which in many cases they are poorly equipped.

In recent months, many health ministries have become unusually aggressive in reacting against their lack of resources, the undeserved label of being consumers rather than producers, and the low priority often given to health considerations within the national political context. The ministries have set up technical advisory committees on AIDS, expanded them to include representatives of other ministries, and managed to gain more attention from the highest government authorities. These changes have happened spontaneously, and in many cases the health services have been faced with a new and serious challenge: taking charge of intersectoral activities very much in the public eye and maintaining close cooperation and collaboration with other sectors that are better equipped and that generally wield more authority. There is an urgent need to provide health personnel who work at the national government, province or district, and community levels with training in the skills they require to carry out leadership and coordination duties, in order to maintain not only the professional dignity of those now responsible for this task but also the credibility of all the health services, public and private.

A final aspect of staff training concerns the need of health workers to learn how to get the community actively involved in prevention and control activities. AIDS came on the scene just when primary health care was successfully being transformed from concept into practice. The disease is daily rising higher on the list of health priorities everywhere in the world. Efforts to prevent its transmission must be concentrated where transmission takes place—in the community. The most affected countries, whether industrialized or developing, favor the idea of community support for AIDS patients, including home treatment with family backup and financial, emotional, social, and religious support. In some countries, the AIDS patient's return to the village will stimulate closer collaboration between health service personnel and traditional practitioners. Knowledge obtained by working to prevent and control AIDS in the community can also be applied to speeding up the implementation of primary health care.

Financial, Material, and Psychological Support

Health personnel must be provided with the necessary support to carry out their tasks. Such support is primarily of a practical nature. Intensive health education cannot be undertaken without the necessary structures, staff, and communication media. It is an expensive and difficult undertaking, and health education units are traditionally among the health services least well provided with human, material, and financial resources. In some national programs today, the budget for AIDS education is ten times the previous budget for all health education activities. This "shot in the arm" for a hitherto undersupported area of endeavor should have many favorable repercussions on health activities as a whole, provided that the sudden expansion is properly planned and that additional financial resources are allocated at the national or international level.

Material and technical support must also include the facilities necessary to detect the virus in donated blood and to sterilize medical and surgical equipment properly, so that health care procedures do not lead to virus transmission. Material and technical support also means providing staff with the equipment and supplies they need for their own protection. National programs in developing countries are having to cope with a dramatic increase in requests for supplies of gloves, reliable and unbreakable laboratory and sampling equipment, and protective clothing, necessitating additional financial resources. Stocking and distribution of supplies and replacement of equipment sometimes occasion major problems; on the positive side, the same precautions used against AIDS will produce substantial gains in the prevention of other viral diseases, especially hepatitis B.

There must be a legal framework as well as internal health service regulations to provide clear guidelines with respect to the rights of individuals and responsibilities of staff regarding such issues as screening for HIV, monitoring virus carriers, and treating patients. This legal and administrative framework provides essential backup for health workers faced with public opposition or hostility when carrying out their prevention and health care activities in the community. For many years, health legislation has received inadequate attention. The advent of AIDS calls for a special effort in this area.

Confronted by a health problem about which knowledge is still scanty, by patients—often very young—whose chances of survival are slim, and (in some communities, at least) by an excessive number of consultations and hospital admissions, health workers are daily exposed to severe psychological stress. It is becoming more and more difficult to persuade staff to remain in departments that see a lot of AIDS cases. Some such departments have granted their staff shorter working hours, others have introduced a system of staff rotation, and others have initiated group dynamics sessions at which staff can discuss problems they have with their patients and in their working environment. All these initiatives need to be followed up rigorously, for the physical and psychological stress to which health personnel are subjected creates conditions that prevent them from providing their patients with adequate support.

Prospects for Further Action

Public and private health organizations have already made significant contributions to the expansion of information available for use by health personnel. The World Health Organization has published a periodic bulletin (*Update on AIDS*), disseminated epidemiological and technical data in the *Weekly Epidemiological Record*, and produced and distributed technical documents on various aspects of AIDS control, such as guidelines for planning national programs and reports on HIV screening criteria (see pp. 271–280), new retroviruses, and international travel. Many other reports are being prepared. The WHO Division of Public Information and Education for Health, strengthened with staff expressly assigned to the Global Program on AIDS, has collected a large quantity of audiovisual material produced in different parts of the world that can be used to develop other materials properly suited to local situations.

Great use has already been made of radio and television to pass on information to the general public and to health personnel in particular. WHO is at present establishing a system that will enable a worldwide user network to have access to an AIDS data bank. Users of the network will need only an ordinary microcomputer connected to a telephone line.

As for training, numerous courses, workshops, and conferences on AIDS have been held during the last few years. These activities have been concerned with varied aspects of AIDS control, ranging from the serological diagnosis of the infection and its clinical and psychological management to information and education. WHO has brought together over 150 specialists in briefing seminars for consultants employed by the Global Program. Two seminars of that type were held in Geneva and one in Australia, during which the consultants who carried out over 300 missions in various parts of the world between February and December 1987 were briefed. Other seminars are being held in 1988 in the Region of the Americas, the African Region, and the Eastern Mediterranean Region. Guides are being prepared for trainers of various categories of personnel who work in health and other sectors.

Although WHO recognizes the advantages of an international exchange of participants in training activities, the Global Program is concentrating its efforts on individual countries. Once the trainers themselves have received thorough training, the specific social and cultural features of national AIDS control programs and the need to train large numbers of people make it essential that training take place in the participants' own environments.

The Global Program on AIDS furnished large-scale support to countries in 1987, allotting to national programs almost US$18 million, or about two-thirds of its total budget. A large proportion of these funds was devoted to strengthening the structures, educational activities, and equipment of the national programs. For 1988, a sum of US$50 million is committed for country activities, and an increasing proportion of national budgets is being assigned to AIDS control by the countries themselves.

The efforts begun so far must be sustained. Provision of information, training, and effective support must be commensurate with the size of the AIDS problem and will require long-term, worldwide mobilization.

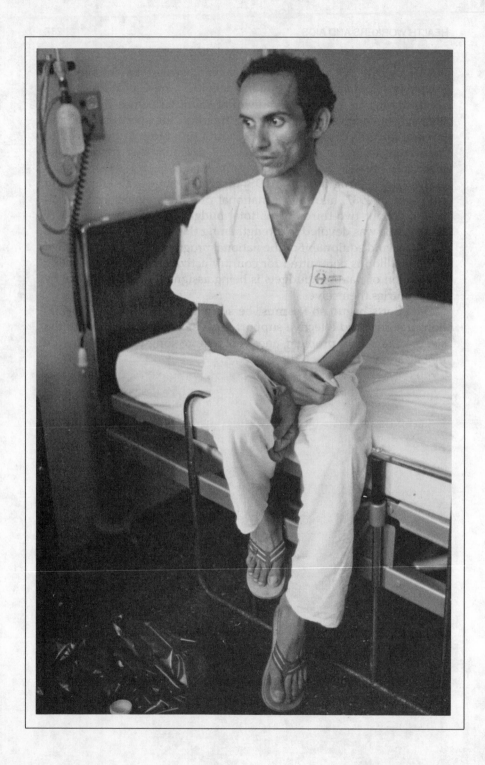

AIDS AND THE WORKPLACE

Human immunodeficiency virus infection and the acquired immuno-deficiency syndrome represent an urgent worldwide problem with broad social, cultural, economic, political, ethical, and legal dimensions and impact.

National and international AIDS prevention and control efforts have called upon the entire range of health and social services. In this process, in many countries HIV/AIDS prevention and control problems and efforts have highlighted the weaknesses, inequities, and imbalances in existing health and social systems. Therefore, in combatting AIDS, an opportunity exists to reexamine and evaluate existing systems as well as assumptions and relationships.

Today there are 2.3 billion economically active people in the world. The workplace plays a central role in the lives of people everywhere. A consideration of HIV/AIDS and the workplace will strengthen the capacity to deal effectively with the problem of HIV/AIDS at the local, national, and international levels.

In addition, concern about the spread of HIV/AIDS provides an opportunity to reexamine the workplace environment. It provides workers, employers and their organizations, and, where appropriate, governmental agencies and other organizations with an opportunity to create an atmosphere conducive to caring for and promoting the

Source: World Health Organization. AIDS and the workplace: consensus statement from the WHO Consultation in association with the International Labor Organization (ILO), Geneva, 27–29 June 1988. *Weekly Epidemiological Record* 63:217–224, 1988.

health of all workers. This may involve a range of issues, and concerns not only individual behavior but also matters of collective responsibility. It provides an opportunity to reexamine working relationships in a way that promotes human rights and dignity, ensures freedom from discrimination and stigmatization, and improves working practices and procedures.

Background

Epidemiologic studies from throughout the world have demonstrated that HIV is transmitted in only three ways: (a) through sexual intercourse (including artificial insemination with semen from an infected donor); (b) through blood (principally blood transfusion and nonsterile injection equipment; also, organ or tissue transplants); (c) from infected mother to infant (perinatal transmission).

There is no evidence to suggest that HIV transmission involves insects, food, water, sneezing, coughing, toilets, urine, swimming pools, sweat, tears, shared eating and drinking utensils, or other items such as clothing or telephones. There is no evidence to suggest that HIV can be transmitted by casual, person-to-person contact in any setting.

HIV infection and AIDS are global problems. At any point in time, the majority of HIV-infected persons are healthy; over time, they may develop AIDS or other HIV-related conditions or they may remain healthy. It is estimated that approximately 90% of the 5–10 million HIV-infected persons worldwide are in the economically productive age group. Therefore, it is natural that questions are asked about the implications of HIV/AIDS for the workplace.

In the vast majority of occupations and occupational settings, work does not involve a risk of acquiring or transmitting HIV between workers, from worker to client, or from client to worker. This document deals with workers who are employed in these occupations. Another consultation to be organized by the WHO Global Program on AIDS will consider those occupations or occupational situations, such as health work, in which a recognized risk of acquiring or transmitting HIV may occur.

The purpose of this document is to provide guidance for persons considering issues raised by HIV/AIDS in relation to the workplace.

Such consideration may involve review of existing health policies or development of new ones. This document focuses upon the basic principles and core components of policies regarding HIV/AIDS and the workplace.

By addressing these issues, workers, employers, and governments will be able to contribute actively to local, national, and international efforts to prevent and control AIDS, in accordance with WHO's Global AIDS Strategy.

Policy

Protection of the human rights and dignity of HIV-infected persons, including persons with AIDS, is essential to the prevention and control of HIV/AIDS. Workers with HIV infection who are healthy should be treated the same as any other worker. Workers with HIV-related illness, including AIDS, should be treated the same as any other worker with an illness.

Most people with HIV/AIDS want to continue working, which enhances their physical and mental well-being, and they should be entitled to do so. They should be enabled to contribute their creativity and productivity in a supportive occupational setting.

The World Health Assembly resolution (WHA41.24) entitled "Avoidance of discrimination in relation to HIV-infected people and people with AIDS" urges Member States:

> "(1) to foster a spirit of understanding and compassion for HIV-infected people and people with AIDS . . .;
>
> "(2) to protect the human rights and dignity of HIV-infected people and people with AIDS . . . and to avoid discriminatory action against, and stigmatization of them in the provision of services, employment, and travel;
>
> "(3) to ensure the confidentiality of HIV testing and to promote the availability of confidential counseling and other support services . . . ."

The approach taken to HIV/AIDS in regard to the workplace must take into account the existing social and legal context, as well as national health policies and the Global AIDS Strategy.

Policy Development and Implementation

Consistent policies and procedures should be developed at national and enterprise levels through consultations between workers, employers and their organizations, and, where appropriate, governmental agencies and other organizations. It is recommended that such policies be developed and implemented before HIV-related questions arise in the workplace.

Policy development and implementation is a dynamic process, not a static event. Therefore, HIV/AIDS workplace policies should be (a) communicated to all concerned, (b) continually reviewed in the light of epidemiologic and other scientific information, (c) monitored for successful implementation, and (d) evaluated for effectiveness.

Policy Regarding Persons Applying for Employment

Pre-employment HIV/AIDS screening as part of the assessment of fitness to work is unnecessary and should not be required. Screening of this kind refers to direct methods (HIV testing) or indirect methods (assessment of risk behaviors) or to questions about HIV tests already taken. Pre-employment HIV/AIDS screening for insurance or other purposes raises serious concerns about discrimination and merits close and further scrutiny.

Policy Regarding Persons in Employment

1. *HIV/AIDS screening:* HIV/AIDS screening, whether direct (HIV testing), indirect (assessment of risk behaviors), or by means of questions about tests already taken, should not be required.

2. *Confidentiality:* Confidentiality regarding all medical information, including HIV/AIDS status, must be maintained.

3. *Informing the employer:* There should be no obligation of the employee to inform the employer regarding his or her HIV/AIDS status.

4. *Protection of employee:* Persons in the workplace affected by, or perceived to be affected by HIV/AIDS, must be protected from stigmatization and discrimination by co-workers, unions, employers, or clients. Information and education are essential to maintain the climate of mutual understanding necessary to ensure this protection.

5. *Access to services for employees:* Employees and their families should have access to information and educational programs on HIV/ AIDS, as well as to relevant counseling and appropriate referral.

6. *Benefits:* HIV-infected employees should not be discriminated against nor denied standard social security benefits or occupation benefits.

7. *Reasonable changes in working arrangements:* HIV infection by itself is not associated with any limitation in fitness to work. If fitness to work is impaired by HIV-related illness, reasonable alternative working arrangements should be made.

8. *Continuation of employment relationship:* HIV infection is not a cause for termination of employment. As with many other illnesses, persons with HIV-related illnesses should be able to work as long as medically fit for available, appropriate work.

9. *First aid:* In any situation requiring first aid in the workplace, precautions need to be taken to reduce the risk of transmitting blood-borne infections, including hepatitis B. These standard precautions will be equally effective against HIV transmission.

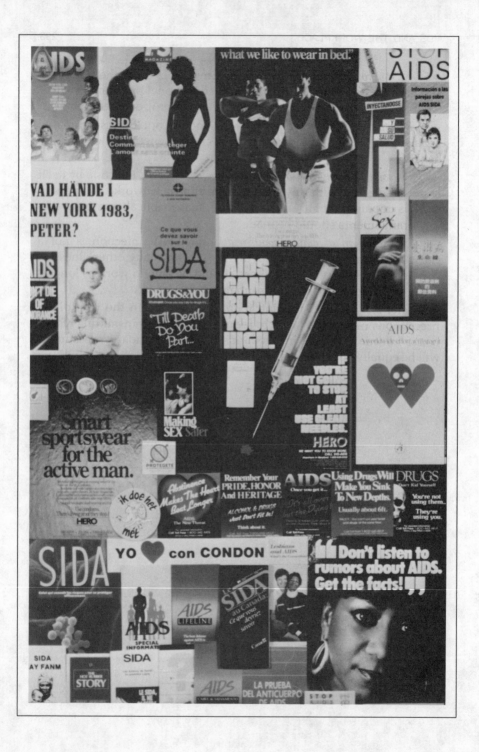

AIDS PREVENTION THROUGH HEALTH PROMOTION: A PLANNING GUIDE

Health promotion can be broadly defined as the systematic attempt to positively influence the specific health practices of large numbers of people by using principles and methods adapted from mass communication, instructional design, health education, social marketing, behavioral analysis, anthropology, and related public health and social sciences. It begins with assessment of the problem, it targets specific actions, and it then develops an action plan that is implemented, monitored, and modified to meet changing conditions. Health promotion is based on the belief that people often behave in ways that seem contrary to what is best for them—but that they have reasons for doing so. Health promotors have the obligation to avoid blaming people for engaging in unhealthy or high-risk behavior, to understand why they choose such behavior, and to develop systems that will encourage voluntary change.

The World Health Organization's Global Program on AIDS is producing a series of publications on health promotion to prevent AIDS. One volume of the WHO Health Promotion Guide is addressed to members of national AIDS committees (NAC) worldwide who plan, implement, and evaluate health promotion activities to prevent the spread of HIV infection. The guide provides a step-by-step review of the major elements and procedures of health promotion. It outlines an approach to selecting the strategies, techniques, personnel, and skills needed to reach the general public and to encourage changes in high-risk practices among specific audiences.

The guide is divided into four chapters that describe the four elements of the health promotion planning process. Chapter One, "Pre-program Assessment," considers what information is needed to develop the Health Promotion Plan, how the community-based information is best collected, and how community-based research techniques are best managed. Chapter Two, "Planning," explains how a health promotion strategy is selected, what behaviors and audiences are targeted for change, and how the targeted changes are best accomplished. In Chapter Three, "Implementation," the practical considerations for implementing an AIDS health promotion plan and the multiple channels and resources used to achieve the targeted changes are discussed. Chapter Four, "Monitoring," deals with what program aspects require monitoring and what community-based methods are most appropriate for effective monitoring.

The guide is not meant to be a textbook but rather an annotated checklist designed to give experienced health educators and communications professionals a comprehensive overview of AIDS prevention through health promotion. What follows is a summary of the information presented in the guide.

Pre-program Assessment

Pre-program assessment is the collection of broad-based information on the disease, the audiences, and the communication channels for the purpose of planning health promotion programs. In order to take the appropriate health promotion actions, solid facts are needed about the AIDS problem—its epidemiology, the natural course of the disease, its psychological impact—and the resources available to solve it. Without assessment, health promoters are dependent upon rumors, hunches, and personal judgment.

An AIDS prevention program requires background information in at least seven areas: (1) the local epidemiology of AIDS, (2) the public image of AIDS, (3) high-risk behaviors, (4) institutional and community resources, (5) service and product availability, (6) communication channels, and (7) anticipated obstacles and constraints. These questions can be answered by either rapid or in-depth assessment techniques. Rapid assessment is the collection of community-based information on the problem, audiences, and channels in order to develop an initial health promotion plan. Some information is collected relating to all seven questions, and the program gets underway quickly. In-depth assessment uses more rigorous sampling techniques involving larger study groups and assesses changes over a longer period of time. In-depth assessment provides more complete and reliable information on a broader range of topics.

All health promotion assessment methods, whether rapid or in-depth, rely on practical community-based information. Theoretical, laboratory, and academic research is not directly relevant to most program planning. Listed below are some of the most common community-based assessment techniques. Different methods that are appropriate for different phases of the assessment and different information needs include the following:

Community surveys—Information is collected on a particular population's knowledge, attitude, and/or self-reported behavior, using formal interviews with a large sample of persons chosen to represent the population. Survey research is most valuable when the information gathered is well-defined and the questions are focused and specific.

Intercept interviews—This form of survey research uses a physical location as the means of selecting respondents. Interviewers are stationed at points frequented by the target audience, and the questions usually take only a few minutes to answer. Intercept interviews can yield a large number of responses in a reasonably short time. They can be a cost-effective means of gathering quantitative data.

Audits—A quantitative inventory is performed to determine if products and services are available. Checklists and simple questionnaires are used to collect standardized information from distribution points in the system, and obstacles to distribution are identified by observation and questioning.

Literature and archival search—Existing written material on the selected topic is reviewed, including clinical and epidemiological studies; media studies; general market research on similar target audiences and products; demographic, health and nutrition, and contraceptive surveys; medical services records; and commercial sales and distribution records.

In-depth individual interviews—Open-ended and probing questions are used to explore an individual's attitudes, knowledge, and reported behavior. These interviews often require lengthy sessions ranging from 20 minutes to two hours.

Focus group interviews—In these interviews, open-ended and probing questions are addressed to homogeneous groups of individuals to explore their attitudes, knowledge, and reported behavior.

Ethnographies—In-depth studies are done of the behavioral environment into which a given health practice will fit. Ethnographies are useful in determining how other cultural aspects can be used to support a new health practice and to avoid cultural taboos.

Observation studies—Trained observers, using checklists and guides, record and analyze behaviors that occur in the natural environment. Observation studies can be useful in determining how widespread a practice or product is, and whether the materials needed to support the practice are in place.

Product and concept testing—These studies can provide information on the probable acceptance of products or concepts by the target audience.

Pilot tests and test markets—A strategy is applied to a small but representative group of the target audience.

Pricing studies—These studies are used to determine what the optimal price for a given product should be, by means of interviews and test markets.

Selection of assessment methods is important. Research is no better than the quality and usefulness of the questions asked. Time should be invested in deciding what information is needed and how it will be used. The best research design includes a variety of community-based methods, since combinations of qualitative and quantitative methods answer broader questions and give more reliable information. Poorly done research can be more harmful than no research at all, since it can give a planner confidence to proceed in the wrong direction.

Community-based assessment techniques require a wide range of staff skills. Quantitative techniques, such as sample surveys and intercepts, require experience in large-scale data management. Qualitative techniques, such as focus groups, in-depth interviewing, and ethnographies, require questioning skills and the ability to probe the meaning of responses. Community-based techniques such as store audits, pricing studies, product tests, and observation studies require practical field experience and keen observation skills. Experience in carrying out, for example, a large sample survey does not qualify an individual to conduct focus groups.

In summarizing and reporting results, it is important to keep findings focused and relevant to specific issues around which the planning process must operate. Some of the most important assessment results will include information on the local epidemiology of AIDS, public attitudes toward AIDS, service and product availability, and the communications infrastructure.

Planning for Health Promotion

Health promotion planning is the process of organizing and sequencing activities to achieve specific health promotion goals. The plan should establish goals for specific audiences. It must describe the messages, concepts, services, and products to be made available. It should list key benefits the audience will perceive as important and show convincingly how these benefits will be presented. The principal channels that will be used to deliver the messages, services, and products must be identified, and the schedule and budget necessary to implement the plan must be outlined.

The written plan need not be lengthy. It should reflect the findings of the pre-program assessment, describe what is being proposed, and relate proposals to the overall AIDS program. It should be organized around the answers to key questions:

- Goals: How will health promotion help reduce HIV transmission? How do health promotion goals relate to the overall goals of the national AIDS program?
- Situation summary: How can the data be summarized to provide the clearest picture of the status of AIDS and HIV infection in the country?
- Target audience: Who, specifically, must change their behaviors in order to reduce HIV transmission?
- Objectives: What specific attitudes, knowledge, and behaviors are to be changed? To what degree? Over what period of time?
- Key benefit: What benefit will the audience recognize as most attractive?
- Support: What evidence will make the program's messages believable to a specific audience?
- Tone: What creative approach will make these messages compelling and convincing to the audience?
- Channels: Which media and instructional networks can reach the audience effectively?

- Materials and logistics: What materials and logistical support (such as condoms, training programs, and travel resources) are needed to achieve program objectives?
- Monitoring: What aspects of the plan will be evaluated to determine if program elements are in place and operating as planned?
- Budget and timeline: How can this plan be accomplished within a given budget and period of time?
- Summary strategy statement: What combination of approaches will best suit particular situations, audiences, and objectives?

The strategy statements should be clear and concise and should encapsulate the plan of action for each significant target audience. Together, the strategy statements form the structure of the national program. A comprehensive national program may include a number of different audience-specific strategy statements.

Implementation

Implementation is the process of putting the health promotion plan in action. It means producing, testing, and distributing the products, materials, messages, and services outlined in the health promotion plan, and includes five tasks.

- Identify the producers and suppliers: Define who will draw the posters, record the radio and TV programs, prepare the curriculum, train the trainers, and so forth.
- Create draft materials: Describe how the training will be structured, what images and words will be used, and who will be the spokespersons in TV ads.
- Pretest and rehearse: Determine how materials and training designs will be tested to ensure that they work for the specific audiences.
- Produce the materials: Select who will do the printing, record the radio and TV programs, and conduct the training workshops.
- Diffuse and distribute: Determine who will deliver and use the flyers, air the radio and TV programs, and provide the face-to-face training and counseling.

People with skills in training, counseling, community organization, and oral presentation are the human contact points for AIDS prevention. Interpersonal programs provide critical face-to-face contact. These programs influence the target audience, develop skills, and provide support, and each of these desired results requires people with slightly different abilities. These persons need educational support and appropriate training.

Health service providers have a crucial role to play in AIDS prevention. Because they are perceived as reliable sources of information, what they tell people about AIDS has special importance. Counseling infected individuals may be difficult for some health workers, and training programs to teach counseling techniques as well as AIDS information, may be needed.

Television spots, radio interviews, posters, flyers, and banners are just a few of the many materials that can by used in health promotion. Creative talent to design the materials must be lined up, and the materials produced must be pretested, finalized, and then distributed. Wise distribution is critical to the success of the program. Technical experts in broadcasting may be needed to advise on distribution plans.

Monitoring

Even well-conceived plans can encounter problems; for example, slogans that seemed clear to planners may confuse the intended audience, posters may never reach distribution points, radio spots targeted at one audience may inadvertently offend another audience segment. Monitoring—the regular measurement of progress during a health promotion intervention—is the means to detect problems in concept or execution so that they can be corrected.

The first monitoring task is to decide what to measure. Many health promotion programs can be evaluated by asking the following six questions:

- Has the target audience been exposed to the message?
- Do they understand it?
- Do they believe or accept it?
- Did they act on it /apply it correctly?

- Have they incorporated it as a routine at appropriate times?
- Has any health benefit resulted?

Monitoring uses many of the same community-based techniques as pre-program assessment, but applies them while a program is underway to determine whether significant problems are occurring during implementation. Like pre-program assessment, monitoring works best when several techniques are used at the same time.

Short questionnaires can be administered at key locations to collect reliable data on a narrow spectrum of information. Small-scale behavioral studies based on observations can help determine whether self-reported data are reliable. Actual behavioral change is frequently difficult to monitor, though some behavioral change is subject to measurement (for example, through tracking of condom sales). In-depth interviewing may be necessary to find out about other types of behavioral change. These studies can be costly to conduct and often can be used for evaluation purposes as well as monitoring.

Results from monitoring can be a powerful tool to attract public attention, foster public support, and influence decision-makers. The news media are generally eager to report new information about AIDS and progress towards AIDS prevention. Results of a health promotion campaign that demonstrate changes in public knowledge, attitudes, and behavior are important news stories. A particular health promotion piece—such as a song or television ad—can become a news item itself if monitoring shows that it was heard or viewed by millions.

A second important by-product of monitoring is its value for the health promoter's professional development. Analysis of monitoring results not only reveals specific program weaknesses or strengths, but also teaches valuable lessons about behavioral change in the society which are applicable to other aspects of the AIDS problem.

Finally, monitoring can have a powerful impact outside the field of health promotion by providing insights into human behavior that can influence overall AIDS policy.

REPORT OF THE CONSULTATION ON THE NEUROPSYCHIATRIC ASPECTS OF HIV INFECTION

Cases of acquired immunodeficiency syndrome are often accompanied by neurologic and psychiatric disorders: 70% of persons who die of AIDS exhibit significant mental and neurologic impairment, and pathologic changes in the central and peripheral nervous system have been reported in the autopsy of up to 90% of AIDS cases (1, 2). Recent reports have also suggested that neuropsychiatric disorders may occur earlier in the course of HIV-1 infection, and possibly even in persons who lack physical symptoms, that is, those classified as Groups II or III according to the U.S. Centers for Disease Control (CDC) classification (see Annex, p. 317). These reports have raised apprehensions concerning possible public health and safety hazards that could result from neurologic, cognitive, or behavioral abnormalities in otherwise asymptomatic infected individuals, particularly those involved in occupations in which mishaps endanger many lives, such as civil aviation or operation of nuclear reactors.

To examine currently available data and formulate appropriate policy responses in this complex area, a four-day consultation was convened in Geneva from 14 to 17 March 1988 by the World Health Organization's Global Program on AIDS and the WHO Division of Mental Health. The consultation was attended by 48 experts from 17

Source: World Health Organization, Global Program on AIDS. Report of the Consultation on the Neuropsychiatric Aspects of HIV Infection, Geneva, 14–17 March 1988. Document WHO/GPA/DIR/88.1. Geneva, 1988.

countries, representing the disciplines of neurology, psychiatry, psychology, neurobiology, epidemiology, social work, occupational health, ethics, clinical research, and health policy.

The first two days of the meeting were devoted to reviewing the available evidence on the neuropsychiatric effects of human immunodeficiency virus type 1 (HIV-1) infection, with particular focus on persons in CDC Groups II and III. The following questions were considered:

- What neuropsychiatric conditions are associated with HIV-1 infection in Groups II and III?
- What is known about the incidence, prevalence, course, and functional impact of such neuropsychiatric effects in these groups?
- How do the incidence and prevalence of such problems among Groups II and III individuals compare with those of neuropsychiatric conditions unrelated to HIV-1 in the general population?

In the second part of the meeting, the policy implications resulting from examination of these questions were identified and discussed.

Neuropsychiatric Diseases and Disorders Associated with HIV-1 Infection

HIV-1 dementia. Individuals with HIV-1 dementia (also known as AIDS dementia complex, HIV encephalopathy, or subacute encephalitis) typically experience forgetfulness, slowed thought processes, poor concentration, and difficulties with problem-solving and reading. They may exhibit apathy, reduced spontaneity, and social withdrawal. In a small percentage of affected individuals, the illness begins atypically as an affective disorder, psychosis, or seizures.

Physical examination often reveals tremor, rapid repetitive movements, imbalance, ataxia, hypertonia, and generalized hyperreflexia, among other signs. Formal neuropsychological testing shows abnormalities on a variety of tests that measure performance under time constraints, problem-solving, visual scanning, perceptual and visual motor integration, and learning and memory.

Although the characteristic symptoms described above strongly suggest a diagnosis of HIV-1 dementia in HIV-1 seropositive individuals or patients with clinical AIDS, other etiologies must be excluded before such a diagnosis can be made. Laboratory and radiographic studies are useful for excluding other causes of dementia in HIV-1–infected individuals.

No data are currently available on the incidence of this disorder. In some studies of AIDS patients, the point prevalence of HIV-1 dementia ranged between 8% and 16% (3, 4, 5, 6). However, in a series of autopsies of cases referred to neurologists, the figure was as high as 66% (2).

It is not currently known what factors may predispose a person infected with HIV-1 to develop dementia, nor whether individuals in CDC Groups II and III who exhibit more subtle neurobehavioral abnormalities (described below) are at any increased risk of developing HIV-1 dementia. Studies are underway to determine whether differences in the manifestations or the course of the disorder exist among different risk groups.

HIV-1 dementia usually progresses quickly to severe deterioration and death. The course and outcome of the disorder in patients without opportunistic infections and neoplasms is not presently known due to lack of data. Also insufficient is evidence regarding the efficacy of antiviral agents in treatment of this disorder. The sole and optimum management strategy at present consists of psychological and social support for patients and their caretakers in order to help sustain quality of life, attenuate the rate of deterioration, and minimize the impact of behavioral disturbance.

Neurobehavioral abnormalities other than dementia. These abnormalities are not specific and can only be related to HIV-1 infection if they cannot be ascribed reliably to any other disorder or etiology after thorough evaluation. Disorders such as adjustment reaction and depression or organic brain dysfunction must be ruled out.

Neurologic, cognitive, and behavioral problems may occur singly or in combination, and include difficulty with concentration, memory, speech, or language; persistent headaches; incoordination; weakness; diplopia; vertigo; apathy; anxiety; or depression. The abnormalities can be detected by history, physical examination, and neuropsychological testing. They are usually mild and are insufficient to establish a diagnosis of dementia by the WHO International Classification of Diseases (10th revision, in press) clinical criteria. Patients report that the problems rarely interfere with job performance in the absence of other AIDS-related illnesses.

The reported prevalence of abnormalities as measured by neuropsychological testing is 9% to 18% for HIV-1 seronegative controls; 20% (2) to 54% (7) for AIDS-related complex (ARC) patients; and 35% (2) to 87% (7) for AIDS patients. There is disagreement about whether the abnormalities measured by such testing occur with increased frequency in CDC Groups II and III individuals. Data from three studies (unpublished data from the ongoing multi-center AIDS cooperative study, unpublished results of the ongoing CDC/San Francisco cohort study, and a study reported by Marshall—4) that involved over 800 men showed no increase in neurologic and neuropsychological abnormalities in otherwise healthy HIV-1 seropositive persons compared to HIV-1 seronegative controls. Data from a fourth study are based on a small sample, but show a higher rate of neuropsychological abnormalities in seropositive persons (7). The weight of current evidence suggests that CDC Groups II and III individuals do not have an increased frequency of neuropsychological abnormalities; however, the existence of divergent findings means that a final conclusion is not possible at present, and further studies are being conducted.

Factors that may increase the risk or predict the onset of neurobehavioral abnormalities in persons infected with HIV-1 are presently unknown. It is also not known whether these abnormalities are transient and reversible, persistent, or progressive, and whether they are predictive of subsequent neurologic or mental deterioration.

Therapy consists of supportive care and referral to psychological specialists when appropriate. Psychogenic factors may account for some of the mild cognitive defects observed, and as such are amenable to psychological interventions. It should be noted that it was the opinion of several participants in the consultation that psychoactive medication such as antidepressants might cause more frequent and severe side effects in HIV-1–infected persons compared with uninfected individuals.

HIV-1–related meningitis. An acute "aseptic" meningitis occurring shortly after infection appears to represent a primary response of the nervous system to HIV-1 infection. The symptoms are compatible with acute meningeal inflammation and include headache, retroorbital pain, meningismus, fever, photophobia, cranial neuropathies, and, rarely, transient encephalopathy (but not progressive dementia). Typically, the acute symptoms are self-limited, require no special treatment, and disappear in one to four weeks.

A milder variant of HIV-1–related meningitis, with only headache and persistent low-grade cerebrospinal fluid pleocytosis, has also been recognized. This type of meningitis can be attributed to HIV-1 infection only after the exclusion of other possible causes.

The incidence of clinically apparent meningitis seems to be low, but no systematic studies have been carried out. It is uncertain whether either acute symptomatic meningitis or "silent" central nervous system involvement (manifested by cerebrospinal fluid lymphocytic pleocytosis, intrathecal synthesis of anti-HIV-1–specific antibodies, and/or HIV-1 isolation) is associated with the later development of progressive dementia.

Vacuolar myelopathy. The clinical manifestations typically include a slowly progressive spastic paraparesis, sensory ataxia, sphincter disturbance, and impaired distal sensation. The myelopathy may be subtle and masked by other neurologic disorders. While this condition is generally associated with HIV-1 dementia, the pathologic changes observed in the two disorders are very different, suggesting different pathogenic mechanisms. It has not been established whether the vacuolar changes result directly from spinal cord infection with HIV-1.

The prevalence of vacuolar myelopathy exceeds 20% among autopsied AIDS cases in New York and New Jersey (8). The lower prevalence rates observed in clinical and autopsy series from other places may be related to case selection or autopsy technique.

Only anecdotal reports have appeared of vacuolar myelopathy in otherwise asymptomatic HIV-1 seropositive persons, suggesting that the incidence of the condition is quite low. More studies are needed to assess the incidence, the course, and the outcome of this condition in CDC Groups II and III persons, the risk factors for its development after HIV-1 infection, and the effectiveness of zidovudine (also called azidothymidine or AZT) or other antiviral agents in the treatment of vacuolar myelopathy.

Demyelinating peripheral nerve disease. This disease is typically either an acute demyelinating motor neuropathy similar to Guillain-Barré syndrome or a more chronic syndrome characterized by motor weakness (9). It may be immune-mediated, representing immune disregulation rather than direct nerve damage from HIV-1. Other viruses, such as herpes group viruses, may also be involved in its pathogenesis.

The disorder is uncommon. Most cases are seen in the early stages of HIV-1 infection (10), and in CDC Groups II and III individuals it may be the first manifestation of HIV-1 infection (11). Risk factors for its development are unknown, and it is unclear whether the syndrome appears in all risk groups. Most patients recover spontaneously.

Mononeuritis multiplex. Several reports have described multiple mononeuropathies in HIV-1–infected individuals, sometimes with accompanying cranial neuropathies and in other cases with central nervous system signs. Several patients have developed a more widespread peripheral neuropathy with features of chronic inflammatory demyelinating neuropathy. The etiology of mononeuritis multiplex in HIV-1–infected persons is unknown and could be related to concurrent infection (for example, with hepatitis B virus).

This disorder is rare in all persons with HIV-1 infection, regardless of group classification. Some cases progress to generalized neuropathy, but too few patients have been studied to generalize about the course of the illness. There is no proven therapy.

Predominantly sensory neuropathy (PSN). This disorder normally involves symmetrical acral paresthesia and dysesthesia, primarily affecting the balls of the feet and the toes. In some patients with PSN, a selective degeneration of the gracile tract in the spinal cord is discovered at autopsy, and it has been proposed that the syndrome represents HIV-1 infection of and damage to the spinal ganglia.

Approximately 20% of patients with AIDS and fewer patients with ARC develop PSN. Since distal symmetrical peripheral neuropathies may be common in the general population, particularly among the elderly, PSN may not be sufficiently characteristic to be considered pathognomonic of HIV-1 infection. PSN only rarely occurs in persons in CDC Groups II and III.

HIV-1–associated myopathy. This syndrome is characterized by a subacute, predominantly proximal muscle weakness with myalgias, excessive fatigue, and an increased serum creatine kinase level. Muscle biopsies may reveal myofiber degeneration and regeneration and perivascular and interstitial inflammation. A self-limited myopathy may also be observed at the time of seroconversion.

The incidence of this disorder in people infected with HIV-1 is unknown, but the clinical syndrome is rare. It is the first manifestation of HIV-1 infection (12) in an unknown percentage of cases. Also unknown are the risk factors for its development and its course and outcome.

Opportunistic infections and neoplasms. A number of opportunistic infections or neoplasms of the central nervous system can affect the patient with HIV-1 infection and immunosuppression. By definition, the presence of these illnesses will result in a diagnosis of AIDS. Thus, while they may arise in CDC Groups II and III patients, once the illnesses have developed the patients are categorized as having AIDS (included in Group IV).

Progressive multifocal leukoencephalopathy (PML) is an unusual infectious central nervous system disease caused by the papovavirus John Cunningham (JC). It causes dementia, blindness, dysphasia, hemiparesis, and ataxia that slowly progress until death. Incidence in AIDS patients has been reported at 0.6% (University of California, San Francisco) and 3.8% (University of Miami). PML may be the initial clinical manifestation of HIV-1 infection in a small number of cases. There are no known factors that increase the risk of developing PML following HIV-1 infection, and there are no known effective therapies. The prognosis is grave; mean survival time after the onset of symptoms is less than two months.

Cerebral toxoplasmosis in AIDS patients results from the reactivation of latent brain infection with the opportunistic intracellular parasite *Toxoplasma gondii*. By October 1987, 838 cases had been reported to the CDC. In a substantial proportion of AIDS patients with cerebral toxoplasmosis, this disease was the first clinical manifestation of illness; overall, however, the percentage of AIDS patients first presenting with cerebral toxoplasmosis is small. Geographic differences in risk for the development of cerebral toxoplasmosis that have been found among AIDS patients in the United States may reflect local endemicity levels of toxoplasmosis, since the illness is a recrudescence of latent infection. Therapy with pyrimethamine and sulfadiazine is effective, but lifelong treatment is necessary in most patients. Survival of up to 18 months has been reported.

Cryptococcal meningitis, caused by infection with the common soil fungus *Cryptococcus neoformans*, is a well-known clinical entity. Symptoms are those of meningitis, including headache, stiff neck, fever, and photophobia. By October 1987, 2,473 cases of AIDS-related cryptococcal meningitis had been reported to the CDC, whose data indicate that 6.1% of AIDS patients have cryptococcal meningitis as their first AIDS-defining illness. Treatment with amphotericin B can alleviate clinical symptoms and control the disease. Use of ketoconazole derivatives for maintenance therapy is under investigation. Lifelong suppressive treatment may be required in most patients.

Primary malignant lymphomas of the brain are rare but well-characterized tumors. CDC data suggest that 1.5% of AIDS patients in the United States first present with central nervous system lymphoma. Epidemiological studies have not revealed risk factors for development of this disease. Although early reports suggested that it was untreatable, one recent study found that tumors of patients in otherwise good general health appear to respond to early aggressive radiation therapy, which may increase the length and quality of life. Without this therapy, mean survival time is about two months.

Severe depressive episode/major depression. Depression is a common mental disorder in most populations and can be reliably diagnosed on the basis of present mental state, personal history, and family history. Depression can occur at any point in the course of an HIV-1 infection, but clinical reports indicate that it is most prevalent in the period following identification of HIV-1 seropositivity and in the initial stage of HIV-1 dementia.

Data on the incidence and prevalence of depressive illnesses among CDC Groups II and III persons are currently lacking. The reported frequency (*13, 14*) among HIV-1 seropositive persons referred to a psychiatric consultation was 15% to 17%. Analysis of the large number of existing observations on HIV-1 seropositive individuals with psychiatric symptoms should permit further estimates of the prevalence of major depression in HIV-1 seropositive populations.

Even if the incidence of depression in persons in CDC Groups II and III is higher than in the general population, the difference (unless excessive) will be difficult to demonstrate in view of the high baseline rate of occurrence of depressive disorders, which may be 5% of the adult population over a six-month period (*15*). Another potential difficulty in attributing mood disorders to HIV-1 infection is the possibility that groups at risk of becoming infected might consist of persons who are more likely to suffer from depression than members of the general population. Additionally, the differential diagnosis of depression in an HIV-1 seropositive individual is difficult because its symptoms may mimic features of ARC (weight loss, sleep disturbance, loss of libido) or dementia (slowing of mental processes, impaired concentration, subjective complaints of memory deterioration). Nevertheless, such differentiation should be attempted because of its important implications for prognosis, treatment, and management.

The risk of depression may be augmented by psychosocial factors, such as lack of social support. Very little is known at present about the course and outcome of depression in CDC Groups II and III persons.

Other affective disorders. There are anecdotal reports of manic episodes in HIV-1 seropositive individuals, but it is not known whether these are causally linked to HIV-1 infection of the nervous system or are the expression of a bipolar affective illness in a person who happens to be seropositive.

Schizophreniform and paranoid disorders. Several case reports (*16, 17, 18*) mention acute psychotic illnesses with hallucination, paranoid or grandiose delusions, and thought disorders in individuals classified as CDC Groups II and III. On the basis of these reports, the etiology of these illnesses cannot be clearly attributed to HIV-1 infection, and further research is needed to establish whether acute schizophreniform and paranoid psychosis could be a neurobehavioral manifestation of HIV-1 infection.

Delirium. This well-defined clinical entity may develop in conjunction with a variety of physical illnesses, infectious and parasitic diseases, and intoxications, and as a complication of head injury. In HIV-1 infection, cases of benign and short-lived delirium have been described in association with the aseptic meningitis that may develop upon seroconversion (*19*). Such cases are probably quite rare in early Groups II and III individuals. Delirium is apparently much more common in HIV-1 dementia (*20*), but estimates of incidence are not available at present. It is not known whether the development of a delirium worsens the overall course of HIV-1 dementia, but this possibility cannot be excluded. Delirium should be regarded, therefore, as a serious complication in the course of HIV-1 dementia.

Other mental disorders. There have been a number of individual case reports of acute illnesses of mixed symptomatology in HIV-1–infected persons (e.g., combinations of delusions and hallucination, affective symptoms, and impaired sensorium). Although such illnesses cannot be classified unequivocally, the etiology is likely to be related to HIV-1. More epidemiological data are required before incidence can be assessed.

An observation of potential significance from Tanzania (*21*) concerns the apparent occurrence of acute psychotic disorders in HIV-1 seropositive individuals. These disorders apparently were the first manifestation of HIV-1 infection, and resulted in rapid deterioration and death within weeks or months, without development of ARC or AIDS. The clinical picture in these cases was not dementia but an acute hallucinatory psychosis with generalized excitement. The nature of these illnesses needs further investigation; no autopsies of affected individuals have been performed thus far.

Adjustment reactions. These reactions are common in persons recently diagnosed with HIV-1 infection. They involve expressions of despair, grief, guilt, anxiety, protest, depression, and hypochondriasis. In type, severity, and duration they are similar to reactions to other major life events or diseases and do not usually lead to chronic functional impairment. Factors such as perceived stigma and the extent of social and familial support have a significant bearing on the severity and duration of such reactions.

Adjustment reactions may occur in up to 90% of persons recently diagnosed with HIV-1 infection. The impact of adjustment problems can be reduced by counseling before and after testing.

Adjustment disorders. Many reports have not differentiated between adjustment reactions and disorders. Adjustment disorders feature chronic functional distress or impairment and involve a morbid (excessive in length and/or intensity) response to the stress of HIV-1 infection identification or diagnosis.

The incidence and prevalence of adjustment disorders in CDC Groups II and III individuals are not known. They may be more frequent in persons with a history of psychiatric problems (*18, 22*). Adjustment disorders may last many months. They are frequently amenable to psychological therapy or medication.

Conclusions and Recommendations

HIV-1 Serologic Status and Job Performance

Persons with AIDS and some of those with AIDS-related complex (ARC) are susceptible to damage or dysfunction of all areas of the nervous system due to HIV-1 or to opportunistic infections or meningitis. However, review of currently available scientific and medical data brought to light no evidence of an increase in clinically significant neuropsychological abnormalities in CDC Groups II and III HIV-1 seropositive persons compared to HIV-1 seronegative controls. The consultation therefore concluded that there is no justification at the present time for HIV-1 serologic screening as a strategy for detecting functional impairment in asymptomatic persons in the interest of public safety. It also recommended that this policy statement be reviewed frequently to take account of the findings of studies currently in progress or planned.

It was recognized that public concern has been aroused regarding issues related to AIDS and HIV infection, and that the public may be excessively influenced by anecdotal or single case reports. Therefore, it was emphasized that single instances and anecdotes cannot and should never replace meticulous analysis of all the available evidence as the basis for conclusions regarding cause and effect and for policy formulation.

On the weight of the data reviewed, it was concluded that asymptomatic HIV-1–infected individuals pose no special problems in occupations with potentially high impact on public safety. The most effective strategy to detect meaningful dysfunction due to any cause (since a wide range of conditions may impair performance, including stress, fatigue, aging, and substance abuse) was felt to be the application of currently recommended performance and functional standards in both industry (e.g., for airline pilots, crane operators, etc.) and the assessment of individual capacity to perform daily activities (e.g., drive a car). Therefore, the effectiveness of performance testing must be reviewed and the correlation between tests of neuropsychological function and actual job performance must be determined precisely.

Given the evidence, denial of access to employment or the freedom to engage in everyday activities for otherwise healthy persons solely on the basis of HIV-1 serologic status would represent a violation of human rights and have broad and detrimental social implications. The consultation pointed out that HIV-1 screening of prospective or current employees might by implemented by employers for reasons other than public safety and unrelated to neuropsychological function, for example, to boost an industry's public relations image by publicizing its concern for public safety, or to exclude HIV-1–infected employees from training programs on the basis of a belief that they have a reduced life expectancy.

In summary, while the continued refinement of functional tests to detect early neuropsychiatric impairment in occupation groups is to be encouraged, there is no justification at this time for the addition of HIV-1 serologic screening to these tests in the name of public safety.

Research

The review of current findings presented to the consultation pointed to the need to define or create a standard neuropsychological test battery for assessing the functional impairment in HIV-1 seropositive persons. Such tests should attempt to measure a broad range of functions, since HIV-1 infection may result in variable nervous system pathology with diverse neuropsychological consequences.

Another problem recognized was the great variation in experimental design of previous studies, which has made analysis and comparison of results difficult. Therefore, the standardization of methodology is of prime importance. In this regard, it was recommended that study populations should be representative of all risk behavior groups, geographic areas, and socioeconomic and cultural groups. The results of studies on patients with differing clinical status should not be lumped together, and it is critical that patients with concomitant psychiatric or neurologic disease be studied separately.

The selection of appropriate control groups is of paramount importance. The lifestyle of many HIV-1–infected persons and the stress associated with a recent diagnosis of HIV-1 infection make comparisons with the general population or any group of uninfected individuals (who do not have the stress associated with the knowledge of HIV-1 infection) problematic. Future studies could use as control groups: (1) HIV-1 seronegative individuals with the same risk factors; (2) HIV-1 seronegative individuals with a recent diagnosis of life-threatening illness; (3) HIV-1 seronegative individuals outside usual risk behavior groups but closely matched in sociodemographic and educational characteristics; (4) HIV-1 seronegative individuals with similar rates of alcohol and drug use; and (5) HIV-1 seronegative patients with other causes of immunosuppression.

Since studies of neuropsychiatric aspects of HIV-1 infection have major public policy implications, it is essential that the data be subjected to the rigorous scrutiny of peer review before they are disclosed. Results should therefore be published in recognized scientific journals. All data collection and analysis must be performed in such a manner as to ensure the confidentiality of information and anonymity of study participants.

Many important aspects regarding HIV-1 dementia and the milder neurobehavioral abnormalities associated with HIV-1 infection remain to be clarified, including their natural history, pathogenesis, and predictors or possible markers of disease. The value of different types of psychological support in the management of HIV-1 dementia needs to be evaluated, as do the value and potential risks of treatment of concomitant psychiatric disorders with antidepressants, neuroleptics, or other pharmacological agents, and the use of anti–HIV-1 agents in its treatment. It is critically important to determine whether the neurobehavioral abnormalities represent distinct disorders or are early symptoms of a progression to HIV-1 dementia, and whether these conditions are permanent or reversible. Potential treatments should be investigated.

Health Care

As the incidence of AIDS increases, an enormous burden of neuro-psychiatric illness will face the health care system in many countries. By 1991, the number of neurologically symptomatic AIDS patients in the United States is expected to be nearly half the number of all epilepsy patients and will far exceed the number of persons with Parkinson's disease. Since that projection relates only to patients with manifest AIDS, it is an underestimation of the impact of HIV-1 infection on neurology services.

Appropriate support and treatment services must be available and accessible not only to individuals with clinical illness but also to asymptomatic individuals as soon as they become aware that they are infected. Health services must be able to respond to those persons experiencing acute adjustment and stress reactions as the result of learning of their seropositive status. Trained psychiatrists, neurolo-gists, psychologists, counselors, and social workers will be required, as will strengthened community services and self-help groups for patients and their families.

Because of the large increase that will occur in the number of affected individuals, it is inevitable that most, if not all, neurologists, psychiatrists, and psychologists will become involved in managing HIV-1–infected persons. Therefore, there is an urgent need for train-ing programs for key categories of health workers. It is essential that all health care workers be aware of the possible range of neuropsychi-atric disorders that may be the initial manifestation of illness or that may develop later, so that they will be able to recognize these prob-lems at the earliest possible stage; to respond with appropriate atti-tudes, understanding, and therapy; and to refer patients for care as required.

In summary, health workers should be made aware of both the wide range of neuropsychiatric conditions associated with HIV-1 infection and the fact that the weight of existing information indicates that functional impairment is not significantly increased over levels found among persons not infected by HIV-1 until or unless patients become clinically ill with ARC or AIDS. Health services need to pre-pare to deal with a large burden of neuropsychiatric illness, much of it severe, in patients with ARC and AIDS, and planning should com-mence immediately.

It was recommended that the report of the consultation be dissemi-nated widely to health workers to help ensure that informed advice is provided to HIV-1–infected persons.

References[1]

1. Gyorkey, F., et al. Human immunodeficiency virus in brain biopsies of patients with AIDS and progressive encephalopathy. *J Infect Dis* 155:870–876, 1987.

2. Price, R. W., et al. The brain in AIDS: central nervous system HIV-1 infection and AIDS dementia complex. *Science* 239:586–592, 1988.

3. Levy, R. M., and D. E. Bredesen. *AIDS and the Nervous System*. New York: Raven Press, 1988, pp. 29–63.

4. Marshall, D. W., et al. Spectrum of cerebrospinal fluid findings in various stages of human immunodeficiency virus infection. *Arch Neurol* 45(9):954–958, 1988.

5. Snider, W. D., et al. Neurological complications of AIDS: analysis of 50 patients. *Ann Neurol* 14:403–418, 1983.

6. McArthur, J. C. Neurologic manifestations of AIDS. *Medicine* 66(6):407–437, 1987.

7. Grant, I., et al. Evidence for early central nervous system involvement in the AIDS and other HIV infections. Studies with neuropsychologic testing and M.R.I. *Ann Intern Med* 107:828–836, 1987.

8. Petito, C. K., et al. Vacuolar myelopathy pathologically resembling subacute combined degeneration in patients with AIDS. *N Engl J Med* 312(14):874–879, 1985.

9. Cooper, B., and H. Bickel. Population screening and the early detection of dementing disorders in old age: a review. *Psychol Med* 14:81–95, 1984.

10. Cornblath, D. R., et al. Inflammatory demyelinating peripheral neuropathies associated with HTLV-III infection. *Ann Neurol* 21:32–40, 1987.

11. Berger, J. R., et al. Neurologic disease as the presenting manifestation of AIDS. *South Med J* 80:683–686, 1987.

12. Dalakas, M. C., et al. Polymyositis associated with AIDS retrovirus. *JAMA* 256:2381–2383, 1986.

13. Perry, S. W., and S. Tross. Psychiatric problems of AIDS in-patients at the New York Hospital: a preliminary report. *Public Health Rep* 99:200–205, 1984.

14. Dilley, J. W., et al. Findings in psychiatric consultations with patients with AIDS. *Am J Psychiatry* 142(1):82–886, 1985.

15. Regier, D. A., et al. The NIMH Epidemiologic Catchment Area Program. Historical context, major objectives, and study population characteristics. *Arch Gen Psychiatry* 41(10):934–941, 1984.

16. Jones, G. H., et al. HIV and onset of schizophrenia. *Lancet* 1:982, 1987.

17. Maccario, M., and D. W. Scharre. HIV and acute onset of psychosis (letter). *Lancet* 2(8554):342, 1987.

18. Thomas, C. S., et al. HTLV-3 and psychiatric disturbance. *Lancet* 2:395–396, 1985.

[1]A more extensive bibliography may be found in the source document.

19. McArthur, J. C. Neuropsychiatric manifestations of HIV infection: results of an initial screening evaluation of homosexual/bisexual men (abstract). Paper presented at III International Conference on AIDS, held in Washington, D.C., 1–5 June 1987.
20. Price, R. W., et al. The AIDS dementia complex: some current questions. *Ann Neurol* 23(Suppl):527–533, 1988.
21. Rweikiza, J., et al. Neuropsychiatric aspects of AIDS as seen at Muhimbili Medical Center Department of Psychiatry. Paper prepared for WHO Consultation on Neuropsychiatric Aspects of HIV Infection, held in Geneva, 14–17 March 1988.

Annex

Summary of CDC classification system for HIV infection.

GROUP I	Acute infection
GROUP II	Asymptomatic infection[a]
GROUP III	Persistent generalized lymphadenopathy[a]
GROUP IV	Other disease
Subgroup A	Constitutional disease
Subgroup B	Neurological disease
Subgroup C	Secondary infectious diseases
Category C-1	Specific secondary infectious diseases listed in the CDC surveillance definition for AIDS[b]
Category C-2	Other specified secondary infectious diseases[b]
Subgroup D	Secondary cancers
Subgroup E	Other conditions

Source: Centers for Disease Control. Revision of the CDC surveillance case definition for acquired immunodeficiency syndrome, *MMWR* 36 (suppl 1S), 1987.
[a]Patients in Groups II and III may be subclassified on the basis of a laboratory evaluation.
[b]Includes those patients whose clinical presentation fulfills the definition of the acquired immunodeficiency syndrome used by Centers for Disease Control for national reporting.

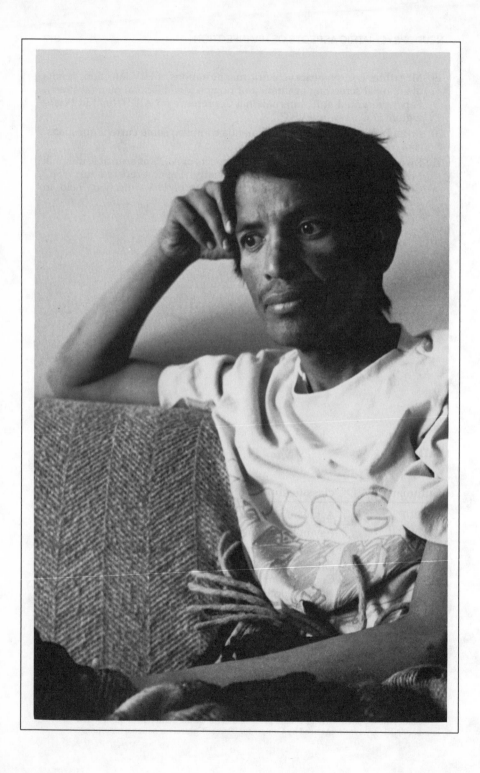

SYMPOSIUM ON NUTRITION AND AIDS

The Subcommittee on Nutrition of the United Nations Administrative Committee on Coordination sponsored a symposium on nutrition and AIDS at its meeting in Geneva, 22–26 February 1988. The purposes of the symposium were to review the current epidemiologic information on the spread of AIDS, to evaluate evidence of possible connections between nutritional status and the initiation or progression of HIV infection, and to consider the nutritional implications of the AIDS epidemic for households, communities, and nations.

The discussion focused on two questions: (1) Does nutritional status or nutritional intervention influence the course of AIDS? (2) Are there indications that the continued spread of AIDS will lead to nutritional problems by reducing supplies and services?

With regard to nutrition and the individual AIDS patient, at present there is no clear indication that poor nutritional status makes a person more susceptible to infection or affects the progression of overt disease, although these possibilities need further study. It was noted that AIDS results in malnutrition, since progressive wasting is a common sign of the disease. Therefore, it is likely that nutritional support for the AIDS patient will improve the quality of remaining life, but it is uncertain whether it will extend life.

In attempting to answer the second question, epidemiologic documentation was reviewed regarding the logarithmic growth of both

Source: United Nations Administrative Committee on Coordination, Subcommittee on Nutrition. Report on the Symposium on Nutrition and AIDS, Geneva, 22–26 February 1988.

HIV infection rates and the number of manifest AIDS cases in all countries now reporting to WHO. The data make it clear that, regardless of any action taken now, the prevalence of clinical disease will continue to rise in the next 10 years. Unless effective methods of controlling the spread of infection or the development of disease are found, the probability exists that the loss of population from the most productive age group (young adults) will lead to major disruptions in production, distribution, and services in at least some countries. Families where one or more breadwinners are affected may face long-term difficulties in obtaining adequate food. This situation would necessitate strengthened local support for families, which might involve some type of food supplementation program.

In countries where the pattern of AIDS transmission is primarily heterosexual (in many developing countries, notably in Africa), an increase in the prevalence of AIDS in the adult population will lead to an associated increase in the prevalence of HIV infection in newborn infants because of transplacental transmission during pregnancy or transmission through blood at delivery. Current information suggests that the fatality rate among these babies during the first two years of life will be high, and in some countries AIDS may negate the reductions achieved in infant, young child, and maternal mortality during the past two decades. Regarding nutrition monitoring and surveillance, it was noted that in countries where the prevalence of AIDS is high, the use of low weight and high mortality as nutritional indicators in children will have to be reinterpreted.

While it is impossible to predict exactly how individual countries will be affected by the growing epidemic, certain scenarios represent strong possibilities. For example, lack of manpower in agrarian societies may lead to reductions in agricultural production. The health systems will surely face major increases in the demand for services and may face this demand with reduced manpower and impaired infrastructures. Any of these outcomes will have major implications for food, nutrition, and health planning, and will increase the need for capital funding while reducing the ability to repay debts. The Subcommittee therefore recommended that governments and the United Nations agencies monitor not only the development of the AIDS epidemic but also the evolution of its structural effects, so that national and international actions can be set in motion to compensate for the wide-ranging impacts on health and development.

MEASUREMENT OF ANTIBODIES TO HUMAN IMMUNODEFICIENCY VIRUS: AN INTERNATIONAL COLLABORATIVE STUDY TO EVALUATE WHO REFERENCE SERA

A. J. GARRETT, V. SEAGROATT, E. M. SUPRAN, K. O. HABERMEHL, H. HAMPL, & G. C. SCHILD

Human immunodeficiency virus (HIV), the causative agent of the acquired immunodeficiency syndrome (AIDS) (1, 2, 3), is transmitted primarily through sexual contact or the injection of contaminated blood or blood products such as anti-hemophilic factors (4). Since 1985, the screening of blood donations for anti-HIV has been instituted in many countries in order to minimize the risk of transmission of AIDS via blood transfusions or treatment with blood products. The detection of antibodies to HIV is also of major importance as a relatively simple and rapid determination of the extent and spread of HIV infections (5), and many commercial and "in-house" immunochemical tests are now in use throughout the world. At present, the most commonly used assays are based on enzyme-linked or radioimmunosorbence, immunofluorescence, immunoblotting, or immunoprecipitation, and variations in the specificities and sensitivities of the techniques reflect inherent differences between the principles of the assays as well as batch-to-batch variations in the preparation of reagents and kits (6, 7). Thus, there is an urgent need for well-characterized reference materials that can be used to define the reliability and sensitivity of the tests, for quality control of batches of kits or reagents, and as common references between laboratories.

Source: Bulletin of the World Health Organization 66(2):197–202, 1988. © World Health Organization.

This report presents an assessment of two proposed reference preparations of sera, one reactive and the other unreactive to HIV, in a collaborative study involving 21 laboratories in 11 countries.

Materials and Methods

Proposed Reference Materials

The preparations of antibody-positive and antibody-negative human sera, freeze-dried in sealed glass ampules, were supplied by Professor K. O. Habermehl (Institute for Clinical and Experimental Virology, Berlin (West)). Each preparation was derived from a single donor; one an asymptomatic carrier of HIV and the other a donor with no known risk factors. Each serum was unreactive when tested for hepatitis B surface antigen (HBsAg) by a standard immunoassay and was heated at 56 °C for one hour before freeze-drying. When reconstituted as recommended (in 0.2 ml water) these preparations had concentrations one-twentieth of the original sera; this dilution factor is not included in the calculations presented in this report.

Coded Preparations

Seven freeze-dried serum preparations, coded A to G, were supplied to each participant. Preparations A and C were duplicate samples of the reactive proposed reference material, preparation E was the nonreactive proposed reference material. Samples D and F were prepared by the Central Public Health Service Laboratory, Colindale, London. Sample D, derived from a single donor, showed weak reactivity in immunosorbent assays. Sample F, derived from sera pooled from several donors, was highly reactive. Samples B and G, which were National Institute for Biological Standards and Control (England) reference preparations freeze-dried from pooled sera in 1973 and 1967, respectively, were both unreactive.

Design of the Study

The study was designed to identify the coded preparations that reacted with HIV antibodies and to ascertain the minimum amount of the reactive samples that could be detected in the methods routinely used by the participants.

The 21 participating laboratories (see Annex) were supplied with duplicate sets of the coded preparations and requested to assay them by the procedures usually employed in their laboratories.

Assay Methods

All but three participants assayed the preparations by indirect or competitive ELISA. Nine different commercial kits for ELISA were used: Abbott, Dupont, ENI, Genetic, Organon, Ortho, Pasteur ("ordinary" and "Rapide"), Travenol, and Wellcome. Two laboratories carried out ELISAs using their own "in-house" methods and one included in its series of assays the Abbott "confirmatory" ELISA, a competitive ELISA based on envelope and core antigens derived from recombinant DNA.

Immunoblots were carried out by 15 laboratories. All except two, whose techniques involved the use of a mouse monoclonal antibody specific for human IgG and labelled with ^{125}I, or protein A labeled with ^{125}I, used peroxidase-linked anti-human IgG for the identification of antigen-antibody complexes. Eight used biotin-avidin amplification of the enzyme system.

One participant used the Karpas method (8) and one used an assay based on particle agglutination (PA).

Method of Analysis

For each test the reactivities of the coded samples A to G and the end-point titers for samples A, C, and F were taken to be those recorded by the participants. End-points were defined as the reciprocals of the highest dilutions of the reconstituted original materials *in normal serum* (not the final dilutions in the assay wells) that gave positive responses in the assays.

Potency ratios of C and F were expressed as ratios of their titers to that of A in the same assays.

Results

Classification of Sera by Reactivity in ELISA and Immunoassays

Samples A, C, and F were found reactive in all tests and samples B, E, and G were reported as negative in all but one test. The exception

Table 1. Assessment of reactivity of sample D by immunoassays.

Assay method	No. of laboratories	No. of assays	No. with stated reactivity		
			+	±	−
ELISA kits:					
Abbott	9	12	9	2	1
Dupont	2	3	3	−	−
ENI	1	2	−	−	2
Genetic	1	2	−	2	−
Organon	3	4	1	1	2
Ortho	2	3	3	−	−
Pasteur[a]	5	8	6	1	1
Travenol	1	1	−	−	1
Wellcome	6	10	8	2	1
"In-house" ELISA	2	3	1	1	1
All ELISAs	18	48	31	9	8
Fluorescence microscopy	4	4	1	1	2
Karpas method	1	1	1	−	−
Particle agglutination	1	2	2	−	−

[a] Includes assays using the "Rapide" version.

was a test based on particle agglutination (PA) in which sample E was judged to be weakly reactive. Sample D was found to be reactive or weakly reactive in 40 of the 48 ELISAs performed, in both the PA and Karpas test, and in two of the four fluorescence microscopy (FM) tests (Table 1). In the eight ELISAs in which sample D was identified as unreactive, it had a higher optical density (OD) than the negative control (although not, of course, as high as the OD of the cut-off limit), and in all but one the ODs were at least twice that of the negative control.

Titration of Samples A, C, and F

Participants carried out single or duplicate assays for individual manufacturers' ELISAs or by their local methods. Some laboratories used several manufacturers' ELISAs; in particular, laboratory 1 used seven different kits. For each kit, the geometric means of the titers for A, C, and F and of the potency ratios for C and F obtained by individual laboratories were calculated. The frequency distributions of these values are shown in Figures 1 and 2. One of the participants using the Abbott kit obtained much higher titers for A and F than did the other participants using both this and other kits. Further, its titers for C were ten-fold and 100-fold lower than those for A. The results from

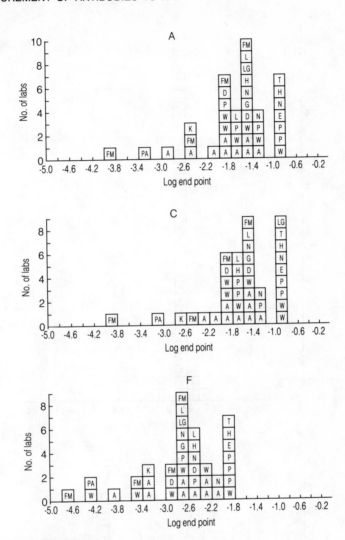

Figure 1. Frequency distributions of the end-point dilutions obtained for samples A, C, and F. Each square denotes an estimate from one test; the letters in the squares refer to the type of assay. A, D, E, G, H, N, P, T, and W denote the following commercial kits of ELISA: A, Abbott; D, Dupont; E, ENI; G, Genetic; H, Ortho; N, Organon; P, Pasteur; T, Travenol; and W, Wellcome. L and LG denote "in-house" versions of ELISA. Letters FM, K, and PA denote the following methods other than ELISA: FM, fluorescence microscopy; K, Karpas; and PA, particle agglutination test.

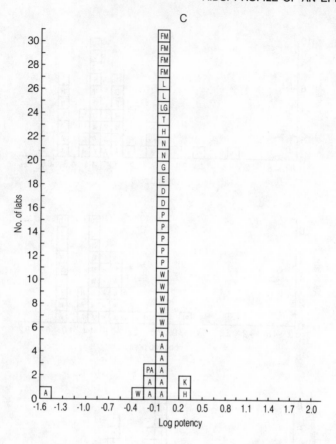

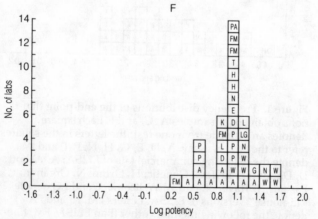

Figure 2. Frequency distributions of the potency ratios of samples C and F in terms of A obtained from individual tests. (See legend in Figure 1 for explanation of the letters in the squares.)

this participant were, therefore, considered atypical and excluded from the subsequent analyses.

The laboratory mean titers varied considerably over about a 20-fold range. There were, however, no obvious differences between the titers from different kits: for instance, the ranges of titers for Abbott, Pasteur, and Wellcome overlapped with each other.

The laboratory mean potency ratios of C, a coded duplicate of A, were mostly unity. All but one laboratory (mentioned above) found the titers of A and C to be within one dilution step (Figure 1), although sometimes these dilution steps were as large as five- and tenfold. The laboratory mean potency ratios for F were more variable than those for C. However, the potency ratios were less variable than the titers (Figures 1 and 2). One laboratory's results gave a potency ratio, based on a single assay, of 256, tenfold higher than the other estimates, and had the highest titer for F (16,384). This titer and potency ratio were, therefore, considered atypical and excluded from the subsequent analysis.

Differences between the laboratories' estimations of titers were found to be significant by analyses of variance, even between those using kits from the same manufacturer. Expressing the reactivities of samples C and F relative to A showed that the differences between laboratories using the same commercial kit were no longer statistically significant. However, there were still significant differences between the potency ratios from different tests. For example, the overall mean potency ratio, i.e., the geometric mean of the laboratory mean potencies, for Wellcome was 22, about three times higher than those for Abbott and Pasteur kits (6 and 7, respectively). The overall mean potency ratios for the other kits fell within this range.

Immunoblots

Fifteen participants tested samples A to G by immunoblot techniques. The results are given in Table 2. The use of control antigens ("mock" antigens) was reported from only two laboratories. Faint reactive bands in the regions of relative molecular mass (M_r) 24×10^3 and 64×10^3 were detected consistently by one participant using "mock" antigen from H9 cells; more information is required on this important aspect of the assays.

The relative molecular masses recorded in Table 2 are those assigned by the individual participants. For convenience of presentation, bands reported within narrow ranges of M_r are not differentiated and are classified in groups (e.g., $(32-34) \times 10^3$ and $(110-160) \times 10^3$).

Table 2. Detection of anti-HIV by immunoblot.[a]

Peptide or glycopeptide	Reactive bands/total reports		
(approximate relative molecular mass $\times 10^3$)	Sample A (C)	Sample D	Sample F
17, 18	11/14	6/14	13/14
24	15/15	13/15	15/15
32, 34	12/14	11/14	11/14
38, 39	9/13	5/14	10/13
41	15/15	6/15	15/15
53, 55	11/14	12/24	14/14
65	13/14	13/14	13/14
110, 120, 160	9/13	7/13	12/13

[a] All participants did not report the presence or absence of each peptide or glycopeptide.

Samples A and C were duplicates of the proposed reactive reference serum. As was hoped, they produced identical results for each immunoblot system and are considered together. One participant reported on the detection of antibodies to peptides p24 and gp41 only. All participants, except one who reported a weak reaction in the p65 region for sample E and another who observed a reaction to p24 antigen in sample G, detected no antibodies to HIV in samples B, E, and G. Of the positive samples, F reacted most strongly in all immunoblots but, except for less frequent detection of antibodies to the envelope antigens gp110–p160 in A and C than in F, samples A, C, and F were qualitatively identical.

All participants detected antibodies to p24, gp41, and p53/55 in A, C, and F; three reported no antibodies to p17/18; and only one reported no antibodies to p65.

Additional Results

Essex and colleagues included in their study an investigation of the reactivity of samples A to G in immunoblots in which the recently isolated strain HTLV-IV was used as antigen. No reactions with any viral antigens were reported for Western blots and only two reactive regions, gp160 for sample A and p24 for sample F, were detected in radioimmunoprecipitation using ^{35}S-labelled HTLV-IV.

Discussion

ELISA kits from nine manufacturers were used in this study. The sensitivities of the various kits were assessed by comparing end-point titers for the highly reactive samples A and F and by whether or not a weakly reactive serum was found "positive" in the tests. This sensitivity varied between laboratories, even between those using the same commercial kit. Expressing the reactivity of sample F relative to A reduced the variation between tests and resulted in agreement between the laboratories using the same kit. Nevertheless, there were still consistent differences between the kits in the comparison of the reactivity of A and F. This possibly reflected the differences in specificities of the ELISA systems.

Overall, immunoblots revealed reactions of sera A (C) and F to all the expected HIV antigens. The presence of antibodies to p24, gp41, and p55 is considered by most workers an important indication of infection with HIV (9, 10, 11). However, for reproducible results the source of antigens, the standardization of electroblotting procedures, and the provision of "control" antigens require careful attention (9); variations of these factors may well explain the differences shown in Table 2.

The results for HTLV-IV confirm earlier findings (11, 12, 13) and emphasize the urgent need for information on the responses of immunoassays to sera from AIDS patients from different geographical areas and for characterization of the genetic and immunological differences between viral isolates. The proposed reference preparation, A, reacted strongly in all ELISAs and related immunoassays and reacted with all the major HIV antigens in immunoblots. Its use will depend on individual requirements, but it may be of value as a qualitative check on the specificity of the assays, to calibrate positive controls included in kits and other assays in arbitrary units, to calibrate detection limits (cut-off) in arbitrary units (as done for HBsAg), and to calibrate immunoblots, particularly for defining the optimal amounts of antigen and for determining the relative mobilities of the major peptides and glycopeptides from HIV. Because the unreactive preparation (E), reconstituted in 0.2 ml water as recommended, represents diluted serum, its use as a reference material will be limited.

The WHO Expert Committee on Biological Standardization reviewed the report of this collaborative study in December 1986 and agreed that preparations A and E would be of value as reference preparations for, respectively, positive and negative anti-HIV sera.

The preparations, under code numbers 86/6302 (reactive) and 86/6238 (unreactive) are available from the Director, National Institute for Biological Standards and Control, South Mimms, Potters Bar, Herts., EN6 3QG, England.

■ ■ ■

Acknowledgment: We thank Jane Bruce for assisting in the statistical analysis of the data from the study.

References

1. Barré-Sinoussi, F. et al. Isolation of a T-lymphotropic retrovirus from a patient at risk for acquired immune deficiency syndrome (AIDS). *Science* 220:868–871, 1983.

2. Levy, J. A. et al. Isolation of lymphocytopathic retroviruses from San Francisco patients with AIDS. *Science* 225:840–842, 1984.

3. Popovic, M. et al. Detection, isolation and continuous production of cytopathic retroviruses (HTLV-III) from patients with AIDS and pre-AIDS. *Science* 224:497-500, 1984.

4. Curran, J. W. et al. The epidemiology of AIDS: current status and future prospects. *Science* 229:1352–1357, 1985.

5. Biggar, R. J. The AIDS problem in Africa. *Lancet* 1:79–83, 1986.

6. Mortimer, P. P. et al. Which anti-HTLV-III/LAV assays for screening and confirmatory testing? *Lancet* 2:873–877, 1985.

7. Petricciani, J. C. et al. An analysis of serum samples positive for HTLV-III antibodies. *N Eng J Med* 313:47–48, 1985.

8. Karpas, A. et al. Lytic infection by British AIDS virus and development of rapid cell test for antiviral antibodies. *Lancet* 2:695–697, 1985.

9. Essex, M. et al. Antigens of human T-lymphotropic virus type III/ lymphadenopathy associated virus. *Ann Intern Med* 103:700–703, 1985.

10. Schupbach, J. et al. Antibodies to HTLV-III in Swiss patients with AIDS and pre-AIDS and in groups at risk for AIDS. *N Eng J Med* 312:265-270, 1985.

11. Biberfeld, G. et al. Findings in four HTLV-IV seropositive women from West Africa. *Lancet* 2:1330–1331, 1986.

12. Clavel, F. et al. Isolation of a new human retrovirus from West African patients with AIDS. *Science* 233:343–346, 1986.

13. Kanki, P. J. et al. New human T-lymphotropic retrovirus related to simian T-lymphotropic virus type III (STLV-III AGM). *Science* 232:238–243, 1986.

Annex

Participating Laboratories

National HIV Reference Laboratory, Fairfield Hospital, Fairfield, Victoria, Australia

Red Cross Blood Transfusion Service, Adelaide, Australia

Laboratory Centre for Disease Control, Ottawa, Ontario, Canada

Laboratoire National de la Santé, Département de Contrôle des Vaccins à Virus et des Produits Dérivés du Sang, Paris, France

Institut Pasteur, Paris, France

Institute for Clinical and Experimental Virology, Free University of Berlin, Berlin (West)

Max von Pettenkofer Institute, Munich, Federal Republic of Germany

Institute for Virus Research, Kyoto University, Kyoto, Japan

Central Laboratory of the Netherlands Red Cross Blood Transfusion Service, Amsterdam, Netherlands

Blood Transfusion Service, Department of Haematology, Singapore General Hospital, Singapore

Centro Nacional de Microbiología, Virología e Immunología Sanitarias, Majadahonda, Madrid, Spain

National Bacteriological Laboratory, Solna (Stockholm), Sweden

North London Blood Transfusion Centre, Edgware, Middlesex, England

Scottish National Blood Transfusion Service, Edinburgh, Scotland

Department of Microbiological Reagents and Quality Control, Central Public Health Laboratory, Colindale, London, England

Department of Haematological Medicine, University of Cambridge, Cambridge, England

Regional Blood Transfusion Centre, Royal Infirmary, Edinburgh, Scotland

National Institute for Biological Standards and Control, Holly Hill, Hampstead, London, England

Department of Cancer Biology, Harvard School of Public Health, Boston, Massachusetts, USA

Division of Virology, Center for Drugs and Biologics, Food and Drug Administration, Rockville Pike, Bethesda, Maryland, USA

AIDS Program, Center for Infectious Diseases, Centers for Disease Control, Atlanta, Georgia, USA

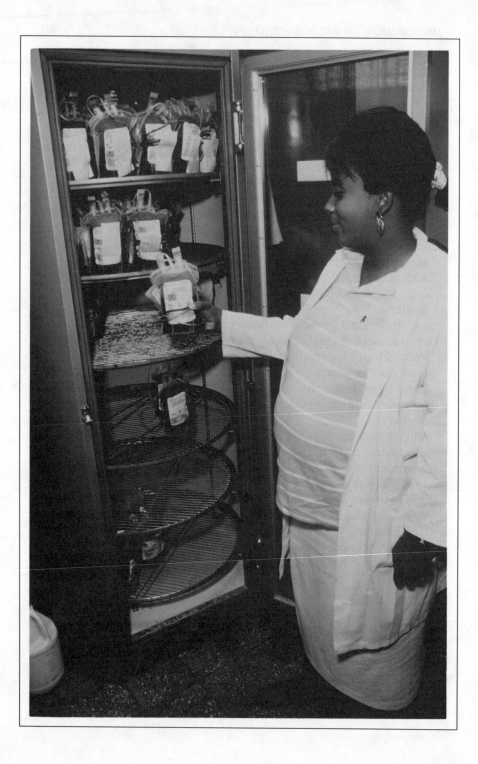

ANIMAL MODELS FOR
HIV INFECTION AND AIDS

HIV is a member of the lentivirus subfamily of the retroviruses. Members of the Retroviridae family, or retroviruses, possess enveloped virions containing an RNA genome. The distinctive feature of these viruses, which gave the name to the family, is the presence in the virus particle of a virus-coded RNA-dependent DNA polymerase, or reverse transcriptase; upon infection, this enzyme transcribes the RNA genome into a DNA provirus, which then becomes integrated into the host chromosomal DNA where it may complete the replication cycle by directing the synthesis of infectious virions, or it may express none or only part of its genetic information in a covert infection. Retroviruses are widely distributed in nature and for many years have been known to infect numerous vertebrate species. Human retroviruses have only been recognized since the late 1970s, and now include the human T-lymphotropic virus types I and II (HTLV-I, HTLV-II) and the human immunodeficiency virus (HIV) (1).

The Retroviridae family is presently subdivided into three subfamilies (Oncovirinae, Spumavirinae, and Lentivirinae), according to their different biological characteristics, which also coincide with different genomic organization. The Oncovirinae subfamily (onco=Greek

Source: World Health Organization. Animal models for HIV infection and AIDS: Memorandum from a WHO Meeting. *Bulletin of the World Health Organization* 66(5), 1988. © World Health Organization. The Memorandum is based on the report of an informal WHO Consultation held in Geneva, Switzerland, on 28–30 March 1988. The names of the participants are given on pages 358–359.

"tumor"), the largest one, includes viruses most commonly associated with lymphoproliferative disorders in many animal species. The Oncovirinae genome consists of the structural genes, *gag*, *pol*, and *env*. The *gag* gene (for group-specific antigen) codes for the internal proteins that constitute the "core" of the virion; the *pol* gene (for polymerase) codes for the reverse transcriptase; and the *env* gene codes for the glycoproteins found in the virus envelope. These three genes are flanked by sequences repeated on both ends of the genome, known as long terminal repeats (LTR), which contain regulatory elements for transcription. Morphologically, oncoviruses have been subdivided into three groups, referred to as type B, C, and D particles. Type C oncoviruses include, among others, the murine, avian, and feline leukemia/sarcoma viruses. Type B oncoviruses are represented by the mouse mammary tumor virus. The Mason-Pfizer monkey virus is the prototype of type D retroviruses, and more recently other type D viruses (simian retroviruses, SRV) have been identified as the etiologic agents of a fatal AIDS-like disease in rhesus macaques, known as simian AIDS or SAIDS. The two other known human retroviruses (HTLV-I and HTLV-II), as well as bovine leukemia virus (BLV) and the simian T-lymphotropic virus type I (STLV-I), are generally considered as members of the oncovirus subfamily, but perhaps they should be placed into a new subfamily, based on their unique genomic organization that includes the presence of at least two regulatory genes.

The spumaviruses (spuma=Latin "foam") comprise a number of viruses from many animal species, including man, which are not associated with any pathological entity and are frequently recognized by their ability to induce the formation of foamy vacuolated syncytia in tissue culture.

Lentiviruses (lenti=Latin "slow") are non-oncogenic retroviruses that induce chronic debilitating diseases following long-term persistent infections. The Lentivirinae subfamily at present includes viruses from ungulates (maedi-visna virus of sheep, caprine arthritis-encephalitis virus (CAEV) from goats, equine infectious anemia virus (EIAV) from horses, and bovine immunodeficiency virus (BIV) from cattle), felines (feline immunodeficiency virus (FIV)), and human and nonhuman primates (HIV, simian immunodeficiency viruses (SIV)). The most outstanding characteristic of the genome of the lentivirus subfamily is the presence of a number of accessory genes with regulatory functions. In addition to *gag*, *pol*, and *env*, at least five other genes (*tat*, *trs/art*, *sor*/Q, 3'ORF/F, and R) have been identified. Some of these accessory genes are required for virus infectivity, and they regulate the expression of the viral structural proteins.

Several animal model systems for HIV infection and AIDS are now available and can be grouped as follows:

(1) infection of nonhuman primates with lentiviruses (simian immunodeficiency viruses);
(2) HIV infection of nonhuman primates;
(3) infection of nonprimate mammalian hosts with species-specific lentiviruses;
(4) infection with nonlentiviruses that induce immunodeficiency; and
(5) new potential models (2, 3).

Simian Immunodeficiency Viruses (SIV)

The simian immunodeficiency viruses are a diverse group of nonhuman primate lentiviruses. Based on their antigenic, genetic, and biological characteristics, they represent the closest known relatives to HIV.

SIV was first isolated in 1985 from diseased captive rhesus macaques in a primate center in the United States. The original isolate was called simian T-lymphotropic virus type III (STLV-III), but it is now designated SIVmac. A serologic survey conducted in 1986–1987 in this primate center showed that only three animals (two rhesus and one cynomolgous macaque) were infected among the 848 monkeys investigated. This low prevalence of SIV infection raises questions as to whether the isolated viruses actually originated from macaques in the wild or whether, perhaps, captive macaques may have acquired their SIV from some other species in the process of importation or while in captivity.

Known SIV Isolates (4–7)

Following the discovery of SIVmac, a number of other nonhuman primate lentiviruses were isolated from:

• multiple species of macaques (*Macaca*)=SIVmac;

- sooty mangabey (*Cercocebus atys*)=SIVsm;
- African green monkey (*Cercopithecus aethiops*)=SIVagm; and
- mandrills (*Papio sphinx*)=SIVmnd.

Natural infection of macaques is rare in captivity and has not been documented in nature, although more extensive serologic surveys need to be conducted to clarify this point. Several isolates of SIVmac have now been obtained in different primate centers, from cynomolgous (*M. fascicularis*), pig-tailed (*M. nemestrina*), and stump-tailed (*M. arctoides*) macaques. Some of these isolations were made from animals experimentally inoculated with tissue samples from a different species of macaque, and their precise origin remains to be elucidated. Macaques from which SIV was isolated very often died with clinical signs and necropsy findings reminiscent of AIDS, including lymphomas and lymphoproliferative diseases.

SIV from sooty mangabeys (SIVsm) was originally identified when rhesus macaques developed immunodeficiency after experimental inoculation with materials obtained from sooty mangabeys. Approximately 75% of sooty mangabeys in a colony were found to be persistently infected with SIVsm, with few manifestations of disease that might be attributed to a lentivirus. On the other hand, infection of mangabeys in their natural habitat in Africa has not been documented, again raising questions as to the origin of this virus.

Early serologic surveys for SIV-reactive antibodies demonstrated that 30% to 50% of green monkeys from Africa harbor a related virus, although a systematic evaluation of the geographical distribution of these antibodies has not been conducted. Curiously, green monkeys present in some islands in the Caribbean, descendants of animals brought to America during the 17th and 18th centuries, have been found to be seronegative. An early putative isolate for African green monkey (STLV-IIIagm) now appears to be a contaminant for SIVmac, but a number of authentic isolates of SIVagm have now been obtained, from animals from Kenya and Ethiopia.

Mandrills also appear to be infected in nature, and SIVmnd has been recently isolated from mandrills in Gabon. Natural or experimental infection with SIVagm or SIVmnd does not seem to result in disease, suggesting a lack of pathogenicity of these viruses.

Antibodies that cross-react with HIV or SIV have been found in several other Old World monkey species, suggesting the existence of other primate lentiviruses that remain to be isolated.

Genetic Relatedness of SIV Isolates (7, 8)

SIVmac is more closely related to HIV-2 than to HIV-1. It shares 75% overall nucleotide identity with HIV-2, and only 40% with HIV-1. Nucleotide conservation between HIV-1 and HIV-2 is approximately 40%, mostly within the *gag* and *pol* genes.

SIVmac isolates derived from a single primate colony display some degree of variation in their nucleotide sequence. Restriction endonuclease mapping of SIVmac derived from five rhesus and one cynomolgous macaques showed that all isolates were closely related, but nevertheless distinguishable from each other, with the isolate from the cynomolgous macaque being the most different.

Antigenic and genetic analysis of SIVagm and SIVmnd have indicated that they are newly identified members of the HIV/SIV group of primate lentiviruses. SIVagm *gag* products are antigenically related to those of HIV-1, HIV-2, and SIVmac. On the other hand, their *env* products are related to those of HIV-2 and SIVmac, but not (or scarcely) with those of HIV-1. Nucleotide sequence analyses have indicated that SIVmac and SIVagm are related, but quite distinct from each other and distinct from HIV-1 and HIV-2.

SIV from mandrills appears to be approximately equidistant from HIV-1, HIV-2, SIVagm, and SIVmac. SIV from mangabeys appear distinct from SIVmac and SIVagm, but precise information is lacking. Likewise, little information is available on the heterogeneity of isolations from a given species or genus done at different locations.

Experimental Inoculations (2, 5, 6, 9)

SIV infection in macaques induces an immunodeficiency syndrome similar to that of human AIDS and is becoming increasingly important as a model not only of infection but also of disease. The two systems that have been most explored are infection of rhesus macaques with SIVmac or with SIVsm.

Infection of rhesus macaques with SIVmac results in persistent infection leading to death in the majority of inoculated animals. The median time of death was 266 days, with a range of 62 to 1,061 days. No correlation has been observed between the dose of virus and clinical outcome, but the ability of macaques to survive correlated directly with the strength of the antibody response. Macaques that died displayed clinical symptoms and necropsy findings similar to AIDS in humans. They exhibited diarrhea, wasting, and decreases in the number of peripheral T4 lymphocytes and mitogen proliferative responses. Opportunistic infections (*Pneumocystis carinii*, cytomegalovirus, *Cryptosporidium*, *Candida*, adenovirus, and *Mycobacterium avium-intracellulare*) have been a common feature. Fifty percent of macaques have died with a characteristic granulomatous encephalitis, similar to that seen in humans.

A new approach to studying the biological properties of SIVmac isolates is the use of infectious molecular clones. At least three such infectious clones have been obtained from SIVmac (SIVmac 251, SIVmac 239, and SIVmac 142), and they may prove to be particularly useful in defining determinants of pathogenicity through in vitro experiments with molecular clones and mutants derived from them.

Experimental infection of the rhesus macaque (an Asian monkey) with SIV from the sooty mangabey (an African primate) demonstrated that this virus, although associated with no apparent disease in its species of origin, can induce an immunodeficiency disease in an alternate host which, in many respects, parallels that of acquired immunodeficiency disease (AIDS) in man. More than 70% of juvenile rhesus monkeys inoculated with a pathogenic strain of SIVsm (delta strain) died within six months of infection. In general, the simian disease parallels AIDS, but with some notable differences. Generalized lymphadenopathy was usually apparent within one month after the inoculation. This condition may persist for months, but usually regresses before the animal's death. The immediate cause of death in the majority of infected monkeys was apparently diarrhea which did not respond to appropriate antibiotic and supportive therapy. Much of the diarrhea associated with SIVsm infection was due to *Shigella* or *Campylobacter*, common pathogens in rhesus monkeys. A retroviral encephalitis morphologically very similar to that observed in AIDS was a frequent finding. B-cell lymphomas associated with an Epstein-Barr–like herpesvirus also occurred in immunosuppressed monkeys. Infection with multiple opportunistic agents was a common finding, with cytomegalovirus being the most frequent viral opportunistic agent observed, often contributing to or being the immediate cause of death. Several protozoan opportunists have also been identified, including cryptosporidia and *Pneumocystis carinii*. Syncytial cells were most commonly found in the lymph nodes and central nervous system of infected monkeys, but have also been seen in other tissues. The presence of giant cells in the tissues of infected individuals appears to be a marker for both SIV and HIV infection, since in monkeys and humans these cells express viral proteins and certain virus particles. Other lesions observed were peribronchiolar lymphoid infiltrates, hepatic lesions, and a prominent erythematous rash.

An interesting observation is that different virus isolates, although related, may vary in both pathogenic potential and the spectrum of disease they induce. Some correlations have been found between the pathogenic potential of these isolates and their ability to productively infect primary monocytes, and one strain was associated with a high incidence of central nervous system infection. As with the SIVmac–rhesus model, pathogenicity is relatively independent of dose. On the other hand, changes in lymphocyte subsets (particularly in the helper-inducer subset of T-lymphocytes), a decline in SIV-specific antibody, and virus-specific antigenemia are prognostic for disease progression. Inoculated animals that remained clinically healthy respond to SIV infection with antibodies to both *gag*- and *env*-related SIV proteins which persist throughout the course of infection. In infected animals displaying immunological alterations, a disproportionate loss of *gag*-specific, relative to *env*-specific, antibodies was observed in the terminal stages of the disease. This decline uniformly coincided with the emergence of viral antigen in serum. These changes are apparent months before any change in the clinical picture can be noted and thus are useful prognostic indicators for disease progression. This observation is consistent with that reported in HIV-infected humans wherein a loss of detectable HIV *gag*-specific antibody coincident with antigenemia was noted in patients progressing from ARC (AIDS-related complex) to AIDS. The striking exception to the SIV antibody response previously described involves animals that develop retroviral-associated encephalopathy. The clinical course of the disease in monkeys with encephalopathy varies from acute (death within eight to nine weeks after inoculation) to chronic (survival for five to seven months). SIV-specific antibodies in all of these animals were either markedly reduced, when compared to other SIV-infected animals, or notably absent, regardless of the time course of the disease. Moreover, lack of detectable SIV antibody corresponds to persistent, recurrent, or progressively increasing levels of SIV antigen in the serum.

Studies similar to those described above have been conducted at another primate center, using a different isolate of SIVsm (strain SMM Yerkes). Twelve rhesus macaques have now been infected for 20 to 33 months, and five of the animals died of an AIDS-like disease between 14 and 28 months after inoculation. Characteristics of the disease in macaques that died following infection include weight loss, diarrhea, lymphadenopathy, pneumonia, hepatosplenomegaly, ataxia, anemia, neutropenia, lymphopenia with preferential loss of CD4$^+$ cells, thrombocytopenia, and hyper- and hypogammaglobu-linemia. Histopathologic analysis revealed that most of the tissues from some animals, including lymph node, spleen, lung, and brain, contained multinucleated giant cells. Following inoculation, most of the animals developed antibodies to *env*- and *gag*-encoded proteins between three and six weeks after virus inoculation and, in agreement with findings in SIV-infected mangabeys, few or no neutralizing antibodies were detected in serum from the rhesus macaques up to 18 months after infection. Loss of antibodies to specific proteins, primarily *gag*-encoded, was detected, but owing to the limited number of animals that have died to date, it has not been possible to determine whether a specific antibody profile will be predictive of more severe disease and death. It was found, however, that cell-free virus can be recovered from the serum of animals that have more frequent and persistent symptoms of disease, but not from those animals that remain well or show only intermittent signs of disease.

SIVsm was also used to inoculate a pig-tailed macaque, which unlike the inoculated rhesus macaques, was found to develop neutralizing antibodies at six months after infection. The pig-tailed macaque had essentially no antibodies to *gag* gene products at any time after infection and was sacrificed 14 months after inoculation because of a deteriorating clinical condition and signs of neurologic disease. At the time of death, virus was recovered from peripheral blood mononuclear cells (PBMC) and from multiple tissues, including the brain. The concentration of cell-free virus increased from 10 fifty percent-tissue-culture-infectious doses per milliliter (TCID-50/ml) at six months after infection to 10^2 TCID-50/ml at 10 months and to 10^4 at the time of sacrifice. Virus isolated at the time of death was used to inoculate additional macaques and SIV-seronegative mangabeys, and resulted in death within 13 days of inoculation in eight out of nine macaques and three out of four mangabeys. The acute deaths were due to severe mucoid diarrhea that led to dehydration and electrolyte imbalance. An interesting observation was that both of two SIV-SMM virus-positive and seropositive mangabey monkeys were protected from the lethal effect of the SIVsm variant (designated SMM-PBj14). Investigations are now being conducted to demonstrate definitively that it is in fact SIVsm that is killing the animals with this rapidity. If validated, the use of a highly virulent strain of SIV may provide a rapid assay system for screening drugs or vaccines for efficacy in the prevention not only of infection but also of disease.

Potential Uses of the SIV Model

The potential use of the SIV model for the study of human AIDS derives from the many similarities of these viruses with HIV. Both viruses have the same morphology and morphogenesis typical of lentiviruses and exhibit tropism for cells bearing the CD4 antigen. Conservation of some critical epitopes of CD4 in a variety of primate species allows the in vitro infection of their lymphocytes with HIV. Infection of CD4$^+$ cells with HIV or SIV can be cytopathic for these cells. As described before, SIV can cause an AIDS-like disease in selected species of nonhuman primates, and the induced disease is remarkably similar to AIDS in humans. However, Kaposi's sarcoma has not been described in SIV-infected primates, and the spectrum of opportunistic agents observed following SIV-induced immunosuppression is slightly different from that in HIV-infected humans. There are many conserved epitopes in the major viral antigens of SIV and HIV, and the existence of these epitopes permitted early serologic identification of the existence of HIV-related viruses in nonhuman primates.

The nucleotide sequence and genomic organization of SIV is closely related to those of HIV-2. However, SIVmac and SIVagm, as well as HIV-2, have an additional gene, X, which is not present in HIV-1. This gene X appears to be expressed in the SIV virus, is immunogenic, and apparently is dispensable for the replication of the virus in vitro. The R gene, which is present in HIV-1, HIV-2, and SIVmac, does not appear to be present in at least one isolate of SIVagm. Comparisons of the genomic structure of pathogenic and nonpathogenic SIV isolates may be important to understanding the molecular basis of the pathogenicity of HIV. Another major molecular difference between HIV-1 and SIV is that SIV (SIVmac and SIVagm) often has a premature stop codon in *env*, resulting in a truncated form of transmembrane glycoprotein. This premature translation termination signal has also been observed in HIV-2.

Continued use of the SIV model will be important in three areas of AIDS research:

(1) To better understand the natural history and evolution of primate lentiviruses. Information is needed regarding species in the wild that harbor SIV as well as the precise genetic make-up of these viruses.

(2) To define the pathogenesis of AIDS, such as mechanisms of persistence, host tropisms, and viral determinants of neuropathogenicity.

(3) To develop AIDS vaccines and treatment strategies. Comparison of vaccine approaches can be more easily achieved using
SIV in readily available macaques than by using HIV in rare
chimpanzees.

Studies in all these areas are dependent on more fundamental
research, including investigations of virus-host interactions and characterization of the immune system of the nonhuman primate host.

HIV Infection of Nonhuman Primates

The ideal model for AIDS would be one in which HIV infects and
induces an AIDS-like disease in a common experimental animal.
Thus far, in addition to humans, only chimpanzees and gibbon apes
have been found to be susceptible to HIV infection. Only very limited
numbers of these animals are available to researchers.

The ability of HIV to infect in vitro the lymphocytes of a number of
primate species indicates that further investigation, particularly with
common New World primates, may be warranted.

Experimental Infection of Chimpanzees (10, 11)

Several groups have demonstrated that chimpanzees can be readily
infected with some strains of HIV-1. Infections are easily established
by intravenous inoculation of human tissue homogenates, HIV-1-
infected PBMC, or cell-free HIV-1, or by application of cell-free virus
to vaginal mucosa. It appears that only small numbers of virus particles are needed to establish infection in chimpanzees, but strain differences may exist. It has been documented that 40 TCID-50 of HIV-1
(strain HTLV-IIIB) established infection in both of two chimpanzees,
but only one of two animals became infected with 4 TCID-50 of the
same pool of viruses.

Within two weeks of inoculation of the LAV-1 strain of HIV-1, virus
can be recovered from PBMC of chimpanzees, irrespective of the
inoculum or route of inoculation, and once an animal is infected,
virus can be recovered on a routine basis from PBMC. In contrast,
cell-free virus has only been obtained from animals during the first six
weeks after infection. Virus has also been obtained from one of two
bone marrow samples, but not from a limited number of saliva or
spinal fluid samples that were tested.

Early after infection (the first two to three months), 10^3 to 10^4 infectious PBMC per 10^7 PBMC can be detected. Over the ensuing months, this number drops to a baseline level of one to 10 infectious PBMC per 10^7 PBMC, which persists for extended periods. Thus, there appears to be an early phase of viremia, corresponding to high numbers of infectious cells, which gradually disappears as HIV-1–specific antibody titers increase; however, the decrease in numbers of infectious PBMC or cell-free virus has not yet been shown to result from immune clearance. HIV-1–specific antibodies are detectable in serum of chimpanzees by enzyme immunoassay (EIA), immunoblot, and radioimmunoprecipitation (RIP) assay within approximately four weeks of virus inoculation. Short-lived low-titered (less than 100) IgM responses to HIV-1 have been detected in about one-half of infected chimpanzees, but IgG titers, as determined by EIA, developed rapidly and stabilized about six months after infection at titers ranging from 25,000 to 500,000. Antibodies to *env* and *gag* gene products are detectable at approximately the same time (three to five weeks after infection) while antibodies to *pol* gene products are delayed by weeks to a few months. More recently, antibodies to the putative regulatory protein encoded by the 3'ORF/F gene have been detected either coincident with antibodies to *env* and *gag* proteins, or even earlier. It is interesting to mention that experimental inoculation of a chimpanzee with the ARV-2/SF2 isolate of HIV resulted in a less-efficient infection, with virus being recovered by PBMC only after five months after the inoculation. In this animal, antibodies to the 3'ORF/F gene product were detected within two weeks after inoculation, whereas antibodies to other proteins were not detected until three months later.

Antibodies that mediate complement-dependent lysis of HIV-infected cells have been demonstrated in infected chimpanzees; these antibodies are generated relatively early after infection and are capable of lysing cells infected with diverse strains of HIV, analogous to cross-reactivity that has been observed for neutralizing antibodies.

All persistently infected animals possess PBMC that proliferate and incorporate thymidine when incubated with purified HIV antigen; this reactivity occurs as a dose-dependent response. In contrast, not all animals have cells capable of lysing HIV-infected cells. Using as target cells autologous or heterologous EBV-transformed B-cells infected with recombinant vaccinia viruses expressing various HIV genes, PBMC from chimpanzees infected with HIV-1 for various periods of time were used as effectors. While PBMC from most infected animals exhibited HIV-specific cytotoxic activity, they killed not only autologous but also heterologous cells to the same extent. These data indicate that the killing may be effected by antigen-specific, non-major histocompatibility complex–restricted natural killer (NK) or lymphokine-activated killer (LAK) cells.

Thus far, no AIDS-like disease has been shown to occur in HIV-1 infected chimpanzees. However, evidence of minimal disease has been documented. During the first six months after inoculation of juvenile chimpanzees, the rate of weight gain in the animals showed a significant decrease. In addition to transient mild thrombocytopenia in one animal, substantial lymphadenopathy was observed in two animals that received large doses of HIV-1. Histopathologic analysis of biopsy material from inguinal lymph nodes of these animals with lymphadenopathy showed marked follicular hyperplasia and irregularly shaped germinal centers, similar to what is seen in human tissue sections from HIV-infected persons. Interestingly, one chimpanzee that had no cellular cytotoxic activity (but whose PBMC did proliferate in response to antigen) has been infected with HIV-1 for four years and has lost antibodies to p24 over the last two years. This animal has exhibited no signs of disease or hematological abnormalities. A second animal, infected for more than three and one half years also has lost antibodies to p24, as determined by radioimmunoprecipitation assay. These animals are being closely monitored to see whether loss of antibodies to p24 in chimpanzees will parallel the human situation where this phenomenon correlates with onset of antigenemia and progression to disease. In addition, a third chimpanzee infected for more than three years has developed persistent lymphopenia with loss of CD4+ cells. Perhaps, as apparently is the case with humans infected with HIV, the major cofactor for the development of AIDS in chimpanzees is time.

Attempts to infect nonhuman primate species with HIV-2 isolates have been partially successful, and some animals have been chronically infected for more than one year. Seroconversion and virus recovery have been documented, but no evidence of hematological abnormality or disease has been observed. Efforts are continuing, by serial passage, to obtain an HIV-2 strain adapted for growth in macaques.

Immunization of Chimpanzees with Prototype Vaccines (12)

Immunization of chimpanzees has been attempted with a variety of antigens: recombinant vaccinia viruses expressing HIV-1 antigens, HIV-1 glycoprotein subunit preparations, purified HIV-1 antigens expressed in different eukaryotic or prokaryotic systems, inactivated HIV-1 virions, and synthetic peptides. Immunization has resulted in the priming of HIV-specific T-cells, and in the development of antibodies detectable by ELISA, immunoblot, and radioimmunoprecipitation. However, sera from the immunized chimpanzees had weak, if any, neutralizing activity against HIV-1. Chimpanzees that were subsequently challenged with HIV-1 were not protected against the development of viral infection.

The following are examples of the approaches being used to develop prototype vaccines which are being evaluated in chimpanzees:

(a) Because the external glycoprotein gp120 specifically binds to the CD4 molecule on the surface of T4-positive cells (the initial event in the infectious process), it is generally assumed that an immune response against this protein may serve to inhibit virus replication. Also, since gp120 is expressed on the surface of virus-infected cells, an effective T-cell–directed immune response to gp120 may be effective in eliminating cells infected with HIV.

Native gp120, purified by immunoaffinity from membranes of cells infected with HIV-1 (strain HTLV-IIIB), has been used to immunize chimpanzees. Precipitating antibodies were maximum at two weeks after subsequent boosters, but rapidly decayed after each immunization. Neutralizing antibodies were produced, but they were only effective against the homologous virus and did not neutralize a different strain of HIV-1 (HTLV-IIIRF). Two chimpanzees were selected for challenge two weeks after a fifth dose of gp120 formulated in alum, receiving 40 or 400 TCID-50. Virus was isolated from both animals and both developed antibodies to p24, indicating an active infection.

(b) It is likely that neutralizing antibodies to HIV, which have been demonstrated in certain HIV-infected humans, may prevent extracellular spread of the virus, but the virus can also spread from infected to uninfected cells by cell fusion and can thereby escape neutralizing antibodies. Antibodies that can lyse HIV-infected cells by antibody-dependent cell-mediated cytotoxicity have recently been detected in healthy HIV-seropositive individuals and in patients who have developed AIDS.

T-cell-mediated immunity, which has been found to be very important in protection against disease or death caused by a variety of envelope viruses in animals, may help eradicate HIV-infected cells which can express HIV antigens before spreading virus to uninfected cells. HIV-specific T-helper cells may produce lymphokines, such as interleukin-2 (IL-2), to expand HIV-specific cytotoxic T-cells or which could activate other effector cells such as natural killer cells or macrophages to lyse HIV-infected cells.

Immunization of nonhuman primates with a recombinant vaccinia virus that expressed HIV envelope glycoproteins did induce HIV-specific T-helper cells in macaques and chimpanzees and also primed HIV-specific cytotoxic T-cells in chimpanzees. T-cells from chimpanzees infected with HIV for three months to three years showed strong proliferative responses to HIV. Some HIV-infected healthy humans also have T-cells that recognize HIV antigens by proliferating and/or by lysing autologous HIV-infected cells. In this regard, it will be interesting and important to determine whether there is an inverse relationship between the level and functional types of HIV-specific T-cell responses with the subsequent development of disease in HIV-infected humans. If this is observed, it will add further rationale for developing AIDS vaccines that can induce strong HIV-specific T-cell–mediated immunity in man, as well as rationale for attempting to augment HIV-specific T-cell immunity in humans already infected with the virus before they develop immunosuppression.

(c) Prototype live recombinant vaccines have also been prepared by inserting the genes encoding either the HIV-1 (strain LAV-BRU) envelope glycoprotein gp160 and/or core proteins p24, p18, or the complete *gag* protein or nonstructural proteins F (3'ORF/F) or Q (*sor*) into a vaccinia virus genome. Resulting recombinant viruses were injected into chimpanzees by the intradermal route or by scarification. The chimpanzees showed a transient but significant proliferative response to HIV or gp160, but not to p24, after two injections of or scarifications with vaccinia virus recombinants. Most animals were also seropositive to HIV-1 by ELISA. Immune responses were enhanced after the boost with recombinant vaccinia virus-infected cells. Antibodies specific for HIV core antigens were also generated.

Prospects for the Future

Experimental infection of chimpanzees with HIV-1 is a reliable model of infection by the human virus. If the evidence suggesting that chimpanzees infected with HIV may develop disease is borne out, it may be possible to identify factors that influence disease progression.

With the development of the simian immunodeficiency model, chimpanzees could be reserved for second-phase testing of more promising candidate vaccines. Preparations with increased immunogenicity, using different immunization vehicles, such as immuno-stimulatory complexes (ISCOMs), are currently being evaluated as possible means for inducing a broader-reacting immune response that is maintained for a longer period of time after vaccination.

Lentiviruses from Nonprimate Mammalian Hosts

The term lentivirus ("slow virus") was applied first to the etiologic agents of maedi-visna disease complex of sheep, the classic example of "slow virus disease." Slow viruses have long incubation periods, with a gradual onset and slowly progressive course of disease that invariably ends in cachexia and death. However, visna virus is not T-lymphotropic and does not cause immunodeficiency.

Other mammalian viruses with biophysical properties similar to maedi-visna virus have been recognized in nature and placed in the lentivirus subfamily. Two recent additions to this subfamily are the bovine immunodeficiency-like virus (BIV) and the feline immunodeficiency virus (FIV; formerly called FTLV). BIV and FIV are distinct from the previously known bovine (BLV) and feline (FeLV) leukemia viruses, which are members of the oncovirus subfamily. The nonprimate lentiviruses are restricted in their host range and are not known to infect primates, including humans.

Visna virus replicates in lymphocytes and macrophages in vivo, resulting in life-long infection in the host. Virus replication continues throughout the infection at a minimally productive rate, a phenomenon that, by definition, emphasizes the ineffectiveness of immunologic mechanisms in eliminating the agents. Enigmas that apply to all lentivirus infections are the nature of the factor(s) that trigger the onset of disease after prolonged periods of subclinical infection and the paradox of virus–host interactions in which the virus replicates at a minimal rate and yet somehow leads to progressive wasting disease.

Pathogenic Mechanisms of Nonprimate Lentiviruses (13)

Studies on the closely-related visna and caprine arthritis-encephalitis viruses suggest that the infection of macrophages plays a pivotal role in the mechanism of virus persistence and in the clinical syndromes that these animals succumb to. HIV also infects macrophages, and as studies on the pathogenesis of AIDS unfold, these cells are coming under increased scrutiny as candidates with probably as great a role in the human disease as they have in the diseases of sheep and goats. The close similarity between the animal lentiviruses and HIV suggests that the interaction between the lentiviruses and host cells may provide relevant information and a better understanding of the biology of the human pathogen.

The lentiviruses show distinct differences in their interaction with macrophages and with nonmacrophage cell types. These latter cells may be fibroblasts in the visna virus system or helper T-lymphocytes in the HIV system. In the visna system, the interactions between virus and fibroblasts and virus and macrophages can be summarized as follows:

(a) *Visna virus/fibroblast interactions.* Visna virus causes fusion of fibroblasts "from without" in a pH-independent manner, reminiscent of paramyxovirus/cell interactions. This suggests that the viral genome is introduced into these cells after fusion of the viral envelope with the plasma membrane of the cell. Initial fusion between virus and fibroblasts is followed by progressive fusion of contiguous cells. Antibodies that inhibit this fusion process usually neutralize infectivity of the virus. However, when antigenic variant viruses are used in these experiments, polyclonal antibodies induced by the parental virus prevent fusion by the variant virus but do not neutralize infectivity of the latter agent. Thus, infection in fibroblasts may occur independently of cell-to-cell fusion. Maturation of progeny virus in fibroblasts occurs at the plasma membrane by a budding process. Treatment of cells with neutralizing antibodies at this stage of the virus life-cycle results in accumulation of virus particles at various stages of budding at the cell surface and "capping off" of these viral aggregates.

(b) *Visna virus/macrophage interactions.* Lentiviruses do not cause "fusion from without" in macrophages, irrespective of the multiplicity of inoculation (up to 10^3 plaque-forming units per cell). This indicates that virus enters these cells by a nonfusing process, perhaps by endocytosis, after binding to a specific receptor, or by random phagocytosis of the particles. Virus preincubated with antibodies is endocytosed faster than non–antibody-treated virus. Both neutralizing and nonneutralizing antibodies accelerate the early events in the virus life-cycle including binding and uncoating of the virus within the macrophage. When neutralizing antibodies are used, virus is internalized and uncoated rapidly, but no RNA transcripts are produced.

Antibodies which bind to viral envelope antigens but do not neutralize infectivity enhance the infection because these immunoglobulins facilitate entry of large numbers of infectious virus particles into the macrophages. This disparity in speed of entry of virus into the cells between antibody-treated virus and virus alone does not occur when F(ab)$_2$ fragments of the antibodies are used instead of intact immunoglobulins. This provides indirect evidence that when virus particles are reacted with antibody molecules, complexes may be endocytosed by macrophages via Fc receptors on the surface of these cells. Thus, infection in the macrophage may occur by three mechanisms: (1) entry into the cell following virus attachment to specific receptors; (2) entry into cells by phagocytosis of virus particles; and (3) entry into cells by phagocytosis of immune complexes via the Fc receptors of the cell. Virus maturation in macrophages occurs within the cytoplasm of the cell by budding off of membranes of intracytoplasmic vacuoles and accumulation within these vacuoles. Only minimal budding of virus particles occurs at the plasma membrane of these cells.

The envelope of lentiviruses consists of a large, heavily glycosylated glycoprotein structure that is encoded by the *env* gene. Oligosaccharide chains with numerous terminal sialic acid molecules are attached to the *env* protein backbone by O and N linkages. These carbohydrate molecules create an outer shell on the virus and cause reduction in the affinity of binding of neutralizing antibodies to virus particles. Treatment of virions with neuraminidase removes the sialic acid molecules, which results in improvement in the kinetics of neutralization. In fact, some sera which have no apparent neutralizing activity (they have infection-enhancing properties) will neutralize neuraminidase-treated virus. The distinction between neutralizing and nonneutralizing antibodies may therefore reside in the avidity of binding between Ig molecules and virus particles. Neutralizing antibodies may bind more tightly to the virus particles than the nonneutralizing antibodies. Since virus neutralization is the net result of two competing systems—virus binding to cells and virus binding to antibodies—any delay in binding between virus and antibodies would increase the chances of infection in the host cell. This is particularly important because the affinity of virus for cellular attachment sites is very high. The mere demonstration of neutralizing antibodies in sera is therefore not enough to indicate protective properties because such antibodies may be "slow" in causing neutralization or even enhance infection in macrophages.

Although virus morphogenesis occurs within the cytoplasm of the macrophages, these cells express viral antigens on their plasma membranes, preceding by two or three days the synthesis of virus particles. One of these antigens is a fusion determinant of visna virus. Cells with receptors for the fusion determinant are readily recruited into multinucleated syncytia. The fusion process represents a potential mechanism for the macrophage to disseminate infectivity by a transfection mechanism. Such a process does not require virus particles to cause infection because viral RNA, transfected into neighboring cells by the fusion process, would be enough to initiate the virus life-cycle without participation by infectious virions. Recent experiments have suggested that high levels of antifusion antibodies (not necessarily neutralizing) may protect animals against massive dissemination of virus in vivo and thus help them to remain clinically normal, albeit infected. A relevant question here is: are anti-fusion antibodies important in protecting against disease? This concept may be important in a vaccine-therapy approach where the idea would be not to prevent infection as a true vaccine does, but rather to boost production of antibodies to the fusion proteins of the virus. The object would be to limit the rate of virus dissemination and thus keep the infection within controllable limits.

Virus-infected macrophages present viral antigens to lymphocytes within restriction limits of major histocompatibility complex antigens. One of the viral antigens is associated with Ia antigens on the surface of the infected macrophage. The viral antigen is distinct from the structural fusion determinant of visna virus and is recognized within the context of Ia by T-lymphocytes of sheep and goats, resulting in production of an interferon. This interferon has a number of effects on the mononuclear cell population, including induction of expression of Ia and production of prostaglandin E2 by macrophages, suppression of proliferation of mononuclear cells, and inhibition of virus gene expression. It has been proposed that maintenance of macrophages in a state of continuous antigen presentation may increase the potential for creating immunopathologic or possible autoimmune reactions.

In summary, lentiviruses have evolved an unusual relationship with the chief defense cell of the body. The infected macrophage not only regulates the amount of virus particles produced during infection, but is also the major disseminator of virus in nature (infected macrophages in colostrum and inflammatory respiratory exudates), for the spread of the virus within the body, and for induction of immunopathologic processes. Therapeutic interventions aimed at preventing infection or reducing the severity of pathologic lesions will have to focus on the infected macrophage in its role as a virus-producing cell and also as an infected antigen-presenting cell. Such interventions will have to be performed with the understanding that this therapy, which may prevent virus replication, may enhance immunologic reactivity and pathology, and vice versa.

Feline Immunodeficiency Virus (FIV) (14)

FIV, previously known as feline T-lymphotropic lentivirus (FTLV), causes a persistent immunodeficiency syndrome characterized by oral, gastrointestinal, and upper respiratory diseases. The pathology most frequently observed is gingivitis, periodontitis, chronic proliferative and ulcerative stomatitis, anorexia and emaciation, chronic diarrhea and dehydration, chronic rhinitis, conjunctivitis, and upper respiratory infections. Other clinical signs observed in the infected cats are lymphadenopathy, neurologic abnormalities, chronic abscesses, fever, and chronic microbial infections.

Serologic surveys conducted in different parts of the world have shown that 14% to 30% of cats with a history of chronic infections are infected with FIV, although coinfection with FeLV is common.

The initial isolation of FIV was derived by co-cultivating peripheral blood lymphocytes (PBL) from infected cats with concanavalin-A (Con-A)–stimulated PBL from specific-pathogen–free (SPF) cats. The virus induced giant cells and cell death in these cultures. The virus isolate replicated in primary T-spleen cells as well as in stimulated thymus cells, feline T-lymphoblastoid cell lines (FL74, LSA-1), and Crandell feline kidney cells. FIV is highly species-specific and does not seem to replicate in a variety of human, canine, and rodent cell lines tested.

FIV has the typical morphology of lentiviruses and possesses a Mg^{++}-dependent reverse transcriptase. In Western blot analysis, FIV antigens do not cross-react with those of SIV, HIV-1, HIV-2, maedi-visna, or caprine arthritis-encephalitis virus. Molecular cloning and detailed analysis of the FIV genome remain to be done.

Experimental infection of SPF kittens resulted in life-long persistent infection. Antibodies are detectable by ELISA or Western blot as early as two weeks after infection. A generalized lymphadenopathy appears in all experimentally infected cats, beginning three to five weeks post-inoculation; peak lymph node enlargement occurs two to eight weeks later, and slowly resolves after two to nine months. An absolute neutropenia, often associated with a leukopenia, occurs in many of the cats, beginning about two to five weeks post-inoculation and persisting for four to nine weeks before disappearing. FIV has been reisolated from the brain, spleen, bone marrow, PBL, mesenteric and submandibular lymph nodes, saliva, and cerebrospinal fluid.

Blastogenic responses to T-cell mitogens are depressed during the initial clinical phase of illness (fever, neutropenia) in experimentally infected kittens. Suppression of lymphocyte mitogenesis lasted for several weeks before reversing itself. Lymphocyte blastogenesis then increased above normal levels during the subsequent two to nine months of the lymphadenopathy stage, and it returned to normal as the lymphadenopathy disappeared. A variable decrease in lymphocyte blastogenesis reappeared in the AIDS phase of the illness.

Attempts to demonstrate experimentally horizontal transmission by prolonged intimate contact have failed. However, FIV appears to be transmitted by bites (through infected saliva).

Bovine Immunodeficiency-like Virus (BIV) (15)

BIV was originally isolated in 1969 from leukocytes of a cow with persistent lymphocytosis, lymphadenopathy, lesions of the central nervous system, progressive weakness, and emaciation. However, the extent of BIV natural infection remains to be determined.

Experimental infection with BIV of colostrum-deprived calves reared in isolation causes a mild lymphocytosis and lymphadenopathy early in the infection (within 3 to 12 weeks after inoculation), which is similar to the persistent generalized lymphadenopathy considered to be part of the AIDS-related complex (ARC). The subcutaneous palpable nodes are of the hemolymph type and are particularly noticeable in the cervical region. Histological examination of these swollen nodes reveals a follicular hyperplasia of the germinal centers without signs of lymphosarcoma. The hyperplasia can be specifically attributed to an increase in the number of small lymphocytes.

BIV can grow in a number of primary cell cultures derived from first-trimester bovine fetuses, although the cell of choice has been spleen. At present, established cell lines of bovine origin have not been permissive for viral replication, but a fetal canine thymus cell line (Cf2th) is susceptible and may provide a good source of antigen for diagnostic tests.

The cytopathic or syncytia-inducing capability of BIV is similar to that seen in HIV and other lentiviruses in their host cells. BIV has a reverse transcriptase which shows a significant preference for Mg^{++}. Electron microscopy of infected cultures reveals virus particles with a lentivirus morphology. Polyacrylamide-gel electrophoresis of concentrated purified virus reveals a major band of relative molecular mass (M_r) 26,000 (p26) corresponding to the major core protein. Preliminary studies of BIV proteins, recognized by bovine antibodies from naturally or experimentally infected cattle, have shown putative transmembrane protein with a relative molecular mass of 32,000 to 42,000 and an exterior envelope glycoprotein as a doublet of M_r 120,000 and 160,000, by radioimmunoprecipitation and Western blotting. Immunofluorescence assays of HIV-infected lymphocytes using polyvalent anti-BIV serum demonstrated the presence of cross-reacting epitopes; these shared determinants were localized in Western blots to the major core proteins, p24 and p26, of HIV and BIV, respectively.

BIV has recently been molecularly cloned, and two infectious proviruses (clones 106 and 127) have been obtained for future detailed studies. Clone 106 has been completely sequenced. Overall, the genome looks much like that of HIV with the exception that it is smaller (8,875 base pairs). The *env* gene region is larger and has a significant number of glycosylation sites. Restriction enzyme comparisons of the two infectious clones suggest a hyperavailability of *env* sequences, as seen in other lentiviruses. There is an intergenic region between the *pol* and *env* genes in which several open reading frames can be found that may functionally correspond to the *sor*/Q, *tat* and *trs/art*, and X genes found in HIV and/or SIV. An additional open reading frame exists at the 3' LTR. Detailed analyses of the structure, function, and relationship of the predicted coding regions are presently under study.

Potential Uses of Nonprimate Lentivirus Models

The nonprimate lentivirus animal models offer several advantages, e.g., they are natural infections common throughout the world and, because of their species-specificity, working with these agents does not require biohazard containment for human protection. These animal models are potentially useful for dissecting the complex biology of HIV infection, including mechanisms for induction of protective immunity.

Once validated, the FIV model has the following advantages: inexpensive, short incubation period, animals available in large supply, various clinical stages from field cases, and specific-pathogen–free animals. This model could also be used for the preliminary screening of large numbers of potentially useful antiviral agents.

Other Viruses and Models

Nonlentiviruses That Induce Immunodeficiency

Included in this category are feline leukemia virus (FeLV) and the macaque type D retroviruses (SRV) associated with simian AIDS (SAIDS).

In addition to subclinical infection and tumors which generally take a long time to develop, FeLV can be responsible for a wide spectrum of chronic nonneoplastic conditions in cats including immunosuppression, wasting, severe diarrhea, and anemia. Similarly, type D retroviruses have been shown to be associated with immunodeficiency and chronic wasting syndromes, opportunistic infections, necrotizing gingivitis, and retroperitoneal fibromatosis in primate colonies.

Experience with several animal retroviruses underpins the rationale for selecting the HIV envelope as the antigen for use in many of the candidate AIDS vaccines. An experimental bovine leukemia virus (BLV) vaccine is being tested, and extensive studies of murine leukemia virus have shown that vaccines incorporating the envelope glycoprotein may prevent infection. A commercial vaccine against FeLV, which includes envelope glycoprotein, protects most cats from FeLV infection and disease.

A killed whole-virus preparation has been shown to confer protection against the type-D SRV infection. This would allow for the comparison of vaccine strategies in this model, using different recombinant and other subunit candidate vaccines. Type-D simian retroviruses are common in macaque colonies, a situation that has to be understood and controlled in order to develop further the more relevant SIV model.

New Potential Models: Transgenic Mice

A characteristic feature of HIV infection is the long asymptomatic phase following initial exposure to the virus. During this period, a positive serology may be the only evidence of infection in an individual with no clinical evidence of disease. It is very likely, however, that multiple copies of integrated provirus DNA are present in infected persons, some of which may be functionally repressed, incapable of performing the production of progeny virions. This latent or persistent phase of HIV infection has been modeled by constructing two types of transgenic mice in which gene expression is regulated by the HIV long terminal repeats (LTR).

The first model consists of the HIV LTR linked to the bacterial gene, chloramphenicol acetyl transferase (CAT). The CAT gene has been ligated to a number of eukaryotic and viral promoter elements and its expression monitored following transfection into mammalian cells. Four founder strains of mice were established carrying two to eight copies of the HIV LTR-CAT construction. High levels of constructive CAT expression were monitored in the thymus, tail, heart, and eye of all four transgenic mouse strains; lower levels were detected in spleen, small intestine, and liver. Although no HIV LTR-directed CAT activity was detectable in circulating lymphocytes or bone marrow-derived macrophages, augmented (20–30-fold) expression was observed when these cells were activated in vitro with mitogens or recombinant cytokines such as IL-2, colony-stimulating factor (CSF-1), and granulocyte–macrophage colony-stimulating factor (GM-CSF). Upon further examination, the elevated CAT expression in mouse tail was localized to the skin. Fractionation of skin constituents revealed very high levels of CAT in epidermal Langerhans cells (LC) and not in keratinocytes. The former are highly differentiated dendritic cells of monocyte macrophage lineage, comprising 2% to 5% of epidermal cells. Functionally, LC are thought to be the most peripheral limb of the immune system, representing the cell type that initially encounters microorganisms/foreign bodies at the portal of entry. LC are considered to be highly differentiated monocytes (macrophages which originate in the bone marrow). Several reports describe the depletion of LC in AIDS patients. It is noteworthy that HIV LTR-directed CAT synthesis occurred in transgenic animals that had never been exposed to the HIV transactivating regulatory protein, *tat*. These findings therefore imply the existence of tissue-specific regulatory factors that are able to modulate the expression of an integrated HIV LTR.

In a second group of experiments, transgenic mice were constructed containing an infectious molecular clone of HIV. Thirteen founder animals, ranging in age from 7 to 16 weeks and containing 2 to 60 copies of HIV, have been obtained. Thus far, all 13 animals are healthy and have exhibited no manifestations of disease. Two animals seroconverted and synthesized antibodies that react with HIV *env* and *gag* proteins. One of these (a female animal), containing two copies of the HIV provirus, was mated to nontransgenic FVB male mice; two litters have been obtained. Approximately 50% (9/19) of F-1 animals developed a unique syndrome and died. The clinicopathologic features of the affected animals include runting, scaling, and fissuring of the skin on the tail, feet, and ears (microscopically characterized by hyperkeratosis and acanthosis), thymic atrophy (about 20% the size of the thymus in nontransgenic littermates), lymphadenopathy, and lymphocytic infiltrates in the spleen, lung, and intestine. Animals developed symptoms at 12 to 14 days of age and died approximately two weeks later. Affected animals invariably carried the HIV provirus, whereas healthy littermates were not transgenic.

Conclusions and Recommendations

The consultation clearly indicated that there are a number of potentially useful animal models for HIV infection and disease. Three major models were discussed: simian immunodeficiency viruses (SIV), nonprimate lentiviruses, and HIV infection of nonhuman primates.

Simian immunodeficiency viruses comprise a diverse group of nonhuman lentiviruses, closely related to HIV. They have been isolated from macaques, sooty mangabeys, African green monkeys, and mandrills. The last two species are known to be infected in their natural habitats. SIV shares a number of molecular and biological characteristics with HIV and causes an AIDS-like disease in selected nonhuman primates. The SIV model will be important to understand the pathogenesis of the disease and will facilitate the evaluation of AIDS candidate vaccines and treatment strategies.

The nonprimate lentiviruses include a number of persistent viruses that cause chronic debilitating diseases and sometimes immunodeficiency in different animal species. These viruses are not known to infect primates, including humans. The nonprimate models, particularly the bovine and feline lentiviruses, could be used for dissecting the complex biology of HIV infection, including the mechanism for induction of protective immunity. A major advantage is that infection with these viruses is common throughout the world, and working with them does not require biohazard containment for human protection. Lentiviruses from small animals could be used for the preliminary screening of large numbers of potentially useful antiviral agents.

Chimpanzees are susceptible to infection with HIV-1 and exhibit a humoral immune response similar to that seen in human HIV infection. At 48 months post-infection, no chimpanzee was found to have developed the clinical features of AIDS, but changes in the HIV antibody profiles, predictive of the disease in humans, are now being observed. Immunization of chimpanzees with a variety of candidate vaccines has resulted in the forming of HIV-specific T-cells and in the development of antibodies, although with little or no detectable neutralizing activity. Immunized chimpanzees that were challenged with HIV-1 were not protected, and more effective immunogens are now being evaluated.

The participants' recommendations to WHO were:

(a) To promote further research on animal models, including HIV, SIV, and nonprimate lentivirus models, with emphasis on the mechanisms of pathogenesis, potential measures for protective immunity and therapy, and studies on the diversity and natural history of primate lentiviruses. Ongoing basic and applied research with SIV should be accelerated and new avenues for its use should be explored.

(b) To assist in the establishment of primate research facilities and in the coordination of international collaborative efforts between investigators in different countries. Critical for this effort is the need for new facilities with adequate biosafety containment.

(c) To continue to facilitate exchange of information pertinent to animal models for HIV and SIV infections through sponsorship of scientific and technical meetings and publication of technical reports.

(d) To assist in efforts to optimize the development and use of primate and nonprimate lentivirus models, including the development of ancillary reagent and test systems, such as a repository of relevant antibodies to characterize viruses and target cells. WHO should facilitate the availability of these reagents by establishing reference centers for animal lentiviruses.

(e) To develop recommendations on the use of relevant animal models for HIV infection in the evaluation of candidate vaccines and therapeutic agents.

■ ■ ■

Participants: L. O. Arthur, National Cancer Institute—Frederick Cancer Research Facility, Frederick, MD, USA; J. Desmyter, Rega Institut, Catholic University, Leuven, Belgium; R. C. Desrosiers, Harvard Medical School, New England Regional Primate Research Center, Southborough, MA, USA (*Co-Rapporteur*); G. R. Dreesman, Department of Virology and Immunology, Southwest Foundation for Biomedical Research, San Antonio, TX, USA (*Co-Chairman*); P. N. Fultz, Yerkes Regional Primate Research Center, Emory University, The Robert W. Woodruff Health Sciences Center, Atlanta, GA, USA; M. Girard, Pasteur Vaccins-1, Marnes-La-Coquette, France; M. A. Gonda, Laboratory of Cell and Molecular Structure, National Cancer Institute—Frederick Cancer Research Facility, Frederick, MD, USA; M. Hayami, Department of Animal Pathology, The Institute of Medical Science, University of Tokyo, Tokyo, Japan; W. Koff, AIDS Program, National Institute of Allergy and Infectious Diseases, National Institutes of Health, Rockville, MD, USA; T. Lee, Department of Cancer Biology, Harvard School of Public Health, Boston, MA, USA; M. A. Martin, Laboratory of Molecular Microbiology, National Institute of Allergy and Infectious Diseases, National Institutes of Health, Bethesda, MD, USA; P. A. Marx, Virology and Immunology Unit, California Primate Research Center, University of California, Davis, CA, USA; M. Murphey-Corb, Delta Regional Primate Research Center, Tulane University, Covington, LA, USA; O. Narayan, Departments of Comparative Medicine and Neurology, The Johns Hopkins University School of Medicine, Baltimore, MD, USA (*Co-Rapporteur*); G. V. Quinnan, Division of Virology, Center for Biologics Evaluation and Research, Food and Drug Administration, Bethesda, MD, USA (*Rapporteur*); G. C. Schild, National Institute for Biological Standards and Control, Potters Bar, Hertfordshire, England (*Chairman*); C. Stahl-Hennig, Deutsches Primaten Centrum, Gottingen, Federal Republic of Germany; J. Weber, Department of Medicine, Royal Postgraduate Medical School, Hammersmith Hospital, London, England (*Co-Rapporteur*); H. Wolf, Max von Pettenkofer Institute for Hygiene and Medical Microbiology, Munich University, Munich, Federal Republic of Germany; J. Yamamoto, Department of Medicine, School of Veterinary Medicine, University of California, Davis, CA, USA; J. M. Zarling, Oncogen, Seattle, WA, USA.

From WHO Secretariat (World Health Organization, Geneva, Switzerland): G. Ada, Special Program of Research, Development and Research Training in Human Reproduction; T. Bektimirov, Assistant Director-General; D. Devlin, Office of the Legal Counsel; J. Esparza, Biomedical Research Unit,

Global Program on AIDS (*Secretary*); J. Gowans, Global Program on AIDS; V. Grachev, Biologicals; E. Karamov, Biomedical Research Unit, Global Program on AIDS; D. Magrath, Biologicals; J. Mann, Global Program on AIDS; J. B. Milstien, Biologicals; H. Nieburgs, Division of Noncommunicable Diseases; H. Tamashiro, Biomedical Research Unit, Global Program on AIDS; G. Torrigiani, Division of Communicable Diseases; R. Widdus, Global Program on AIDS; P. Wright, Expanded Program on Immunization.

Selected References

1. Biberfeld, G. et al. WHO Working Group on characterization of HIV-related retroviruses: criteria for characterization and proposal for a nomenclature system. *AIDS* 1:189–190, 1987.

2. Desrosiers, R. C. Simian immunodeficiency viruses. *Annu Rev Microbiol* (in press).

3. Desrosiers, R. C., and N. L. Letvin. Animal models for acquired immunodeficiency syndrome. *Rev Infect Dis* 9:438–446, 1987.

4. Schneider, J., and G. Hunsmann. Simian lentiviruses—the SIV group. *AIDS* 2:1–9, 1988.

5. Murphey-Corb, M. et al. Isolation of an HTLV-III-related retrovirus from macaques with simian AIDS and its possible origin in asymptomatic mangabeys. *Nature* 321:435–437, 1986.

6. Fultz, P. et al. Isolation of a T-lymphotropic retrovirus from naturally infected sooty mangabey monkeys (*Cercocebus atys*). *Proc Nat Acad Sci USA* 83:5286–5290, 1986.

7. Fukasawa, M. et al. Sequence of simian immunodeficiency virus from African green monkey, a new member of the HIV/SIV group. *Nature* 333:457–460, 1988.

8. Kestler, H. W. et al. Comparison of simian immunodeficiency virus isolates. *Nature* 331:619–621, 1988.

9. Zhang, J. Y. et al. SIV/delta-induced immunodeficiency in the rhesus monkey: correlation of the humoral immune response with virus-specific antigenaemia. *J Infect Dis* (in press).

10. Fultz, P. et al. Persistent infection of chimpanzees with human T-lymphotropic virus type III/lymphadenopathy-associated virus: a potential model for acquired immunodeficiency syndrome. *J Virol* 58:116–124, 1986.

11. Fultz, P. et al. Superinfection of a chimpanzee with a second strain of human immunodeficiency virus. *J Virol* 61:4026–4029, 1987.

12. Zarling, J. et al. Proliferative and cytotoxic T cells to AIDS virus glycoproteins in chimpanzees immunized with a recombinant vaccinia virus expressing AIDS virus envelope glycoproteins. *J Immunol* 139:988–990, 1987.

13. Narayan, O. et al. Lentiviruses of animals are biological models of the human immunodeficiency virus. *Microb Pathog* (in press).

14. Yamamoto, J. et al. The pathogenesis of experimentally induced feline immunodeficiency virus (FIV) infection in cats. *Am J Vet Res* (in press).

15. Gonda, M. et al. Characterization and molecular cloning of a bovine lentivirus related to human immunodeficiency virus. *Nature* 330:388–391, 1987.

WORLD AIDS SUMMIT IN LONDON

The World Summit of Ministers of Health on Programs for AIDS Prevention was held in London from 26 to 28 January 1988. The conference was attended by health ministers from 148 countries, representing 95% of the world's population. The meeting, jointly sponsored by the World Health Organization and the British Government, marked the first time that so many nations had come together to discuss the topic of AIDS on a political, rather than scientific or medical, level.

In a series of short speeches and informal discussions, the health ministers shared statistics on the incidence of infection in their countries and reviewed the programs for public information, prevention, and treatment that they had developed. Among the messages brought to light were (1) that the spread of AIDS can be prevented through national information programs, (2) that health care workers must be educated for the struggle against AIDS, and (3) that effective means must be sought to inform and educate specific groups whose behaviors place them at high risk of infection.

According to Dr. Halfdan Mahler, WHO's former Director-General, the most important contribution of the conference was that political and medical leaders had adopted the "revolutionary" concept that

Sources: Karen DeYoung, Global AIDS conference ends with call for action, *The Washington Post*, 29 January 1988; *and* London Declaration on AIDS Prevention, World Summit of Ministers of Health on Programs for AIDS Prevention, 28 January 1988.

the spread of information can slow the spread of the disease by persuading people to alter high-risk behaviors. Until recently, Dr. Mahler said, ''information and communication had been to a large extent stonewalled by the health professionals, including myself. We now have to relearn that communications is decisive in fighting such a global threat as AIDS.'' In a declaration that was issued at the close of the three-day conference, the representatives agreed that information and education about AIDS were the most important components of national control programs, in the absence of a vaccine or cure.

Dr. Jonathan Mann, head of the WHO Global Program on AIDS, said that the most important aspect of the declaration adopted by the delegates was its rejection of discrimination against those infected with the virus or suffering from the disease. In addition, Dr. Mann and others at the conference argued that there is no evidence that widespread screening for the infection, particularly on a mandatory basis, would contribute to stemming its spread.

The text of the declaration, which was endorsed by all the delegations, is presented below.

London Declaration of Ministers of Health

The World Summit of Ministers of Health on Programs for AIDS Prevention, involving delegates from 148 countries representing the vast majority of the people of the world, makes the following declaration:

1. Since AIDS is a global problem that poses a serious threat to humanity, urgent action by all governments and people the world over is needed to implement WHO's Global AIDS Strategy as defined by the Fortieth World Health Assembly and supported by the United Nations General Assembly.

2. We shall do all in our power to ensure that our governments do indeed undertake such urgent action.

3. We undertake to devise national programs to prevent and contain the spread of human immunodeficiency virus (HIV) infection as part of our countries' health systems. We commend to all governments the value of a high-level coordinating committee to bring together all government sectors, and we shall involve to the fullest extent possible all governmental sectors and relevant nongovernmen-

tal organizations in the planning and implementation of such programs in conformity with the Global AIDS Strategy.

4. We recognize that, particularly in the absence at present of a vaccine or cure for AIDS, the single most important component of national AIDS programs is information and education, because HIV transmission can be prevented through informed and responsible behavior. In this respect, individuals, governments, the media, and other sectors all have major roles to play in preventing the spread of HIV infection.

5. We consider that information and education programs should be aimed at the general public and should take full account of social and cultural patterns, different lifestyles, and human and spiritual values. The same principles should apply equally to programs directed toward specific groups, involving these groups as appropriate. These include groups such as:

- policy makers;
- health and social service workers at all levels;
- international travelers;
- persons whose practices may place them at increased risk of infection;
- the media;
- youth and those that work with them, especially teachers;
- community and religious leaders;
- potential blood donors; and
- those with HIV infections, their relatives, and others concerned with their care, all of whom need appropriate counseling.

6. We emphasize the need in AIDS prevention programs to protect human rights and human dignity. Discrimination against, and stigmatization of, HIV-infected people and people with AIDS and population groups undermine public health and must be avoided.

7. We urge the media to fulfill their important social responsibility to provide factual and balanced information to the general public on AIDS and on ways of preventing its spread.

8. We shall seek the involvement of all relevant governmental sectors and nongovernmental organizations in creating the supportive social environment needed to ensure the effective implementation of AIDS prevention programs and humane care of affected individuals.

9. We shall impress on our governments the importance for national health of ensuring the availability of the human and financial resources, including health and social services with well-trained personnel, needed to carry out our national AIDS programs, and in order to support informed and responsible behavior.

10. In the spirit of United Nations General Assembly Resolution A/42/8, we appeal to all appropriate organizations of the United Nations system, including the specialized agencies; to bilateral and multilateral agencies; and to nongovernmental and voluntary organizations to support the worldwide struggle against AIDS in conformity with WHO's global strategy.

11. We appeal in particular to these bodies to provide well-coordinated support to developing countries in setting up and carrying out national AIDS programs in the light of their needs. We recognize that these needs vary from country to country in the light of their epidemiological situation.

12. We also appeal to those involved in dealing with drug abuse to intensify their efforts in the spirit of the International Conference on Drug Abuse and Illicit Trafficking (Vienna, June 1987) with a view to contributing to the reduction in the spread of HIV infection.

13. We call on the World Health Organization, through its Global Program on AIDS, to continue to:

 (i) exercise its mandate to direct and coordinate the worldwide effort against AIDS;

 (ii) promote, encourage, and support the worldwide collection and dissemination of accurate information on AIDS;

(iii) develop and issue guidelines on the planning, implementation, monitoring and evaluation of information and education programs, including the related research and development, and ensure that these guidelines are updated and revised in the light of evolving experiences;

(iv) support countries in monitoring and evaluating preventive programs, including information and education activities, and encourage wide dissemination of the findings in order to help countries to learn from the experiences of others;

 (v) support and strengthen national programs for the prevention and control of AIDS.

14. Following from this Summit, 1988 shall be a Year of Communication and Cooperation about AIDS in which we shall:

- open fully the channels of communication in each society so as to inform and educate more widely, broadly, and intensively;
- strengthen the exchange of information and experience among all countries; and
- forge, through information and education and social leadership, a spirit of social tolerance.

15. We are convinced that, by promoting responsible behavior and through international cooperation, we *can* and *will* begin *now to slow the spread of HIV infection.*